Enduring Issues in American Nursing

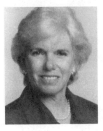

Ellen D. Baer, RN, PhD, FAAN, is the Wallace Gilroy Visiting Professor of Nursing at the University of Miami and Professor Emeritus of Nursing at the University of Pennsylvania, where she held the Hillman Term Professorship in Nursing and where she remains an Associate Director of the Center for the Study of the History of Nursing. Dr. Baer's research and writing in nursing history have been recognized by the Centennial Nursing Heritage Award from the American Nurses' Association, the Lavinia L. Dock Award from the American Association of the History of Nursing, the Distinguished Nurse Researcher Award from the Foundation of the New York State Nurses' Association, the Agnes Dillon Randolph Award from the University of Virginia, and distinguished alumni awards from New York University and Columbia University.

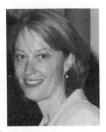

Patricia D'Antonio, RN, PhD, is an Adjunct Associate Professor of Nursing at the University of Pennsylvania, a Fellow at the Center for the Study of the History of Nursing at the University of Pennsylvania, and the Associate Editor of *Nursing History Review.* She is currently working on a book about psychiatric care in early nineteenth-century Philadelphia.

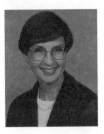

Sylvia D. Rinker, RN, PhD, is Associate Professor of Nursing at Lynchburg College in Lynchburg, Virginia. She is Chair of the Strategic Planning Committee of the American Association for the History of Nursing, archivist for the Xi Upsilon Chapter of Sigma Theta Tau at Lynchburg College, and on the Advisory Board for the Center for the History and Culture of Central Virginia. Dr. Rinker was the Associate Director of the Center for Nursing Historical Inquiry at the University of Virginia from its founding in 1991 until 1998. Her highly regarded historical scholarship was recognized by the Teresa Christy Award from the American Association for the History of Nursing. She is currently developing a women's history course entitled "Women at Work: Medieval to Modern."

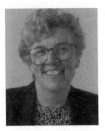

Joan E. Lynaugh, RN, PhD, FAAN, is Professor Emeritus of Nursing at the University of Pennsylvania where she held the History of Nursing and Health Care Term Professorship. Dr. Lynaugh was the Founder and Director, now Associate Director, of the Center for the Study of the History of Nursing and the Associate Dean and Director of Graduate Studies at the University of Pennsylvania School of Nursing. She currently chairs the Board of Trustees of the Visiting Nurse Association of Greater Philadelphia. A prolific researcher, writer, and editor, Dr. Lynaugh's distinguished career in nursing has been recognized by the Centennial Nursing Heritage Award from the American Nurses' Association, the Lavinia L. Dock Award from the American Association of the History of Nursing, the Hannah Lectureship of the Canadian Association for the History of Nursing, the Agnes Dillon Randolph Award from the University of Virginia, and the Distinguished Alumni Award from the University of Rochester.

Enduring Issues in American Nursing

Ellen D. Baer, RN, PhD, FAAN

Patricia D'Antonio, RN, PhD

Sylvia Rinker, RN, PhD, and

Joan E. Lynaugh, RN, PhD, FAAN

Editors

 Springer Publishing Company

Springer Publishing Company, Inc.
536 Broadway
New York, NY 10012-3955

Acquisitions Editor: Ruth Chasek
Production Editor: Jeanne W. Libby
Cover design by Susan Hauley

02 03 04 / 5 4 3

Cover Photo: Top left—Susannah Fisher, Class of 1891, at work in the Philadelphia General Hospital, circa 1890. Bottom right—Intensive Care for a very small infant, circa 1985. Courtesy of Center for the Study of the History of Nursing, University of Pennsylvania.

Library of Congress Cataloging-in-Publication Data

Enduring issues in American nursing / Ellen D. Baer . . . [et al.], editors.
    p. cm.
    Includes bibliographical references and index.
    ISBN 0-8261-1373-7
        1. Nursing—United States—History. 2. Nursing—United States—History.
    I. Baer, Ellen Davidson.

    RT4.E53 2000
    610.73'0973—dc21   00-063528

Printed in the United States of America

Contents

Contributors

Douglas O. Baldwin, PhD, Professor of History, Acadia University, Nova Scotia, Canada.

Karen Buhler-Wilkerson, RN, PhD, FAAN, Professor of Community Health Nursing and Director, Center for the Study of the History of Nursing, University of Pennsylvania. **Carole A. Estabrooks, RN, PhD,** Assistant Professor of Nursing, University of Alberta, Edmonton, Canada.

Julie Fairman, RN, PhD, FAAN, Assistant Professor of Nursing, University of Pennsylvania.

Diane Hamilton, PhD, RN, Associate Professor of Nursing, Western Michigan University.

Darlene Clark Hine, PhD, John A. Hannah Professor of History, Michigan State University.

Janet Wilson James, PhD, late Professor of History at Boston College and co-editor of *Notable American Women.*

Judith Walzer Leavitt, PhD, Ruth Bleier WARF Professor of the History of Medicine, History of Science and Women's Studies, University of Wisconsin-Madison.

Susan M. Reverby, PhD, Professor of Women's Studies, Wellesley College.

Margarete Sandelowski, RN, PhD, FAAN, Professor of Nursing, University of North Carolina at Chapel Hill.

Linda V. Walsh, CNM, PhD, Associate Professor of Nursing, University of San Francisco.

Preface

The purpose of this book is twofold. First, its purpose is to identify and explain dilemmas with which nursing has struggled throughout its history. Second, it is to expose nursing students, practitioners, faculty, and administrators to the helpfulness of using history to understand and deal with persistent dilemmas.

The most powerful conflicts the editors identified in nursing concern the very heart and identity of nursing, its power and authority, its level of dependence or independence, and its requirement for structured knowledge. And, while it is understandable that nurses have blamed legislators, physicians, administrators, and sundry other groups for the practical, educational, and administrative dilemmas in nursing, we must also recognize that nurses have made many of the choices that led to these conflicts. One of the strengths of historical analysis is that it fosters the type of debate and examination needed to illuminate these issues.

For almost two decades the editors of this book have observed and participated in the growing interest in nursing history from nurses, nursing students, health policymakers, women's historians, and other people interested in the history of health care. In the early 1980's the American Association for the History of Nursing (AAHN) was founded, followed by an important conference on nursing history at the Rockefeller Archive Center, that brought together nurse historians, social, labor, and women's historians. Soon thereafter, established research journals and university presses published important papers in nursing history, and nurses around the nation began to retrieve and collect archival materials in several highly regarded nursing history centers. In 1993, AAHN launched its excellent journal *Nursing History Review*, now published by Springer.

The merging of these interests in a book like this one seems almost preordained. As teachers, the editors struggled yearly to create course outlines and book packs that represented an appropriate sampling of ideas, discussion, and debate about the issues we believed to be vital to nursing's well-being. This book grew from those yearly efforts and is directed at everyone interested in the possibilities and problems of nursing over time. Certainly we expect a good number of readers will be faculty and students of all varieties, such as all the health field and nursing undergraduate and graduate students seeking understanding of the background for many of nursing's continuing problems. And we expect readers in clinical practice, practitioners confronting daily the issues raised in this book. But, additionally, we anticipate readers in nursing history, health policy, nursing issues and trends, clinical majors at the master's level, and doctoral students studying various research methods. To them all, we send an articulate reminder of the powerful nature of nursing's work, spoken by Alice Fisher, Philadelphia Hospital Nursing Superintendent (1884–1888):

> *"I am sure that of all the means by which it is possible to gain daily bread, there is none more irksome, more trying, nay, more positively revolting than the charge of the sick, if the nurse have not that inborn love of the work which is given, alas, but to a few. But, on the other hand, if it so happens that she [or he] have this love in addition to the other necessary mental and physical qualities, no calling can be found which offers so happy a life, or where labour brings so quick or inevitable a reward, or which, in spite of many undeniable anxieties, secures such absolute peace of mind."[1]*

Ellen D. Baer, for the Editors

---

1. Alice Fisher quoted in Stephanie A. Stachniewicz and Jill K. Axelrod. *The Double Frill* (32). Philadelphia: Stickley, 1979.

SECTION 1

CONTEMPORARY ISSUES
IN HISTORICAL CONTEXT

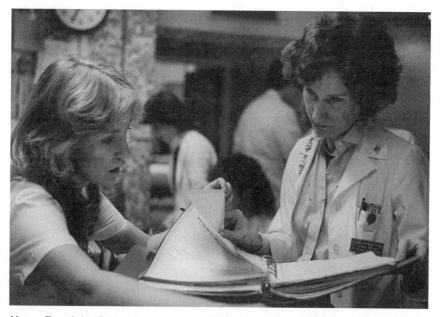

Nurses Examining Patient Record, Hospital of the University of Pennsylvania, circa 1985. Courtesy of the Center for the Study of the History of Nursing, University of Pennsylvania.

Introduction

Ellen D. Baer

Although nursing is as old as the world, modern nursing developed as a response to the social changes of the 19th century. From the outset, nursing faced challenges in its acceptance as legitimate work performed (in those times) by single, lay women, for pay, outside of their homes. Although eager to embrace the safety, comfort, and care provided to family members by nurses, society worried about the social consequences of the women's activities. Nurses lived away from their families; attended lectures and demonstrations; provided intimate bodily services to strangers, eventually even males; traveled alone around cities and towns visiting the sick and the homebound; earned their own salaries, paid their own expenses, made their own decisions, and supported their own independent life choices.

To allow such revolutionary behavior from single, lay women during the Victorian Era, society extracted certain compromises. Nurses could live away from their families, but only in supervised, restricted, almost cloistered environments, wearing modest clothing and adopting humble behaviors. They could care for the bodies of strangers, but only under the watchful gaze of parental substitutes, physicians and matron nurses. They could earn their own salaries, but only pittances that kept them dependent on hospital lodgings or group housing. Nurses accepted these requirements in order to gain access to work, self-sufficiency and more independence than was otherwise available to women. But the nurses' choices marked nursing from the outset, and remnants of these choices follow nursing into the millenium, causing conflicts for nursing within its own fold and between it and other health care groups.

NURSING CONFLICTS

The Victorian beginnings of nursing eventually became honored traditions, with nurses choosing to continue many of the restricted options

3

by the early 20th century. As our first two readings describe, nurses maintained gender and racial controls, merged training programs with practice needs, continued class distinctions and competition among various training schools, sustained allegiance to symbols and badges of dress, and nourished suspicions regarding university education and research-based practice. Most of these arrangements were originally constructed by the male and female philanthropic supporters of nursing in agreement with early nursing leaders. But by the mid-20th century, practicing nurses demonstrated their support for these choices. My own research[1] suggests certain recurring themes among these traditions, that have, in many cases, produced conflict or divisiveness in nursing.

Nurses' Ideals Nurses tend to assume that other groups share nurses' ideals about patient care, and that assumption is false. Nursing's ideal is that patients are at the center of health care practices and that caring for patients is the primary objective of health care. However, different health care participants (such as insurance companies, government agencies, for-profit institutions, religious groups, research scientists and other health professionals) may have different goals that are based on different ideals. This variation in ideal does not involve right or wrong. It is a variation in perspective with which nurses must learn to deal.

Gender In the very societies that established nursing as a female occupation, women's work is generally devalued. In the case of the United States, non-sentimental, entrepreneurial enterprises and marketable products are the honored occupational characteristics. So, what possible status can there be for personal care services that generate few income dollars? In case there is any doubt about this point, consider the response of business managers when health care became a major investment target in the 1990s. Administrators and managers immediately sacrificed nursing assets and budget lines to gain profit, proving how little they valued nursing's work.

Status and Exclusion In search of that elusive goal, status, nurses have always practiced exclusion within their own group. Needing bodies to do the work of nursing, various nursing educational facilities often accepted students of less than optimal talent. Recognizing this, nurses applied standards of excellence after the fact, limiting participation in honored organizations of people already called 'nurse' to those who met some additional criteria, such as additional degrees, certification, or workshop participation. Other professions practice exclusion at the entrance to their professions, limiting admission to only those applicants deemed excellent prospects.

Merging Education and Practice From the outset of modern nursing, nurses had three connected, competing and overlapping obligations: caring for patients, educating the students who would deliver the actual patient services, and managing many of the bureaucratic and administrative details in the institution. As nurses' roles divided, so did their loyalty, professional perspective, and beliefs about educational preparation and practice. As a result, nurses competed with each other for students' time, institutional resources, and professional status, creating conflicts and divisions within the profession.

Prolonged Apprenticeship Other professions, reared in the apprenticeship model at the same time as nursing, moved to university education in the early decades of the 20th century. Nursing did not. Nursing leaders resisted losing command of the schools. Practicing nurses feared that "book learning" would replace carefully crafted clinical skill, and that graduates of less powerful training schools would be ". . . sacrificed to the hope of professionalization" and a search for "status" on the part of the nursing elite.[2] Hospital administrators believed that the loss to the hospital of student labor would necessitate training a new "hospital helper" in replacement. In consequence, nursing education became institutionalized as different, and less respected, than other forms of professional education. In addition, parochial attitudes engendered in the training schools created rigidity in educational practices, small-mindedness in dictating the details of students' lives, and petty jealousies among the various schools.

ENDURING ISSUES IN AMERICAN NURSING

As the twenty first century begins, nurses still struggle to attain autonomy for their profession, control of their practice, the right to independent decision-making, the determination of appropriate knowledge, education and licensure for various levels of nursing practice, nurse staffing levels that ensure patient safety and comfort, and salaries commensurate with nurses' responsibilities. The editors of this book have separated these various problems into thematic categories that address identity, the meaning of nursing, the nature of power in nursing, and the nature of knowledge needed in nursing. Within each section, we have selected previously published articles or book chapters that demonstrate the specific area of struggle for nursing. Although each chapter stands alone, each one also provides a piece of the overall puzzle that is nursing and reflects its possibilities. Each section of the book has an introduction which focuses on the concept or issue being addressed in that section. The introduction describes how each chapter provides a different view of the stated issue, draws together themes, and explains why authors wrote in particular ways.

Each chapter tells a real story, experienced by real nurses at various points in our (approximately) century and a half of modern existence.

These stories are not the usual celebrations of great events or inspired leaders that often populate nursing history books. While nursing history is certainly full of such material and people, they are not the focus of this book. Rather, our purpose here is to present articles that interpret, analyze and evaluate the decisions and actions taken by real people struggling in real situations within real contexts, and having the mixed results that come with such real life experiences. Our hope is that, in the reports of problems and possibilities presented here, readers will see their own stories, gain insight into their own circumstances and, in consequence, manage their own situations with wisdom and success.

Nursing History

Because these nurses' stories occurred in the past, they fall into the broad category of nursing history. But they are not merely narrative reports of a chronology of nursing events. Rather, they are databased articles, carefully researched and written by qualified historians, and selected by peer review for their initial publication. As in all research disciplines, history has various schools of thought and study. While all historians pay attention to the impact of major social events and great leaders on the actions of human beings, different historians emphasize different themes. Therefore, in analyzing nursing data, women's historians, such as Susan Reverby, emphasize the impact of genderized work patterns, employment relationships and economic configurations on the decisions and actions of nurses. Intellectual historians, such as Diane Hamilton, analyze the development of the ideas of nursing and ask what do nurses think. But most of the historians presented in this book share the common focus of social history, or "history from the bottom up," which focuses on the actions and decisions of everyday, ordinary people. In other words, social historians focus less on what was proclaimed from on high and more on what was actually done by the workers in the field.

As one example, Joan Lynaugh's introductory article emphasizes the social context in which nurses decided and acted, such as war, depression, our dependence on hospitals and insurance, the rise of science and the growing dominance of technology. But overlap and interaction among types of research also frequently occur, with the merest flavor of difference among avenues of thought evident in some cases, and outright disagreement apparent in other cases. The editors have sought to capture this debate in our selection of studies. Compare, for example, the views of Hamilton and Reverby on the ideas of nursing or the perspectives of Leavitt and Rinker on obstetric nursing. We hope the selections make for a wonderfully rich brew of intellectual stimulation to help us sort out the ongoing problems and possibilities of nursing.

The articles presented do not capture all aspects of scholarship in nursing history. But all do, to some degree or another, attend to the predominant influence of gender, race and class in nursing's development. We cannot estimate accurately the impact, for good or for ill, of these three variables on nursing's course. For, even as we know that nurses dealt (and still deal) daily with the negative aspects of discrimination based on one or the other of their demographics, we also know that, on the positive side, nursing gave the opportunity for work, independence and self-actualization to women, minorities and members of the working and immigrant classes long before such possibilities existed in other occupations and professions. However, in our search for articles to examine discrimination in these three areas, we have faced the fact that there is little published work on discrimination against men and minorities in nursing. In the end, therefore, our selections do reflect the entrenched historical legacy, that our profession was originally designed to be a profession of and for white women, almost all, but not completely, of the middle class. Our profession had a place for working class women, if they wanted to improve their lot in life. It had a smaller place for men if they would confine themselves to particular occupational niches. And, it had an even smaller place for African Americans and other women of color if they kept to their place in a segregated society. We hope our selections and our discussion help confront this history and ensure the profession's commitment to change in the future in order to make our membership as diverse as the patients we treat.

HISTORIANS AS CLINICIANS

Readers unacquainted with history as a method may ask Why History? Why turn to the past when attempting to build nursing's future? We could resurrect George Santayana's famous dictum that "Those who cannot remember the past are condemned to repeat it."[3] But as nurses who are both historians and clinicians, the editors of this volume have an additional reason. Just as a nurse can make little progress caring for or curing a patient's presenting problem without knowing the patient's physiological, psychological, and cultural history, so it is for a nurse trying to make sense out of the persistent problems and possibilities in nursing and health care. To make good decisions in planning nursing's future in the context of our complex health-care system, nurses must know the history of the actions being considered, the identities and points of view of the major players, and all the stakes that are at risk. These are the lessons of history.

History, both as a clinical tool and as an intellectual method, embraces complexity even as it analyses, interprets and deduces meaning from it.

In a practice setting, nurses fuse clinical knowledge, personal experience, and particular theoretical perspectives with those of their patients, families, or communities to arrive at qualified assessments of what interventions the patient needs. So it is with history. The historian investigates past experience, examining assumptions, attitudes, interests and points of view so that past events can be carefully understood, present possibilities accurately assessed, and future interventions appropriately undertaken.

CONCLUSION

To ground the reader in the basic chronological and thematic "facts" of nursing history, we close this introductory section with one article by Joan Lynaugh and a second by Darlene Clark Hine. Both papers present good synopses of major events and people in nursing in the 20th century. Lynaugh's article was selected to give the reader an introduction to the overall course of nursing's history. Hine's chapter was selected to give the reader an introduction to several important themes in nursing's history and in the history of the whole health care industry: race, class, and gender.

In addition to preparing readers for subsequent readings, these two papers serve as a useful introduction to the various footnoting and bibliographic styles contained in this book. As readers know, writing styles vary among disciplines. For brevity and succinctness, nursing and nursing journals prefer the writing style developed and published by the American Psychological Association (APA). Historians and history journals, however, employ the (University of) Chicago style. The Chicago style offers scholars the opportunity to put additional information in the footnotes that expands upon data presented in the text and comments on the sources cited. Because of the length of such footnotes, they are represented by numbers and often appear at the end of the text (end notes) rather than at the foot of the page (footnotes). However, many nurse historians publish in the general nursing press, where they are required to use APA format. Our opening two papers represent such cases. The styles of subsequent articles presented in this volume vary according to the writing style prescribed for their original publication. We hope that readers will take the time to review and appreciate the merits of each style.

NOTES

1.   Ellen D. Baer, "American Nursing: 100 Years of Conflicting Ideas and Ideals. *Journal of the New York State Nurses Association* 23, no. 3 (1992): 16–21. See also, Ellen D. Baer, "'A Cooperative Venture' in Pursuit of Professional Status: A

Research Journal for Nursing." *Nursing Research* 36, no. 1 (1987): 18–25. See also, Ellen D. Baer, "Nursing's Divided Loyalties: An Historical Case Study." *Nursing Research* 38, no. 3 (1989): 166–171. See also, Ellen D. Baer, "Nursing's Divided House: An Historical View." *Nursing Research* 34, no. 1 (1985): 32–38.

    2.   Barbara Melosh, *The Physician's Hand: Work Culture and Conflict in American Nursing.* (Philadelphia: Temple University Press, 1982.) 42–3.

    3.   George Santayana, "Reason in Common Sense" in *The Life of Reason* I (1905–6).

1

Nursing's History: Looking Backward and Seeing Forward

Joan E. Lynaugh

Søren Kierkegaard, the 19th century Danish philosopher and theologian, assayed pragmatic but common justification for studying history with this aphorism: ". . . . life can only be understood backwards, but, it must be lived forwards". In that spirit this essay offers a historical interpretation of American nursing as we find it now. It is hoped that it will provide a useful framework for conceptualizing the shape of our discipline and its place in our society for the rest of this decade and beyond.

CREATING AMERICAN NURSING

Human beings know that sickness, injury, birth, and aging are inevitable, unavoidable human experiences. To preserve individual lives and social stability, caregivers are charged with the work of helping others through these periods of dependency. For all of recorded time, this caring work has been primarily a function of the family, the basic structural unit of social life. In some cultures, certain aspects of the caring work has fallen to persons outside the family, usually religious or benevolent groups. We do not find the beginnings of formalized, secular nursing—that is, systematic, widespread delegation of nursing work to nonfamily workers— until the 19th century. Beginning in the 1830s and then with more conviction in subsequent decades, people began to consider total reliance on family caregivers in times of sickness to be dysfunctional. Clearest expression of this new thinking was found in the urban and increasingly secular societies of the Western world. Between 1860 and 1880, the idea

Note: This chapter was originally published in *Charting Nursing's Future*, eds. Linda Aiken and Claire Fagin, 435–447. Philadelphia: Lippincott, 1991. Reprinted with permission.

10

of moving some part of the work of caring from the domestic setting of the family to the nurse and the hospital finally took root, spawning new institutions and new occupations.

Influential experiments in modern nursing first appeared in Germany, then in England, France, the United States, and Canada (Hampton, 1949; Poplin, 1988; Woodham-Smith, 1951). Rapidly industrializing economies in Europe, England, and America, which needed their workers gathered together in factories, mines, and shops, proved a fertile environment for change. As the people of these industrializing countries left rural farms and villages and moved to cities, their traditional communities, their way of life, and their methods for coping with the exigencies of daily experience, including sickness and childbirth, were forever altered. Thus industrialization, combined with urbanization, helped set the stage for the "invention" of nursing as we know it today.

Nineteenth-century American nurses watched over hospital patients, gave them food, bathed them, kept order in the wards, and dispensed medicine. They collaborated with hospital board members to reform the hospital so as to match the idealized middle-class home, that is, a place of safety, cleanliness, and respectability where healing would be possible. Nurses established routines in hospitals that made the execution of medical regimens feasible; thus they persuaded physicians to send patients to hospitals instead of relying on family care at home. The hospital and nurse training school guaranteed their constituents that care would be available to them when needed and that the hospital could safely substitute for home in times of sickness (Long & Golden, 1989).

Nursing was reformist, not revolutionary; it accommodated both traditional and novel views of women's social role. For about 30 years, the idea of nursing as "every woman's work" coexisted with the idea of nursing as a specialized social task requiring a defined education. The classic example of this duality is Florence Nightingale's influential book, *Notes on Nursing*, published in 1860 in the United States. Addressing not nurses but a general audience of literate women, Nightingale argued that all women of intelligence needed to understand basic nursing principles. Similarly, the first Philadelphia training school for nurses, organized by physician Ann Preston at Woman's Hospital in 1861 and financed by Philadelphia benefactor Pauline Henry, opened its nurses' classes to all women of Philadelphia who wished greater proficiency in their domestic responsibilities (O'Brien, 1987).

Hospital nursing caught on quickly; it became a durable new strategy to deal with social dislocation and upheaval of custom in work and family life. By the 1890s, we find the phrase "trained nursing" integrated into the language of American life. The nurse, whether depicted in a "Gibson girl" profile or as serenely vigilant at the bedside, symbolized an optimistic modern response to the problems of caring for dependent members of society. Equally important, she did it within existing boundaries of domestic propriety so that middle class Americans could accept and support her new work.

Nursing, a distinct occupation requiring specified skills and knowledge, carved out its niche in the world of work outside the domestic sphere and attracted women to its hospital training schools for several reasons. It was a respectable, interesting occupation that seemed to fit the ideal of individual productivity espoused by a growing middle class. Further, nursing as paid work was economic salvation for many women. It offered a way to make a living to women who found themselves redundant and unemployed in an industrializing economy. And it merged easily with a wide range of late 19th century moral and progressive philosophies that stressed "usefulness" for women as a modern substitute for piety and commitment to family (Baer, 1985; Vicinus, 1985).

Nursing's assignment, that is, caring for dependent, sick Americans, could hardly have been carried out without significant social and political change. Gradual erosion of 19th century laissez-faire political attitudes toward dependency and poverty allowed a few new social services to emerge at the beginning of this century. Lillian Wald and Lavinia Dock are the best remembered of many nurses who worked to change the social agenda through public health, education, school and industrial health, and settlement house work. The Children's Bureau, protective labor legislation, venereal disease programs, the antituberculosis campaign, and the progressive income tax were products of progressive and populist activists trying to ameliorate some of the harsher aspects of our capitalist system through political change.

Nursing, now redefined as an occupation based on formal training (instead of "every woman's work"), developed at the same time as teaching, library science, engineering, forestry, dentistry, veterinary medicine, accounting, telegraphy, history, and many more specialized occupations. Some of these occupations metamorphosed into professions, some became extinct, and some, like nursing, are still self-consciously debating questions of entry to the work, standards of practice, and professional status. The point is that nursing, among many other occupations, evolved in an industrial, urban context that supported, and indeed required, specialization of work and workers.

Nursing leaders were energized by a variety of motivations. For some, like Linda Richards, it was religious commitment; for others, like Lillian Wald, it was the opportunity for real reform; and for many, it was the excitement of learning new things and doing important, paid work in careers that freed them from traditional domestic, family dependence.

In the early years of the 20th century these new nurses focused on solving the patient care problems confronting them and on sustaining their schools in the face of extreme financial hardship (Nutting, 1984). They banded together into alumnae associations to counteract the loneliness of a practice life isolated by private duty nursing in their patients' homes. Later, thousands joined the American Red Cross and went off to World War I. If they married, their nursing careers usually stopped, not to resume unless they were widowed or otherwise thrown back on their own resources.

Nursing education and practice took direction from sweeping intellectual changes in science and medicine. Radical change in 19th century medical thinking eventually altered the way the general public conceived of disease. Theories of specificity of cause and treatment of disease drove out earlier concepts of general causation based on compatibility or incompatibility between the person and environment. These ideas of specific causation and the search for specific treatments became even more popular when late 19th century revelations based on the germ theory led to the discovery of specific pathogens such as the tubercle bacillus. Confidence in medicine, inspired by these new achievements, helped fuel the growth of hospitals and nursing (Rosenberg, 1987).

Hospitals, Nurses, and the Health Marketplace

Nurses were enthusiastic about 20th century scientific and technologic strategies for dealing with sickness. Indeed, nursing made the remarkable proliferation of community hospitals possible. Their patients' requirements for intensive personal care, combined with new technology that both saved and created labor, served to shape the work of nurses. The operating rooms, the new x-ray machines, the laboratories, the scientific diet kitchens, and the pharmacies—all were managed by nurses. They also washed the patients, the beds, the floors and walls, and all the equipment—anything that might carry infection, the still dreaded, although better understood, bane of the hospital experience. The amount of physical labor required to conduct the hospital of 1900 was prodigious. By then, hospitals had electricity, telephones, flush toilets, and elevators. Desperately ill, febrile patients needed to be bathed and fed, however. Every surgical item was sterilized and wrapped by nurses' hands, nurses mixed and poured every medication, and they folded and stored every piece of linen.

By 1910 nearly every community in the United States had at least one hospital and probably more, depending on the size and ethnic and/or religious composition of the population. All these hospitals (the number peaked near 7000 in 1920) needed nurses. What emerged between 1890 and 1940 was a collection of small, local enterprises operating in

the private sector. The majority of these were organized as voluntary charities, somewhat competitive along ethnic, religious, and local lines, but
because they were charitable projects, they were not governed either by
public authority or by marketplace rules (Long & Golden, 1989).

What many of these hospitals did have in common was cheap help—
the student nurses in the training schools. The availability and persistence of exploitative student labor, a system created and sustained by the
problems of underfinanced hospitals, corrupted the education of nurses.
American procrastination in solving this problem also undermined hospitals' early promise as purveyors of general health care to their communities. One can argue that the reliance of hospitals on cheap student
labor not only prevented Americans from facing the real personnel costs
of institutional care but stunted the development of broad-based community services. The use of untrained and constantly changing pupils
made it necessary to centralize patient care so that the pupils could be
closely supervised by a small number of experienced nurses. Notwith-
standing pupils' limitations, for the hospital managers it was essential
that a constantly renewed supply of low-cost general workers compen-
sate for institutional dependence on uncertain charity and variable revenues from paying patients (Lynaugh, 1989b; Rosner, 1982).

Hospital popularity among the American middle class coincided, at
the turn of the 20th century, with educational decisions that called for
eight years of universal public education for all children. Communities
taxed themselves to support public education, but Americans chose not
to make general care of the sick a tax-funded service. People who sought
professional health care for themselves or their families expected to pay
cash to both physicians and hospitals. If they could not pay, they cared
for themselves. If that became impossible, they were forced to seek charity, either from local hospitals or from other benevolent groups in their
communities. For a variety of cultural and economic reasons, the idea
of any level of personal health care as a tax-supported right did not take
root during the period of rapid hospital development.

Instead, Americans restricted government responsibility for health to
marginal care of the desperate poor, the insane, those with dangerous
infectious disease, and later to childhood immunization against contagious disease. Except for scattered public health service hospitals and
military installations, the federal government played no role at all in
health care. Insane asylums, city and county hospitals for the sick poor,
and tuberculosis hospitals were supported by local or state revenues.

Hospital expansion went forward in an environment of economic
uncertainty. Voluntary hospitals, the vast majority of successful community hospitals, depended on patient fees, benefactors, and local donations for their entire income; importantly, after the turn of the century

they did get special tax relief in most communities. Nevertheless, many failed when benefactor generosity and stringent management did not keep up with costs. The local, religious, and ethnic segmentation that characterized hospital development guaranteed that many hospitals would be small and, therefore, vulnerable to financial exigencies (Lynaugh, 1989b).

Even though the American market-oriented economic system seemed poorly suited and even hostile to financing and delivering social services, we managed to build a complicated structure of voluntary hospitals and agencies. These coped, as best they could, with the fundamental incompatibility between demanded health services and unfettered free enterprise (Stevens, 1989). It seems clear that Americans wanted and needed hospitals in their communities, even though they could not solve the problem of how to make hospitals fit into normal ways of doing business.

Most American nurses were introduced to their life's work in the voluntary, local hospital system; thus, the first 60 years of nursing history were dominated by private values and local custom. Decisions about nursing practice and education were essentially insulated from public debate. Even compliance with early 20th century registration laws regulating nursing practice in the states was voluntary (Tomes, 1983).

It would be decades before Americans grappled with the immutable fact that sick people run out of money, cannot work, and cannot pay their bills for health care or anything else. Americans could not reach a consensus on European ideas of public spending for general health care. The debate over universal access to health care began around 1915 in the United States. It was set aside with the advent of World War I but raised repeatedly in subsequent years, and the argument continues today.

The first major move toward collective responsibility for health and social services came in Franklin Roosevelt's administration with the Social Security Act of 1935. National health insurance was part of the original Social Security proposals, but it was abandoned when Roosevelt concluded that the American Medical Association's opposition to "socialized medicine" could scuttle the whole idea of Social Security. Nevertheless, the 1935 legislation signaled that Americans would support social programs. Although Social Security relied on an insurance concept, it was a firm step toward some measure of collective responsibility for individual welfare. In the meantime, also in the 1930s, Americans began to buy individual hospital insurance in the form of locally controlled Blue Cross and Blue Shield plans and a variety of commercial insurance plans.

After 1900, voluntary community hospitals began to use their beds mostly for surgical patients and for those with acute medical illnesses; they also opened wards for maternity patients and children. Throughout these years hospital boards came to believe that if they filled their beds with people who could not pay and the chronically ill who would not get better, the resulting losses would ruin their institutions. As one hospital board member from a voluntary hospital in Kansas City remarked in 1917, "[we must] develop this institution to a high plane of efficiency; taking it away from the invalid home idea; also from the [image of a] high-class boarding house for chronic cases" (Lynaugh, 1989b).

Visiting nurses and public health nurses were influenced by the American enthusiasm for community hospitals. Their practice in the neighborhoods of cities and towns and in rural counties, which had been accelerated by the social reform climate early in the 20th century, was independent of hospitals. But as Karen Buhler-Wilkerson has shown, their work eventually was affected by the growing dominance of hospitals in the American health care system (Buhler-Wilkerson, 1989). In fact, the success of hospitals in garnering the major production of new dollars through health insurance in the late 1930s may have undermined the earlier potential of visiting nurse and public health services to ameliorate gaps in health services, especially for the poor and chronically ill.

Many nurses, physicians, and other health care leaders understood the folly of limiting hospital responsibility to short-term, treatable ills. Interest in the chronically ill and the aged as well as efforts to improve general health among the population continued throughout the first four decades of this century. Experiments with neighborhood health centers and expanded health department services found some support. Public enthusiasm and medical confidence, however, combined to focus more and more attention and money on scientific medicine and the search for cures. In the decades after World War I, planners visualized the hospital as the institutional center from which health services would assuage the ills of each community.

However, since the insurance plans devised in 1930s were designed to cover only acute care services, the chronically ill and the aged, who were not protected by insurance coverage, found themselves outside of community hospital interests. The poor remained the responsibility of local government or private charity. Hospitals, in Charles Rosenberg's cogent phrase, clung to their "inward vision" of scientifically based, curative medicine (Rosenberg, 1979).

RECREATING AMERICAN NURSING

American confidence in health and health care underwent profound alteration in the general economic depression of the 1930s, followed by worldwide war in the 1940s. These cataclysmic events marked our gradual turning away from reliance on highly localized, private approaches to health care. World War II was a watershed event for nursing, for the general social and world consciousness of Americans, and for the health care system.

Nursing leaders in the 1940s deliberately exploited the war emergency to seek a new deal for nursing. They pushed for better education, better standards of nursing service, and better pay. They merged five weak national nursing organizations into two stronger units, and they gained some accrediting control over the nursing education system. The National Nursing Council for War Service, a voluntary committee of nursing leaders, collaborated with nurses in the United States Public Health Service; they used foresight and political acumen to lever nursing out of its isolated and fragmented localism (Goostray, 1969; Lynaugh, 1990).

The problem for nursing before World War II was how to improve nursing education within impoverished hospitals and deliver safe nursing care using mostly student caregivers. The problem after the war was how to create both a new nursing education system outside the hospital and a safe nursing care system using mostly paid caregivers.

Focusing the history of the first 60 years of nursing this sharply is not intended to deny the existence of university nursing education before World War II. However, the impact of collegiate programs and graduates was small. Nor should the importance of visiting and public health nurses and the reforms in which they participated be diminished. Rather, emphasis is placed here on the dominance of hospitals in 20th century nursing history. Delivering safe nursing care in hospitals and relocating nursing education away from hospitals into colleges and universities, two linked problems, absorbed the energies of postwar nurses.

Delivering Safe Nursing Care

Delivering safe care using paid staff instead of an all-student work force was very much complicated by the postwar expansion of hospitals. Demand for hospital services was up, partly because of successful labor negotiations for better health insurance in Americas burgeoning postwar economy. The Hill-Burton Act of 1946 financed new hospitals and the reconstruction of old hospitals. New hospitals and more beds helped to exacerbate the already existing severe shortage of nurses after the war. Intregrating nurses' aides, practical nurses, and student nurses into teams led by professional nurses (team nursing) was the strategy of the day. But because of the protracted shortage of professional nurses and increasing demand for hospital beds, team nursing often degenerated into an assembly line type of functional hospital nursing care system. Head nurses and supervisors with prewar experience and limited educational preparation were accustomed to relying on student workers in large numbers. Students were getting scarcer for two reasons—the rising operating expenses of hospital schools and restrictions on exploiting student labor by accrediting agencies.

Care of patients inside hospitals clearly needed redesign to cope with different caregiver personnel and rising acute illnesses among hospital patients. It took about 15 years of struggle and readjustment through the 1950s before staff nursing by graduate nurses replaced reliance on students and broke away from the rigid, novice-oriented assignment systems of prewar hospitals. Imitating the 1940s idea of the postoperative recovery room, geographic clusters of the sickest patients were created to try to use professional nurses more efficiently and better guarantee the safe care of patients.

Nurses and hospital administrators altered traditional uses of space, i.e., wards and private rooms, to cope with the influx of seriously ill people and the intensive postoperative care problems created by more invasive surgical procedures. They put certain types of less physiologically stable patients into intensive care units and changed staffing patterns to improve the patient-nurse ratio. New treatments and new technologies were spurred by popular concern about heart disease, a leading cause of death. Federal funding in the 1960s assured that patients with coronary artery disease got special attention in coronary care units. A few years later, passage of the 1965 Medicare/Medicaid legislation ensured a constant flow of patients and dollars into hospitals.

The motive for reorganization of nursing practice was to conserve nurses and assure hospital patients of protection from neglect. And, in fact, anecdotal evidence suggests that the problem of poor care for unstable hospital patients (i.e., patients being left alone with signs and symptoms unattended) is much less severe 30 years later.

But there is a history lesson here—the lesson of the unintended outcome. The intensive or special care unit, which was devised to conserve the number of nurses needed to care for the most seriously ill patients and to put the "best" nurses with the sickest patients, did accomplish the latter goal. However, the strategy increased rather than decreased the demand for nurses. At the risk of oversimplifying a complex series of events, what seems to have happened is that the intensive care unit, instead of reducing the total number of nurses needed to staff hospitals, proved to be a breeding ground for experts. Expert nursing in intensive care units made it possible to deploy technology successfully and to try more vigorous treatments, and more progressive therapy made nurses even more in demand as well as more expert (Lynaugh & Fairman, 1990).

Our experience with critical care nursing, as it is now called, is reflective of the history of all of nursing. The advent of trained nurses made hospitals possible—made it feasible to cluster the sick in large numbers and care for them safely and efficiently. One hundred years later, the advent of critical care nurses made it possible to create and expand intensive care units—made it feasible to cluster extremely sick people and care for them more effectively.

In both cases—the 19th century hospital and the 1960s intensive care unit—we instituted change to solve specific problems. We could not foresee where those changes would lead us. Creation of intensive care units led to complete renovation of the interior of hospitals. Patients now are grouped according to the stability of their physiologic condition. No longer are they assigned a bed by 1950s categories such as sex, ability to pay, or the identity of the admitting physician.

The hierarchy of nursing changed as well. Specialized clinical nursing expertise now ranks with or above administrative position as a measure of professional status. The clinical nurse specialist in many institutions either supersedes the head nurse or supervisor or shares the same status.

Paralleling this massive investment in high technology and intensive care in the 1960s and 1970s was a strong movement to enable all Americans to have access to ordinary medical care under its new rubric—primary health care. Proponents of primary health care argued that each person should be able to obtain service from a general health care provider without restriction owing to income or place of residence.

It became evident to primary health care advocates that no such policy could be implemented if the credential for all primary health care providers remained a medical degree. The idea of the nurse practitioner and the physician's assistant was born, along with an effort to restore the general medical practitioner, renamed the family physician. The nurse practitioner movement of the 1970s became an avenue to advanced clinical expertise for nurses working with the chronically ill and with children as well as those providing care in the areas of minor illness, public health, and health education.

The political promise of access to care for all proved ephemeral in the political and economic turmoil of the late 1970s and the 1980s. Nevertheless, nurse practitioner practice evolved successfully and encompassed responsibility for delivering health services to a wide spectrum of the population. Growing dependence on nurse practitioners is verified by their success in winning direct reimbursement for their services, thus breaking through the monopoly on insurance payment for direct patient care enjoyed by physicians since the 1930s.

These two practice arenas, critical care and primary health care, exemplify the responsiveness of nursing to societal demands for certain services. Although some nurse leaders argue that nursing is altogether too responsive to social pressure, critical care nurses and primary care nurse practitioners are just the most recent examples of an occupation willing and able to change itself as its environment changes. Seen in this light, these recent movements are logically correlative with the renaissance of American midwifery under nursing's auspices and turn of the century public health nursing.

Creating a New Educational System

Creating a new nursing education system outside the hospital proved just as difficult as restructuring nursing practice. The associate degree nursing education strategy was proposed in 1950 by nurse educator Mildred Montag to prepare "technical" nurses in the rapidly expanding community colleges of the nation. Planners expected that graduates from associate degree nursing programs would replace hospital school graduates. Other new nurses would come from the expanding baccalaureate nursing programs. In the original concept outlined by Montag and others (Montag, 1951; Montag, 1959) baccalaureate nursing graduates would be accountable for patient care and would direct the work of the nurse technician. That is not what happened.

Hospitals were starved for nurses; neither they nor state boards of nursing made distinctions between graduates of associate degree, baccalaureate, or diploma programs. It was easier for hospitals and state regulators to assume that all nurses were the same in terms of registration, assignments, pay, and advancement. Inability to differentiate levels of nursing practice responsibilities on the basis of educational preparation or any other abstract standard has proved to be one of the most intractable problems of 20th century nursing.

Although it is beyond the scope of this chapter to detail the problems of nurse supply, demand, and quality in our current health care system, it is possible to outline the debate for the last 50 years. Historically, there are at least two and possibly three sets of enduring conflicts. First, nurse leaders' efforts to upgrade preparation for practice and to restrict numbers often conflict with social desires to contain cost in providing nursing care. Second, differentiation of nursing practice to improve quality through specialization conflicts with institutional needs for flexible generalist nursing staffs. And finally, nurse-controlled practice and differentiated practice, such as that of nurse practitioners and nurse midwives, creates competitive fears among physicians.

Redesigning nursing practice and nursing education during the three decades after World War II dominated nursing's attention. In the background, however, a dramatic, slow-moving shift changed the context of the education debate. More and more nurses were going to college. Nurse veterans coming out of service went to college on the GI Bill; later, other nurses found support for higher education under the federal Nurse Training Acts of the 1960s.

The postwar revolution in American higher education—i.e., access of the middle and working classes to college—finally enabled nursing, with its members largely drawn from those classes, to realize its longstanding educational agenda. Nurses began to earn baccalaureate degrees, master's degrees, and doctoral degrees in substantial numbers.

The tuition dollars these nurses paid were lifesaving for small, struggling nurse education programs in colleges and universities. From 1964, when federal funding for nursing education stood at $9,900,000, through and beyond the peak year of 1973, when $160,000,000 was appropriated, nurse education programs in colleges and universities grew at an unprecedented rate. Once those nursing schools in colleges and universities attained a viable size through the influx of financially aided students, they could begin to attend to the training of clinical specialists, well-prepared faculty, and researchers. Direct federal aid for students leveled off in the 1970s, but the infusion of funds in the decades following World War II proved crucial to the movement of nursing education out of hospitals and into mainstream higher education.

In the United States, higher education is one proxy for class. In our polyglot, immigrant society, we use college education and accumulated wealth to substitute for inherited status. Of course, there always had been nurses of middle class and even upper middle class origins. From the beginning, daughters of clergy, bankers, wealthier physicians, and university professors made their careers in nursing. But the majority of nurses were from the working class; their hospital training gave them a new opportunity to make a living but did not change their class status.

Under the double handicap of gender and class, it is somewhat surprising that nurses have been able to control the fate of nursing as much as they have. Part of nurses' social authority stemmed from the essential and intimate nature of the work and their complex relationships with patients. Nurses are taught to adopt a "nursing character," to use Susan Reverby's phrase, which allows them to transcend class barriers in the care relationship (Reverby, 1987b). This means that in the nurse-patient relationship the nurse is able to keep control of the encounter even when differences in class, gender, or race might suggest otherwise. But when nurses operated outside the care relationship, e.g., in negotiations with hospital boards, university presidents, or physicians, their "nursing character" lost its effectiveness. To be in the places where health policy decisions were made meant breaking through class barriers. Before the educational revolution of the second half of this century, class handicaps, along with gender, prevented all but a few nurses from attaining sufficient social authority to be full participants in the negotiations that determined and managed the fate of their profession.

In addition to gaining access to higher education, nurses benefited from the civil rights achievements of the 1960s women's movement. Lavinia Dock and women's rights advocates of the pre-World War I era constantly reiterated one basic tenet: nurses' rights and women's rights are inextricably linked. Present-day nurses, although still socially conservative, seem much more in tune with women's rights than were Dock's colleagues during the first women's rights campaign. Nursing, in its relationship with society, is more pragmatic and confrontational and less deferential and altruistic than it used to be. In that sense nursing is now more integrated and less isolated from the larger society.

CONCLUSION

When sick, injured, and dependent people first gathered together in hospitals, chaos resulted because clustering the sick in hospitals elevated ordinary domestic and medical problems to herculean proportions. Nursing, practiced at a relatively simple but resolute level, reduced chaos to order as nurses, to again use a Reverby phrase, were "ordered to care" and they did (Reverby, 1987b). At the same time, a peculiar hospital-based nursing education system helped subsidize the rapid growth of America's hospital system.

Beginning in the 1930s and resuming after World War II, a protracted and sometimes stumbling effort to change the staffing system in hospitals ultimately produced a safe, responsive level of nursing practice using fully trained nurses. It is clear, however, that constant reconceptualization and revamping are required to deliver safe nursing care both inside and outside institutions.

Nursing education is no longer dominated by hospitals, but it is still tightly linked to nursing practice. With all its problems, the nursing education system is remarkably well developed, although it is chronically underfunded. Nursing still faces thorny issues of licensure and credentialing of its basic practitioners and specialists as well as severe disadvantages in reimbursement. Probably the most difficult educational problem for nurses will be to agree on and plan for an appropriate mix of levels of nursing personnel.

Since the beginning of nursing history, leaders in nursing have been slow or unwilling to acknowledge and take responsibility for aides, attendants, and similarly trained personnel. These auxiliary personnel are often feared as threats to quality of care or as competitive to nurses. Moreover, nursing educators who teach at different levels such as master's, baccalaureate, associate degree, practical nursing, and in continuing education communicate with each other with difficulty and rarely plan together. Possibly, as nurses become more certain of the nature of advanced practice and more confident about nursing's research and place among the professions, they may be able to cope effectively with demands for more basically trained caregivers.

The major deficit in the American health care system continues to be citizens' access to health care services. Access problems range from lack of insurance, which excludes needy persons from acute care, to a preponderance of low-quality, high-cost nursing home care. These problems persist in spite of enormous expenditures (600 billion dollars in 1990) and unrelenting political attention. What Americans want is what we seem to have always wanted—a responsive community of health-related services. A significant proportion of demanded services today is nursing's responsibility. Given this country's history of restless, short-term problem solving, it is going to be extremely difficult for Americans to rethink health care, but it seems likely that inexorable pressure for fiscal reform and renewed concern about problems such as high rates of infant mortality and the crisis of acquired immunodeficiency syndrome will drive change.

The issues remain much the same as they were when nursing was invented: how, where, and how much care should be given when people cannot care for themselves; how should care be paid for; how will the work of care be divided; where will caregivers come from; and how much knowledge and skill should caregivers have?

As we search for answers to these questions, we should not forget one important difference between the 19th century and now. Nursing is very much with us, with its expertise in devising care systems, its holistic care orientation complementing medicine's specificity, its flexibility and resilience, and its two million members. Although born in the 19th century, nursing grew to maturity in the tumult of the 20th century. We can hope that our experience, seasoned knowledge, and commitment will be sufficient to the task of restructuring American health care for the 21st century.

REFERENCES

Baer, E. (1985). Nursing's divided house—An historical view. *Nursing Research,* *34*, 32–38.

Buhler-Wilkerson, K. (1989). *False dawn: The rise and decline of public health nursing 1900–1930.* New York: Garland Publishing, Inc.

Goostray, S. (1969). *Memoirs: Half a century in nursing.* Boston: Nursing Archive.

Hampton, I. (1949). *Nursing of the sick 1893.* Reprint. New York: McGraw-Hill Book Company.

Long, D., & Golden, J. (Eds.) (1989). *The American general hospital: Communities and social context.* Ithaca & London: Cornell University Press.

Lynaugh, J. (1989a). *The community hospitals of Kansas City, Missouri, 1870–1915.* New York: Garland Publishing, Inc.

Lynaugh, J. (1989b). From respectable domesticity to medical efficiency The changing Kansas City Hospital, 1875–1920. In D. Long & J. Golden (Eds.), *The American general hospital: Communities and social contexts* (pp. 21–39). Ithaca & London: Cornell University Press.

Lynaugh, J. (1990). Stepping in. *Nursing Research, 39,* 126–127.

Lynaugh, J., & Fairman, J. (1990). History of care of the critically ill since 1940. Unpublished data.

Montag, M. (1951). *The education of nurse technicians.* New York: G.P. Putnam & Sons.

Montag, M. (1959). *Community college education for nurses.* New York: McGraw-Hill Book Co.

Nutting, A. (1984). *A sound economic basis for schools of nursing and other addresses.* Reprint. New York: Garland Publishing, Inc.

O'Brien, P. (1987). "All a woman's life can bring": The domestic roots of nursing in Philadelphia, 1830–1885. *Nursing Research, 36,* 12–17.

Poplin, I. (1988). *A study of the Kaiserswerth Deaconess Institute's Nurse Training School in 1850–1851: Purposes and curriculum.* Unpublished doctoral dissertation, University of Texas at Austin.

Reverby, S. (1987a). A caring dilemma: Womanhood and nursing in historical perspective. *Nursing Research, 36,* 5–11.

Reverby, S. (1987b). *Ordered to care: The dilemma of American nursing, 1850–1945.* Cambridge: Cambridge University Press.

Rosenberg, C. E. (1979). Inward vision and outward glance: The shaping of the American hospital, 1880–1914. *Bulletin of the History of Medicine, 53*(3), 346–391.

Rosenberg, C. E. (1987). *The care of strangers: The rise of America's hospital system.* New York: Basic Books, Inc.

Rosner, D. (1982). *A once charitable enterprise: Hospitals and health care in Brooklyn and New York, 1885–1915.* Cambridge: Cambridge University Press.

Stevens, R. (1989). *In sickness and in wealth: American hospitals in the twentieth century.* New York: Basic Books, Inc.

Tomes, N. (1983). The silent battle: Nurse registration in New York State, 1903–1920. In E. Lagemann (Ed.), *Nursing history, new perspectives, new possibilities* (pp. 107–132). New York: Teachers' College Press.

Vicinus, M. (1985). *Independent women: Work and community for single women, 1850–1920.* Chicago & London: University of Chicago Press.

Woodham-Smith, C. (1951). *Florence Nightingale 1820–1910.* London & Glasgow: Fontana Books.

2

The Intersection of Race, Class, and Gender in the Nursing Profession

Darlene Clark Hine

Nurses are among the most critical components of the entire health care delivery team. Physicians, hospital administrators, social workers, and community leaders are quick to attest to the significance of the nurse as a key professional involved most directly in hospital patient care and in health care delivery in general. In spite of the strategic importance of nurses' special skills there continues to exist a chronic shortage of nurses. No racial-ethnic community or geographic region has escaped the many adverse consequences of an inadequate pool of trained nurses. Moreover, since the 1960s an ever-expanding number of communities has wrestled with severe problems of dilapidated hospital facilities that have forced many closings across the country. In addition, the alarmingly short supply of physicians has especially exacerbated health care delivery problems in poorer rural and urban inner city areas.

Contemporary economic exigencies, gender stratification, and a history of racial exclusion have interacted in ways that shape and sustain the current nursing and medical personnel crisis. In recent years increased media attention has heightened our sensitivity to the external, or societal, and internal, or professional, forces that result in high incidence of "nurse burnout." Articles, reports, and surveys have delineated all the variables contributing to "burnout," including low pay, long and irregular hours, and the demeaning subservient roles nurses are expected to play in the medical and hospital hierarchies. Further, as nurses seek

Note: This chapter was originally published in *Critical Issues in American Nursing in the Twentieth Century: Perspective and Case Studies,* 59–68. New York: Foundation of the New York State Nurses Association, Inc., 1994. Reprinted with permission.

advanced educational credentials the profession itself has been forced to confront a deepening stratification along racial and ethnic lines.

Racial-ethnic and working-class White women occupy the lowest rung in the professional nursing hierarchy. Supervisory positions in hospitals and private agencies, and the nursing professoriate remain, with few exceptions, the exclusive preserve of middle-class White women. The nursing profession is a potent laboratory for the study of the convergence of factors and forces that helped to create the structural under-representation or exclusion of women and men of color from virtually all of the controlling institutions and learned professions in this country. More specifically, against the backdrop of nursing, it is possible to examine the historical difficulties that Black Americans have encountered in their struggle for greater access to the medical and legal professions throughout the first half of the twentieth century.

In my book, *Black Women in White: Racial Conflict and Cooperation in the Nursing Profession, 1890-1950* (1989), 1 examine the struggle of Black nurses to win integration and acceptance into the mainstream of American nursing. Fully one half of the book, however, traces the establishment and evolution of the institutional infrastructure of Black health care, that is, hospitals, nursing training schools, and collegiate programs in nursing. In two works in progress, one a history of Black physicians, and the other, a history of Black lawyers in the 20th century, 1 continue this line of investigation, but with a slightly different shading. I move from a horizontal to a vertical level of analysis as I probe the ways in which the Black struggle for professional integration helped to lay the basis for the emergence of the modern civil rights movement during the 1950s and 1960s.

Infusing all of my work on the history of Blacks in the professions is the desire to demonstrate how essential it is for scholars of women's history to incorporate race as a category of analysis, and for Black Studies scholars likewise to pay greater attention to the construction of gender roles within the Black communities that they investigate. And, of course both Black and women's history scholars should be ever mindful of class, or where people in any given group stand in relation to the means of production, and differences growing out of regional location. Finally, when examining those groups considered or relegated to marginal status by the larger society, it is critically important to use agency as an analytical category. Agency can be variously defined either as a consciousness of resistance or as a process whereby subordinate groups acquire the skills needed to effect social change, modification, or reform.

In sum, I am urging my colleagues in both areas, and reinforcing those who already do, to employ more sophisticated multi-dimensional conceptual categories in their analyses of Black and women's subjects. The categories or concepts that work for me are race, gender, class, regionalism, and agency. Only by employing them and probing their intersection was I able to approach more comprehensive understanding of the conflict and cooperation that permeated the nursing profession and that punctuate the past and present of Black women.

The contours of Black nurses' struggle for acceptance and recognition, like those of the Black doctors and lawyers, were shaped by factors as diverse as regional location, economic depression, and the catastrophe of war. The decades between the world wars witnessed first a hardening and then eventually a softening of racial animosities between Black and White nurses. Racism was a pervasive ideology during the period from the 1890s through the 1950s. This ideology of Black inferiority and White supremacy dictated the subordination of Blacks in every key area of American society.

Although slave women had for generations provided nursing care for both Blacks and Whites, when the first nursing schools opened their doors in 1873 few administrators expressed interest in training Black women. The New England Hospital for Women and Children in Boston was an exception. In 1879 the school graduated the first Black professional nurse in the United States, Mary Eliza Mahoney (1845-1926). But even here, the reception of Black women was restricted. The charter of this pioneering nursing school stipulated that only one Negro and one Jewish student be accepted each year. No school in the southern states admitted Black women.

The conflict and tension, as reflected in the attempts of White nurses to bar Black women from entry into the profession, to deny them appointments to supervisory positions, to exclude them from membership in professional organizations, to restrict their access to training schools and post-graduate education, and to ensure that they received less pay for the same work go beyond racist ideology. White nurses feared economic competition with Black nurses who, for understandable reasons, would sometimes work for less money and perform household tasks shunned by their White counterparts. Further, Black women's long association with domestic service provoked status anxiety among those White nurses who labored to distance the profession from any taint of servitude.

While investigating the history of Black women in the nursing profession my attention soon focused on the larger political arena in which they worked. In order to affect social change and to improve their status in the nursing profession, Black nurse leaders had to cultivate the necessary organizational skills, and had clearly to articulate an integrationist political agenda. Simultaneously, they had to create a consciousness of resistance to demeaning stereotypes of themselves as women and as nursing professionals.

The leadership of Black nurse Elizabeth Carnegie captures well this consciousness of resistance so essential to survival and self-esteem. In keeping with long-established patterns of racial etiquette, all the White administrators, physicians, and nurses at St. Philip Hospital in Richmond, Virginia addressed White nurses as "Miss" and Black nurses as "Nurse." In the 1930s this practice was, as Carnegie notes, "a step up from being addressed by first names." As if to compound Black subordination within the hospital hierarchy, Carnegie recalls, "Not only were Negro nurses addressed this way by the White nurses and doctors, they were instructed to address each other and refer to themselves in this manner." Refusing to acquiesce to this social affront and professional slight, Carnegie, then a new clinical instructor, exhorted her Black co-workers, "You can't control what someone else does, but you can control what you do." She admonished the Black student nurses to "address themselves and each other as 'Miss'." She insisted that the Black students extend this courtesy and show respect by addressing all their Black patients as "Miss, Mrs., or Mr.," in spite of the fact that White nurses and doctors also addressed the Negro patients by their first names (Jones, 1988, p. 178).

Nursing, a predominantly female profession, existed in the shadow of the male-dominated medical establishment. Early dreams of an autonomous profession of women health care providers had quickly faded into a subordinate reality. Within ten years of the founding of the first nursing schools, hospital administrators dominated virtually every aspect of nursing training. Two factors, insufficient capital and endowment, and the demand for more scientific-based instruction, enabled hospital administrators quickly to gain hegemony in nursing education.

Through the opening decades of the twentieth century, White nursing leaders had no alternative but to leap into the political fray. They struggled to gain control over admission standards, curriculum, work practices within the hospitals, and nursing licensing and registration. When male hospital administrators, motivated chiefly out of a desire to secure an obedient, subservient, cheap labor force to clean the hospitals and care for the patients, accepted impoverished, poorly educated, unrefined women into their diploma programs, nursing leaders objected. As long as the young women lured into nursing came from impoverished backgrounds hospital administrators enjoyed absolute control over their dominions. Nurse leaders rightly reasoned that the convergence of traditional female subservience, and class disparity between student and administrator, nurse and physician, actually strengthened and secured male authority over the nursing profession.

As early White nursing leaders devised strategies to raise the status of nursing, they ignored the adverse consequences that their actions and policies had upon the career aspirations of Black women. Thus, White leaders emphasized the need to attract the "superior type" of woman into the training schools. Obviously this "superior type" mirrored the Victorian ideal of true womanhood: middle-class, native-born, White, unmarried, and protestant. The vision of the ideal nurse excluded Black women who not only suffered the legacy of slavery but were, as a rule, members of the class of working poor.

The efforts of nurse leaders to recruit "superior types" converged with the modernization of American hospitals. By the turn of the century administrators recognized the need for a more reputable and efficient supply of cheap labor to maintain the hospital and to attend to the demands of a growing middle-class patient clientele. Not surprisingly, the class lines initially drawn in the late nineteenth century hardened considerably during the early decades of the twentieth century.

As a second strategy to raise the status of the nursing profession, White nurse leaders organized professional associations. In 1894, spurred by the call of Isabel Hampton, superintendent of the Johns Hopkins School of Nursing, nurse leaders formed a body which subsequently became the National League of Nursing Education (NLNE). Soon thereafter, American and Canadian graduate nurses organized what would be renamed in 1911 the American Nurses' Association (ANA). The leaders of the NLNE, ANA, and the many other emergent national societies fought to upgrade the status of nursing and to transform a "calling" into a profession. Again, Black women, in the absence of specific provisions that would have overcome the racial exclusion practiced by southern state organizations, were, with few exceptions, denied membership in these national associations, and thus rendered professional outcasts.

In this respect the experiences of Black women in nursing parallel those of Blacks in both medicine and law. Two medical schools, Howard Medical School in Washington, D.C. founded in 1868 with support from the federal government, and Meharry Medical School in Nashville, Tennessee, bore the responsibility of training over eighty percent of all Black doctors in the country prior to the modern civil rights movement. While Howard and Meharry effectively preserved the presence of Black men in medicine, so effective were the exclusionary practices and sexually discriminating policies of the vast majority of medical schools that women, especially Black women physicians, all but disappeared by the advent of the Great Depression.

In 1890 there were 909 Black physicians, approximately 90 of whom were Black women. By 1920 the figure had jumped to a total of 3,885, but the number of Black women doctors declined to only about 65 by 1925. A similar reduction is also true for White women. It is reasonable to suggest that Black women desiring health care careers turned in larger numbers to nursing.

That Black women did secure a place, albeit a negligible one, in the early nursing profession reflects the self-determination, sacrifice, and self-denial of hundreds of Black community residents and the leaders who founded the hospitals and nursing training schools. Beginning with Chicago's famed Black physician, Daniel Hale Williams, who in 1891 founded Provident Hospital, scores of Black professionals, educators, and Black women's clubs launched a veritable "Black Hospital and Nursing Training School" crusade. Under the leadership of Booker T. Washington, the Tuskegee Institute School of Nurse Training in Tuskegee, Alabama opened in 1892. In the same year the Hampton Nurse Training School and Dixie Hospital in Hampton, Virginia accepted its first class. In 1894, Williams was instrumental in creating another Black nursing school, the Freedmen's Hospital and Nurse Training School in Washington, D.C. Two years later, in October 1896, Black women of the Phillis Wheatley Club founded the only Black hospital and nursing training school in New Orleans, which eventually became the Flint Goodridge Hospital and School of Nursing.

By 1920 there existed 36 separate Black nursing training schools. Of course, in 1926 there were 2,150 predominantly or exclusively White institutions. It is difficult to exaggerate the extent to which Black communities, with their meager resources and hand-made supplies, sustained these fledgling and perpetually struggling institutions. Many of the hospitals and nursing schools courted financial disaster and seemingly always existed on the brink of collapse. The community contributions to their survival ranged from cash donations to that of an elderly Black woman who in 1905 donated to Douglass Hospital in Philadelphia, "a mince pie, 1 leg of lamb, 3 cakes of hard soap, and 4 pounds of grits" (Rudwick, 1951, p. 52). Organized groups of Black clubwomen raised funds to purchase linen, food, equipment, and to repair physical plants.

Any discussion of Black women in the nursing profession necessarily involves an examination of the institutions that trained, and to a limited extent, employed them. These early Black nursing schools were, for the most part, as deficient in quality and standards as were many of their White counterparts. In keeping with prevailing practices the student nurses were exploited as an unpaid labor force. In every institution they performed all the domestic and maintenance drudgery, attended the patients, and dispensed medicine. The trials and tribulations endured were such that many student nurses at Tuskegee Institute in Alabama required extended leaves of absence to recover from damage done to their health while working in the hospital. It was not inconsequential, therefore, that one of the early Tuskegee catalogues noted that the major admission requirement into the nursing program was a strong physique and stamina to endure hardship.

Clearly the most oppressive aspect of Black nursing training at some of these early schools involved the hiring out of student nurses to supplement the hospital's income. At the Charleston, South Carolina Hospital and Nursing Training School, the student nurses were required to turn over to the hospital the dollar-a-day they earned on private cases. These students also managed the hospital's poultry operation, tended the vegetable gardens, and organized public fund-raising activities. At Tuskegee the extensive hiring out practices and unrelieved toil in an unhealthy environment provoked a student nurse revolt and a threatened mass walk-out. The embattled hospital administrator, physician John A. Kenney, eventually persuaded Booker T. Washington to accede to some of the students' demands. Kenney later blamed this unique demonstration of belligerence on women who were, as he maintained, "not prepared for the serious study of nurses" (Kenney, 1909).

The meagerness of primary sources prevents a detailed analysis of the Tuskegee Training School's culture that made such an organized expression of discontent possible. A letter from a 1918 graduate of Tuskegee Institute, Bessie Hawse, does, however, shed some light on the kinds of services the student nurses were expected and able to provide upon completion of the training program. Hawse wrote to John A. Kenney:

I shall tell you of an experience of which I am very proud. Eight miles from Talladega (Alabama) in the back woods, a colored family of ten were in bed and dying for the want of attention. No one would come near. I was glad of the opportunity. As I entered the little country cabin, I found the mother in bed. Three children were buried the week before. The father and remainder of the family were running a temperature of 102–104. Some had influenza, others had pneumonia. No relatives or friends would come near. I saw at a glance I had work to do. I rolled up my sleeves and killed chickens and began to cook. I forgot I was not a cook, but I only thought of saving lives. I milked the cow, gave medicine, and did everything I could to help conditions. I worked day and night trying to save them for seven days. I had no place to sleep. In the meantime, the oldest daughter had a miscarriage and I delivered her without the aid of any physician. I didn't realize how tired I was till I got home. I sat up at night alone, and one night with a corpse in the house. The doctor lived about twenty miles away. He came every other day. He thought I was very brave. I didn't realize till it was over just how brave I was. I did feel happy when they were out of danger. I only wish I could have reached them earlier and been able to have done something for the poor mother. (Kenney, 1919, pp. 53–58)

In spite of the attendant hardships and the mediocre instruction, hundreds of Black women like Hawse were graduated from these segregated hospital nursing programs and proceeded to render invaluable service to the Black sick. It is little wonder that given the service they provided, and the fact that they were often the only available health care professionals, Black nurses enjoyed a high level of respect and esteem within the Black communities. Indeed, many Black hospital administrators and physicians agreed that the Black nurse had helped rural Blacks to overcome their abhorrence, often justified, of hospitals. Physician J. Edward Perry founded the small proprietary Wheatley Provident Hospital and Nurse Training School in Kansas City, Missouri. In a particularly candid appraisal of the nurse, Perry declared that "The nurse is a co-partner of the doctor. Without her, in many instances, his efforts in the battle of disease would be futile." Perry admitted that "since the inception of the work of Wheatley Provident Hospital the nurses have played a conspicuous part." He confided, "But for their loyalty and devotion, the institution would early have been grounded upon a sandbar of disaster and chaos" (Perry, 1947, pp. 376, 382).

One caveat is in order at this juncture. Few of these Black institutions would have been able to survive without the substantial financial contributions of White philanthropists. Throughout the first half of the twentieth century White philanthropic foundations, most notably the Chicago-based Julius Rosenwald Fund, and a Rockefeller trust, The General Education Board, provided sums for building construction and renovation. Foundations established graduate and post-graduate fellowships for nurses and physicians, granted salary supplements for special personnel, offered operating expenses for clinics and training programs.

The role of the philanthropic foundations in the overall struggle to provide adequate health care for Black Americans is a complex one. On the one hand philanthropic donors could not escape the charge that their contributions to Black hospitals and nursing training schools actually strengthened racial discrimination and preserved segregation. To the extent that Blacks maintained and operated parallel institutions their demands for admission into White or public institutions fell upon unsympathetic ears. While it is tempting to interpret philanthropic largesse in simple altruistic terms, here again the underlying motivations are more complex.

Between 1929 and 1942 the Julius Rosenwald Fund distributed over a million and a half dollars to Black health care enterprises. Rosenwald explained that improving Black health was the only way to protect and preserve the health of the White population. He advised all to heed that "It is well to remember that germs recognize no color lines and the disease in one group threatens the health of all" (Rosenwald, 1928). Certainly mindful of his admonition, the General Education Board (GEB) launched an ultimately doomed million-dollar experiment. The GEB attempted to entice the University of Chicago to cooperate with Provident Hospital to provide clinical experiences for the University's Black medical students who were not allowed to work in the institution's own hospital. A 1922 interoffice memo gives additional insight into beliefs and assumptions underlying philanthropic benevolence:

> *The GEB's interest is neither sentimental nor merely humanitarian, it is practical. The Negro race is numerous and widely scattered; it is with us to stay. Aside from any concern which on humanitarian grounds might be felt for the Negro for his sake, it is clear that the welfare of the South, not to say the whole country—its prosperity, its sanitation, and its morale—is affected by the condition of the Negro race. (Fosdick, Rose, & Dillard, 1922)*

Here it is important to underscore that racism within the health care professions not only restricted the numbers of Black men and women who became physicians and nurses but it also endangered the health of African Americans in general. The most tragic example of the disregard for Black health and life was reflected in the infamous Tuskegee Syphilis Study conducted at Tuskegee, Alabama under the aegis of the United States Public Health Service. The experiment, begun in 1932, doomed approximately 400 Black sharecroppers who were deliberately denied treatment for their syphilitic infections in order that researchers could study the course of the disease.

Historian Allan M. Brandt pointed out the two essentially racist percepts undergirding the experiment. He declared, "First, the doctors who designed the study believed that virtually all southern Blacks were infected. Second, they contended that the men involved would never be treated anyway." During the forty-year duration of the study, the Public Health Service, as Brandt notes, "actively sought to prevent the men from receiving therapy, all the while telling the subjects that they were being treated by government doctors. Many of the men—perhaps more than 100—died as a result of tertiary syphilis" (Brandt, 1987, pp. 157–158).

As indicated, Black leaders and communities with White philanthropic allies created institutions that provided Black men and women the opportunity to become physicians, nurses, and even lawyers. But earning the nursing diploma, the medical or legal degree did not signal acceptance into the professions. Most professional associations, including the American Medical Association, the American Nurses' Association and the American Bar Association, denied membership to Blacks. In order to belong to these hierarchically structured groups, nurses, physicians, and lawyers first had to win membership in local affiliates. Of course, all southern-based affiliates prohibited Blacks from becoming members.

Left with little alternative, Black professionals embraced the ideology of self-determination and commenced in the late 1890s the arduous task of creating a separate network of professional associations. Black physicians meeting in Atlanta, Georgia in 1895 founded the National Medical Association. In August 1908, fifty-two Black nurses met at St. Mark's Episcopal Church in New York City to found the National Association of Colored Graduate Nurses (NACGN). And finally, in 1925 Black lawyers established the National Bar Association at a meeting in Des Moines, Iowa. To be sure, the separate associations played a significant role in the ongoing struggle against racial exclusion and segregation. One of the most important contributions these associations made was the promotion of positive self-esteem among the Black professionals. Their annual conventions and deliberations enabled Black professionals to build networks, make business contacts, share information and sharpen leadership skills. Still, not all Black professionals approved of the separate Black organizations and institutions. Some northern Black professionals, especially those who had been trained at elite White institutions, argued that the existence of separate Black units took the pressure off Whites to integrate. Black nurses rarely seemed to participate in this debate.

In 1912 the NACGN had 125 members and by 1920 it boasted a membership of 500. Beginning in 1934, at the height of the Great Depression, under the leadership of NACGN President Estelle Massey Riddle and Executive Director Mabel K. Staupers, with funds provided by White philanthropic foundations, especially by the Julius Rosenwald Fund, the organization launched a sustained attack against discrimination and segregation in the nursing profession. At this juncture, White nurse leaders, perhaps alarmed by the possibility that Black nurses would accept the invitation of Black physicians to become an auxiliary of the National Medical Association, for the first time seriously entertained dropping exclusionary barriers to membership in the American Nurses' Association. Under no circumstances, they reasoned, should any group of nurses affiliate with the male-dominated medical profession. Such action would set a precedent injurious to the autonomy of the nursing profession.

It was this decades-long and often frustrating quest for integration that distinguished the Black nurses' engagement in the process of professionalization from that of their White counterparts. Riddle's and Staupers' relentless struggle against the discriminatory quotas imposed by the military establishment during the World War II years eventually won for Black women full integration into the mainstream of American nursing.

The struggle for acceptance and recognition impelled Black nurses to develop a finely tuned political consciousness and to devise innovative battle plans. They had to nurture relations with an array of public agencies, civil rights organizations, media representatives, and prominent individuals outside the boundaries of the profession itself. The inescapable reality of entrenched racism within and without nursing, therefore, necessitated and reinforced in them a dual consciousness. At a fundamental level their professional struggle simply mirrored the larger war for first-class citizenship waged by Black people across the centuries.

In 1951, their integration goal achieved, Black nurse leaders took an unprecedented step. They dissolved the NACGN. Never before had any male—or female—dominated Black professional or civil rights protest organization deliberately folded. Ironically, in 1971, a new generation of Black nurses, dissatisfied with the limitations of the integration meted to them, created the National Black Nurses Association, and in so doing, suggested that the earlier dissolution had been premature. Nevertheless, the existence of the National Black Nurses Association bears witness to the resilience and intransigence of racism that infect not only American nursing but the entire society. In sum, the trials and tribulations of Blacks in the learned professions mirror the larger war for a truly diverse and pluralistic society where the content of one's character is the only viable measure of worth.

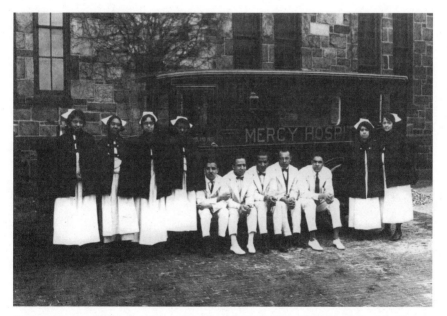

Student Nurses and Doctors, Mercy Douglass Hospital, circa 1935. Courtesy of the Center for the Study of the History of Nursing, University of Pennsylvania.

REFERENCES

Brandt, A. M. (1987). *No magic bullet: A social history of venereal disease in the United States since 1880* (expanded ed.). New York and Oxford: Oxford University Press.

Fosdick, R., Rose, W., & Dillard, J. H. (October 6, 1922). Interoffice memo on Negro education. General Education Board Papers. Rockefeller Archive Center, Pocantico Hills, North Tarrytown, NY.

Hine, D. C. (1989). *Black women in white: Racial conflict and the nursing profession, 1890–1950.* Bloomington: Indiana University Press.

Jones, A. H. (Ed.). (1988). *Images of nurses: Perspectives from history, art, and literature.* Philadelphia: University of Pennsylvania.

Kenney, J. (February 4, 1909). Memorandum to executive council. Booker T. Washington Papers. Library of Congress, Washington, DC.

Kenney, J. (1919). Some facts concerning Negro nurse training schools and their graduates. *Journal of the National Medical Association, 11,* 53–38.

Perry, J. E. (1947). *Forty cords of wood; Memoirs of a medical doctor.* Jefferson City, MO: Lincoln University Press.

Rosenwald, J. to Finney, J. M. T., Jr. (September 25, 1928). Julius Rosenwald Papers. University of Chicago, Chicago, IL.

Rudwick, E. M. (1951). A brief history of Mercy Douglass Hospital in Philadelphia. *Journal of Negro Education, 20,* 52.

SECTION 2

IDENTITY:
THE MEANING OF NURSING

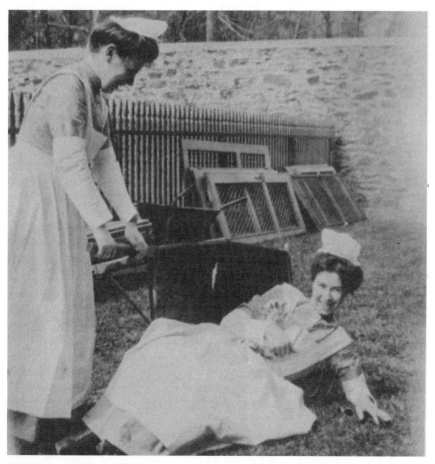

Pupil Nurses in Their Off Hours, circa 1915. Courtesy of the Center for the Study of the History of Nursing, University of Pennsylvania.

Introduction

Joan E. Lynaugh

How is it that a person takes on the persona of a nurse? And, how does the personal meaning behind that identification take root, change over time, and respond to place and custom? In spite of a natural inclination to identify ourselves with our predecessors—in effect, to link ourselves with a heroic past—historians are learning that the professional identity assumed by nurses varies with time, place and custom. Nurses mirror the culture wherever they reside. But still, when we look at any given time or place, we see nurses participating in a shared identity or, as Bernard Anderson would put it, building an imagined community.[1]

For instance, as historian Janet James explains in the first article in this section, Isabel Hampton invested her great energy in creating an identity in which the women of her time could wrap themselves. In Hampton's imagination women represented a superior moral force. Shared loyalty and discipline among nurses, she believed, would enable them to leave the protection of their homes and go out to work in the world. Her concept of nursing identity relocated women's domestic probity and productivity to the new, institutional venue called the hospital. In this way, Hampton intertwined the nurse's identity with her hospital where she trained to become a member of the new turn-of-the-century nursing community. Pride in one's school, badges of distinction, uniforms and caps, all served to link novice and graduated nurses together in a "little world of our own."[2]

But, when we turn to Douglas Baldwin's story of Mona Wilson, we find this idealized world viewed from the bottom up. And, a very different world it is! Young, middle-class Canadian Mona Wilson, arrives at Johns Hopkins to live and learn to become a nurse in the protected but isolating system created by Isabel Hampton and her colleagues. Mona finds a way to cope with the rigors of nurses' training by identifying with her new friends. In a way somewhat reminiscent of soldiers in combat, Mona and her friends accept the nursing school's 'molding' demands for obedience, loyalty, and much hard work. At the same time, they discover and sustain their own real world of trust and support by identifying with each other. In these two accounts we can readily see, first, a public nursing identity designed to frame and protect a new woman's work in a hostile environment, and second, a very personal nursing identity built on shared experiences, affection, survival of hardship and camaraderie.

Sylvia Rinker's study of obstetric nursing carries the matter of nursing identity into the complex world of nursing practice. Here we see the tension between nurses' self-identification as nurturers and their aspirations for taking up the scientific tools of 20th century patient care. Can nurses merge the identities of mother surrogate and healer? In the 1920s and 1930s this question perplexed nurses trying to reconcile the standardizing demands of aseptic efficiency with their ideal of patient-oriented compassionate care. Historian Rinker argues that the rigid, scientific obstetric nursing developed by 1940 conflicted with the individualized and sympathetic care desired by patients and idealized by nurses. Of course, this was problematic on humane grounds but, as Rinker observes, when rigidity overcame compassion, it also undermined nurses' relationships with patients—threatening a crucial source of their nursing identity and authority. Nowhere is nursing identity more complex and potentially conflicted than when nurses are negotiating the difficult tasks of selecting and giving needed care while, at the same time, trying to nurture individual human needs and relieve suffering.

Finally, in the last paper in this section, Linda Walsh examines the identity of professional women who are wives, mothers, and neighbors. Using the life stories of Philadelphia midwives she reveals the family support systems, the community respect, and the financial remuneration she argues were essential to sustain enduring caregiver identity. Walsh's midwives viewed themselves as professional and financially self-dependent practitioners. They were esteemed for their work and, following the pattern of professional women, they expected and received domestic help from husbands, children, other relatives and sometimes neighbors. Most nurses of their times left the paid workforce when they married or certainly did so on the birth of their first child. That these midwives remained in life-long practice suggests a clear identification with work that transcended social expectations for women's behavior. In this case the cultural prestige of their practice validated, both for them and for their family and community, a life that relied on alternative approaches to meet domestic demands.

We find in all four of these articles both the nucleus of nurses' identity and the impact of environment, knowledge, friendship and community respect on nurses' self-perception. Although the characteristics of professional identity change over time, identification as a nurse remains a powerful force granting the lone individual participation and sustenance within a larger group. History suggests that it is this sought-after and shared identity that adds meaning and significance to life and work.

NOTES

1. Bernard Anderson, *Imagined Communities*. (London and New York: Verso, 1983.)
2. Nancy J. Tomes, "Little World of Our Own": The Pennsylvania Hospital Training School for Nurses, 1895–1907." In *Women and Health in America*, ed. Judith Walzer Leavitt, 467–481. (Madison, Wisconsin: The University of Wisconsin Press, 1984.)

3

Isabel Hampton and the Professionalization of Nursing in the 1890s

Janet Wilson James

In the fall of 1889 a young woman in Chicago and another in Baltimore took up jobs which were to have a major impact in the interlocking worlds of social welfare and health care, as well as on the status of women. Jane Addams opened the doors of Hull House; Isabel Hampton took charge of the new school for nurses at the Johns Hopkins Hospital, which had opened the previous spring. At the time, Miss Hampton and her training school were more in the public eye. The Johns Hopkins Hospital, sixteen years in the planning and building, was widely expected to inaugurate a new era in medical research and education, as well as in hospital construction, administration, and patient care. Miss Addams and her project for a social settlement had become somewhat familiar to Chicagoans but were unknown outside the city. Time was to reverse the spotlight. Today Jane Addams is a historical figure of the first rank, while Isabel Hampton, who led the movement that still continues for the professional independence of a major occupation for women, is buried in seldom-read histories of nursing to be found only in nursing school libraries.

Hampton's relative obscurity owes something to the fact that her effort took place within a social structure over which she had little control, and hence was only partly successful. Jane Addams, on the other hand, was an entrepreneur in what her contemporaries called philanthropy, who independently fashioned an institution. Yet the two had much in common.

Note: This chapter was originally published in *The Therapeutic Revolution: Essays on the Social History of American Medicine*, eds. Morris J. Vogel and Charles E. Rosenberg. Philadelphia: University of Pennsylvania Press, 1979. Reprinted with permission.

Both were feminists of a nondoctrinaire sort, who, in their girlhoods of the 1870s, had absorbed some sense of the opportunities appearing in the world outside the confines of the Victorian home. Evading marriage, each cast about for wider spheres of influence. Industrial society at the time was beginning to institutionalize women's traditional domestic functions, both economic and nurturing. Without much risk of criticism, women willing to try something new in an urban setting could be guardians of culture in libraries, uplift the poor in charity organizations and settlement houses, or nurse sick paupers in hospitals that were being made safe and respectable through sanitary reform. Jane Addams determined to "study medicine and 'live with the poor,'"[1] but lost her enthusiasm for science in medical school and found another way to benefit the lowly. The less affluent Isabel Hampton fled from teaching district school into nursing and discovered a struggling new women's field without standards or leadership.

The Johns Hopkins Hospital Training School for Nurses was Hampton's opportunity. In the hospital, professionalization was in the air, and feminism was politely knocking at the gate. A group of well-to-do Quaker women in Baltimore, several of them daughters of the trustees, had enlisted friends in other eastern cities together with a number of well-known female physicians in an ambitious effort to secure funds for establishing the long-awaited Johns Hopkins University School of Medicine. The ladies attached two conditions: that entrance standards be raised above those in existence anywhere else, and that admission be open to women. The conditions were not so welcome as the money. The first caused the medical staff a moment of panic. Yet the central purpose of the Hopkins plan had always been to raise the standards of the medical profession and medical care through the striking example of a hospital which should function as a laboratory for teaching and research; it was not hard for them to raise their sights a bit higher. The second condition occasioned more misgivings, for they had not envisioned women as part of the select company who would lead the way into modern medicine.[2]

After the fund had reached the $100,000 mark, the hospital trustees gave a luncheon for the donors. The speaker was Dr. Mary Putnam Jacobi of New York, whose professional attainments surpassed those of all other medical women and most medical men of her day. Dr. Jacobi declared that two ruling ideas animated her group—one, that medical education was "an intellectual matter," and the profession "not a mere trade, to be practiced for pecuniary profit"; the other, that "women are to participate to the full in this intellectual aspect of medicine."[3] The luncheon was held at the Nurses' Home at the hospital, where everyone met on common ground, so to speak, for on the propriety of training women as nurses, all were agreed.[4] A training school had been a feature of the farsighted plans for the hospital from the beginning, at a time when no such schools existed in the United States except in a few women's hospitals staffed by women physicians. Such a school, constituting a skilled labor force of apprentices directed by experienced head nurses and a woman superintendent, was an essential part of the concept of the modern hospital as defined by Florence Nightingale, along with pavilion-style wards, and elaborate provision for hygiene, through sanitation and ventilation. A model of hospital design, the Johns Hopkins was prepared to set the pace for the training of nurses, also.

This intention was clear at the ceremony inaugurating the training school in October 1889. "A large and distinguished audience" was on hand, including the mayor of Baltimore, James Cardinal Gibbons (archbishop of this oldest American diocese), President Daniel Coit Gilman of the Johns Hopkins University and Mrs. Gilman, hospital trustees and medical staff, several superintendents of nursing schools from Philadelphia hospitals, and the Sister Superior of Baltimore's Mount Hope Retreat, together with about a hundred interested local ladies. Isabel Hampton hailed the progress of nursing ("of the various professions opened to women during the past few years, none have made more sure and rapid growth nor met with greater public favor than that of the Trained Nurse"). She pointed out that the Hopkins school had already attracted women of "superior attainments," and promised that "as the University and Hospital are looked to from all quarters for what is best in science, so . . . this School may be looked to for what is best in nursing." The hospital's superintendent, Dr. Henry M. Hurd, assured the gathering that in this training school, "service in the Accident Department and in the Dispensary; in the Medical, Surgical, Gynaecological and Pay Wards" would be accompanied by "carefully devised courses of study and systematic mental training. . . . In the eyes of the Trustees," he added, "nursing the sick is not to be considered a trade but a learned profession."[5]

The speakers' emphasis on the word "profession" is striking, since the question of whether nursing is a profession in any strict sense of the word is still moot today. It is true that the term, then as now, was commonly applied to vocations which, if less exacting and autonomous than medicine, for example, could be considered equally altruistic. Hurd and Hampton could simply have been indulging in rhetoric intended to enhance the status of nursing. Nor did the term, in 1889, have today's sociological denotations; medicine itself had not become a profession in the full modern sense.

On the other hand, the speakers had the confident air of heralds of progress, and the place and the company gathered there were significant. At Johns Hopkins, President Gilman had created the American prototype of the modern university, with its research orientation and its facilities for graduate training. Thus he was already a prime mover in shaping modern professional standards and distinctions. At the request of the hospital trustees, the majority of whom also served as trustees of the university, Gilman had personally set up the hospital's administration and sought out its key personnel, including Dr. Hurd and Miss Hampton. Furthermore, if the female fund-raisers for the prospective medical school succeeded with their plan, the school's entrance requirements would set new standards for the medical profession. At the same time, admission of women medical students would be a striking advance for their sex.

Looking back at that day from the viewpoint of our own, one may wonder why there was no thought at Johns Hopkins of bringing the training of nurses into the university structure at some level. The social psychologist Anselm Strauss calls this "a curious paradox," although he correctly observes that not even Isabel Hampton envisioned such a connection for nursing.[6] To imply, however, that the group at Hopkins refused to seize a genuine opportunity for the advancement of nursing and women is to raise a false issue and one that distracts attention from the real significance of the plans for the training school. College education for nurses (as for 95 per cent of the American population) was not a social necessity in 1889, any more than it was for teachers, who constitute a more appropriate reference group than physicians. The training school was and would remain a part of the hospital, not of the university. But the Johns Hopkins was to be a new kind of hospital, in which patient care would be closely related to medical teaching and research. The nurses would be part of a community of science, and the elaborate ceremony opening the school signified a deep interest in and high expectations for this important department of the new institution. The talk of professionalism was not idle. The major impetus for the professionalization of nursing in the United States was to come, in the decade of the 1890's, from the Johns Hopkins training school and its successive women administrators, with some assistance from their male associates.

Lavinia Dock, who was Isabel Hampton's associate superintendent of nurses at Johns Hopkins, learned from hard experience, and from the example of British nurses of her generation, the peculiar problems of professionalization in her field. Dock's nursing career made her a feminist, and the themes of independence, autonomy, and self-determination resound through her account of what the historian today might call the "modernization" of nursing.[7] She knew well the tension, classic in the modern history of health care, between efforts to raise standards of education and practice on the one hand, and, on the other, the controls exerted over women by society in general, and over nurses by the medical and hospital professions. In the early years at Johns Hopkins this tension had somewhat abated, and the atmosphere was unusually favorable to professional growth. We must begin, therefore, by separating out the historical elements in that atmosphere.

The hospital and the school had their roots in Baltimore's Quaker community, and its traditions of humanitarianism and the equality of the sexes. Both the founder, Johns Hopkins, and Francis T. King, president of the board of trustees, had a lifetime interest in medical charities. Hopkins, a survivor of the cholera epidemic of 1832, had retained from that experience a shocked memory of the dearth of medical and nursing care and hospital facilities. For many years he and King served on the board of the Maryland Hospital in Baltimore. They were therefore acquainted with the state of such institutions in mid-century America: charitable shelters for the sick poor, where "nursing" was a low-paid, low-status job for laboring class women, who, over a twelve-hour day, attended to the physical needs of the patients while doing the heavy domestic work on the wards. In 1867 Hopkins, King, and the other board members reported that the hired nurses at the Maryland Hospital lacked "method, order, invention, or energy" and were not "sufficient in number or intelligence to perform their duties." That was the year when Hopkins secured an act incorporating a new hospital and set up its board of trustees, with King at the head. To found this institution and a university, he left his fortune of $7 million, the largest sum any American had yet bequeathed for philanthropic purposes. In his final letter of instructions, written in March 1873, Hopkins made it clear that a "training school for female nurses" was to be established "in connection with" the hospital, a facility intended, in his sober words, to "compare favorably" with the best in Europe or America.[8]

Behind the specifications of Hopkins's letter lay not only his own experience as a local hospital trustee but some lessons of recent history. The mortality from disease among soldiers in the Crimean War and the American Civil War had drawn public attention both to glaring deficiencies in army hospital and medical care and to the capabilities of women in organizing at least partial remedies—from the towering figure of Florence Nightingale to America's lesser heroines in hospital service and in the work of the Sanitary Commission. It seems likely, from his choice of words, that Hopkins had in mind the model training school for nurses which Miss Nightingale had established in 1860 at St. Thomas's Hospital in London. The school had certain feminist aspects. Except for orders regarding the care of patients, the Nightingale plan rejected medical administration of nursing services in favor of an independent, women's nursing organization, the training school, "connected with" the hospital but having its own funds, a separate nurses' home, and a lady superintendent. The Nightingale model thus in a sense restored to women, in a secular framework, a measure of the autonomy they had lost in Protestant countries with the decline of the religious nursing orders.[9] In response, nursing in England had begun to regain status and to attract more intelligent and dedicated women. One may surmise that this reform made a strong appeal to Hopkins and King. After Hopkins's death, King journeyed to England in 1875 to see the Nightingale school at first hand. He had "lengthy interviews" with Miss Nightingale and after his return sat "night after night" (as his daughter recalled) talking about her work.[10]

Meanwhile other Americans in large cities, activated by the same concerns, and led by women veterans of wartime volunteerism, had also been studying the training school at St. Thomas's. In 1873, the first three American "Nightingale schools" for nurses opened in connection with hospitals in New York, Boston, and New Haven. As King and his fellow trustees (the majority of them also Quakers) carefully proceeded with the planning and construction of the Johns Hopkins Hospital over a period of fifteen years, they were able to observe the progress of these pioneering experiments.

At Bellevue in New York, for instance, "pupil nurses" replaced the "hired nurse" of a former day. These trainees, recruited from "a better class of women" and working under the direction of a woman superintendent, did give the patients more humane and conscientious care, and introduced cleanliness and order into institutions where these had been lacking. Nevertheless, the long hours, heavy work, and working class image hung on. The "training" was mostly hard experience under scanty supervision by the superintendent and by head nurses who were themselves only second-year students. Once a week, in the evening, after twelve hours or longer on the wards, the nurses were exposed to an elementary lecture by a physician; as a young lecturer at the Bellevue Medical School, Dr. William H. Welch, who would become chief of pathology at Hopkins, had delivered such talks to classes of weary young women hardly able to keep awake. In the second year of training school, "pupils" were sent out to nurse in private homes, their pay going into the school or hospital treasury. At the end of the two-year course they "graduated" and left the hospital for a career of live-in private duty nursing, caring mostly for obstetrical or "fever" (typhoid or pneumonia) cases in the homes of those sufficiently well-to-do to afford such a luxury.

The Bellevue training school produced most of the nursing leaders of the next generation, including Hampton and Dock; it also inspired them to strenuous efforts toward more radical improvements. The school's founders had done their best, but even the combined resources of this group of aristocratic women, most of them veterans of war relief work who had turned to reforming public charities in New York, could raise standards no further. Municipal officials and the medical staff were satisfied with things as they were. The pupils, receiving room and board and a meager wage called an "allowance" for personal expenses, provided nursing service at low cost. The more visible abuses of the old system had been removed, and the quality of nursing service was adequate, especially for a patient population whose medical care was an act of charity. The greater respectability of the pupil nurses, and the glamour shed upon nursing by Florence Nightingale, concealed from the public, from hospital administrators, and from the pupils themselves the fact that they were as much an exploited female labor force as the old hired nurses had been.

In planning the nursing for the Johns Hopkins Hospital, its trustees began afresh, rethinking nursing in the context of a new kind of institution. As their chief medical adviser they chose John Shaw Billings, of the United States Army Medical Corps. Essentially a sanitarian of the Nightingale era, Dr. Billings was convinced that buildings were the key to the problem. Not only would correctly designed structures eliminate contagion and cross-infection, but in a hospital intended "to assist in educating physicians, in training nurses, in promoting discoveries in medicine," they would also attract "proper and suitable persons to be the soul and motive power of the institution" by providing a favorable environment for growth.[11]

As an admirer of Miss Nightingale's principles of hospital design, Billings had supposed that her training school for nurses would also provide the model for the school at Hopkins. But a tour of hospitals all over Europe, followed by an inspection of the American schools and a study of the literature on the subject (almost all of it "favorable to . . . the Nightingale system"), completely changed his mind. The essentially feminist plan of the Nightingale school he found personally exasperating and administratively unsound. He could not advise the trustees "to establish an independent female hierarchy, which will consider from the very commencement, that one of its main objects is to endeavor to be independent of all males, who are to be considered as the natural enemies of the organization." The superintendent of nurses would have her hands full "teaching the women how to nurse"; she should report to the hospital authorities.[12]

As an army man Billings was accustomed to nursing by hospital orderlies; he was reluctant to see nursing become an entirely female occupation and would have liked the trustees to "try the experiment of training a few, say half a dozen, male nurses."[13] Nevertheless he agreed that in general women made better nurses and had no doubt that "an educated, properly trained female nurse," in many cases "as important to the success of treatment as a competent doctor," was essential "in a properly conducted hospital ward."[14] On this ground all could agree.

One problem remained, and Billings, not given to beating around the bush, approached it directly. Promiscuous sex had been part of the folklore surrounding the hired nurse, but Florence Nightingale and the women advocates of trained nursing believed that the superior character of the trained nurse would banish immorality from the wards. Billings, remarkably free of the conventional Victorian assumptions about female sexuality, was skeptical. "If a female nurse is a properly organized and healthy woman," he declared, "she will certainly at times be subject to strong temptation under which occasionally one will fall, and this occurs in all hospitals in which women are employed without any exception whatever."[15]

Billings now returned to the drawing board. To "remove opportunities" for temptation as much as was practicable, the nurses' quarters would be located not in the hospital but, as Miss Nightingale advised, in a separate home, though on the hospital grounds. Francis King was insistent that the home be "a model of excellence and of sanitary perfection." Billings exerted himself and produced "a large and handsome building," as he described it at the hospital's opening exercises, "separated from the others, and exclusively appropriated to the female nurses, where each can have her comfortable room," along with "a common parlor, library, dining-room, bath-rooms, and, in short, the arrangements of a first-class hotel. . . . The intention is that when the nurse has finished her . . . tour of duty with the sick, she shall come quite away from the ward and all that pertains to it, and take her rest and recreation in a totally different atmosphere."[16]

Such surroundings could be expected to attract women qualified to be nurses not only for the new medicine but for an expanded patient population. It was already evident that with increased powers of healing, hospitals in the future would no longer be merely charitable shelters for the sick poor but centers of scientific care for all. Voluntary hospitals had always made some provision for the upper classes—travelers, for instance, who might fall ill in a strange city. Following Johns Hopkins's wish, Dr. Billings included "special accommodations" for "pay and private patients" in his earliest plans. Fourteen years later, when the hospital opened, he took pains to assure the well-to-do "that when they are afflicted with certain forms of disease or injury they can be better treated in a properly appointed hospital than they can be in their own homes, no matter how costly or luxurious these may be."[17]

Though Billings's rejection of independent status may have been a loss for the training school, Daniel Coit Gilman's plan for the administration of the hospital proved a gain. As Dr. William Osler told the story, the manager of the Fifth Avenue Hotel in New York, a friend of Gilman's, gave him a tour of its operations, from which he emerged with the idea of organizing the hospital "in departments, with responsible heads, and over all a director," each unit being "the exact counterpart of one of the sub-divisions of any great hotel or department-store."[18] The training school thus acquired an equal standing among components of the hospital that served to enhance the superintendent's authority.

There remained the major administrative appointments, for the head of the training school and the director of the hospital. Gilman's choice for the latter post, Dr. Henry M. Hurd, was an experienced administrator of asylums for the insane. Dr. Hurd cared about the quality of hospital life. Though he was in agreement with Billings on the importance of "strict accountability for the performance or neglect of duty," he had a distaste for the stiff military approach. To Hurd the prime consideration was "the development of kindly instincts and humane methods of thought among all employees." Discipline ought to be "sustaining in its nature and calculated to develop the individual." Far from a mere "avocation, a trade, a preparation for getting a living," the nursing of the sick should be infused with "sympathy, kindly feeling, enthusiasm and personal interest," the nurse "happy and contented in her chosen calling."[19]

As a man of science, however, Hurd saw other aspects of the nurse's role besides nurturing. He had realized from the beginning that the school "must inevitably feel the influence of the great University to which the Hospital is so nearly allied."[20] Soon after his appointment, the trustees despatched him on a tour of training schools in Boston, New York, New Haven, and Philadelphia. He returned with the recommendation "that careful attention should be given to the more purely intellectual part of the nurse's training," with studies "systematized and extended beyond what is at present attempted in any existing school."[21] Sympathetic from the beginning to nurses' aspirations, Dr. Hurd became a willing speaker at training school graduation exercises, on which occasions he was wont to assay the professional status of nursing and urge a forward step. His description at the opening of the Hopkins school of "the hands of the nurse" as "a physician's hands *lengthened out* to minister to the sick" was to become a favorite quotation of Isabel Hampton's when explaining her profession to the public.

For the post of superintendent of the training school there had been "scores of applicants," including the heads of most of the major existing training schools.[22] King, Dr. Billings, Gilman, and Dr. Osler, hospital physician-in-chief, interviewed the four leading candidates. Osler recalled later that "as Miss Isabel Hampton left the room, Mr. King looked approvingly at Mr. Gilman, who smiled assent at Dr. Billings. I whistled gently the first two bars of the tune of '*Conquering kings their titles take—from the foes they captive make*'; as it was quite plain that a commanding figure, a sweet face, and a sweeter voice had in the short space of fifteen minutes settled the election of the Head of The Training school." Osler did add that "of course, the fact of two years experience at Chicago was taken into consideration."[23]

The four men had interviewed a young woman of twenty-nine, unusually tall at five feet ten inches, with fair hair, high coloring, blue eyes, and an ample figure, in the Lillian Russell style of the day. Her feminine attractions and air of authority may have swept the field, but the interviewers also sensed other qualities that fitted her to play a key role in their undertaking. Francis King, his daughter remembered, came home that day and said, "I have found an administrator." Like the staff physicians, Hampton had gone beyond a mastery of the existing knowledge and skills in her field to conceive broad and ambitious plans for its future, with which she had identified her own career. Like them, she had a strong physique and a vivid personality—in her case, a combination of dignity, charm, and enthusiasm and a maternal sense that evoked a strong positive response from patients, colleagues, and students alike.[24]

At New York's Bellevue Hospital she had seen the best and worst of hospital nursing in the 1880's. Some fellow pupils later remembered her as something of a nuisance, determinedly precise and methodical, despite the pressure of work in the busy wards, and constantly asking questions. Others, who, like her, were dissatisfied with their scanty instruction, met in her room in the evenings after the long working day to study anatomy and physiology out of medical books they bought themselves. When *Century* magazine in 1882 published a major article on the "new profession for women," it was illustrated by a sketch of first-year pupil Isabel Hampton measuring out medicines in a Bellevue ward.[25]

After graduation came two years of nursing at an Episcopal home in Rome for sick English and American travelers. There she gained social experience, a love for Italy and the arts, and a cosmopolitan outlook unknown in the small Canadian town of Welland, Ontario, where she had grown up. She came to Hopkins from three years (Osler's memory erred) as Superintendent of Nurses at the Illinois Training School in Chicago, whose pupils staffed wards in the Cook County Hospital. There she had worked well with the women's board of the school, won over hostile doctors to cooperation, and even, by "judicious engineering," induced the commissioners to make "long-needed improvements" in the hospital.[26]

Within the Illinois school, Hampton extended the instruction, meager though it was, into the second year, introducing for the first time in a training school something like a graded course of study. In addition, she abolished the practice of sending senior pupils out to work in private homes, and arranged an affiliation with the private Presbyterian Hospital where they might have supervised experience in the care of private patients.[27] Already her determination to eradicate the old image of

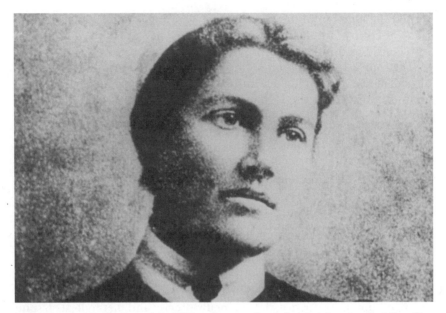

Isabel Hampton Robb. Portrait by William Sergeant Kendall, Administration Building, The Johns Hopkins Hospital.

the nurse was evident. A former pupil of this era later recalled that as Miss Hampton made rounds with the pupil head nurses, she gave little talks impressing "the fact that nursing is womanly work and we need lose no refinement in doing it. That one who became coarsened and hardened by her experience must blame herself, not the work. And in a last talk she expressed the hope that her pupils might marry and have homes and children."[28]

Hampton's ideal was to produce nurses who would meet the best British Victorian standards of womanhood. Perhaps even more than the moderately feminist American-born leaders of her generation, she took seriously the religious, moral, and cultural responsibilities assigned to her sex. She saw in nursing an opportunity for individual development and social service. Only a slight shift from the domestic scene would be required. Nurses, whether pupils or graduates, caring for rich or poor in home or hospital, were performing a nurturing function essential to human welfare. At the same time, modern medicine, hygiene, and dietetics were opening up new vistas of health. In her position close to the family, the nurse could exert enormous influence. As Lavinia Dock later recalled, Hampton held "the highest belief in the mission of women as the superior moral force, and in the possibility of universal happiness."[29]

Ontario, in the 1880's, had provided no outlet for her energy and ambition. A static provincial economy, her sex, and her social position as the daughter of a tradesman barred the way upward. Adelaide Nutting, her successor at Hopkins, who worked with her longer than anyone else, reflected at Hampton's death in 1910 that "had she been a man and in the business world, nothing could have kept her from an active and controlling share in some of the great organizations and combinations of which the world now hears so much."[30] In the United States, she saw an opportunity to improve society and make a career for herself by expanding woman's influence through a role already prescribed for her—to make nursing work "second to none done by women" through what has since come to be called professionalization.[31]

By the time Miss Hampton took up her job in Baltimore, the reputation of the Johns Hopkins Hospital, already widespread even before its opening, had attracted inquiries about the training school from a group of young women of strong educational background and social position. A comparison with the first and second generations of pupil nurses at the Boston Training School (one of the schools of the Nightingale model founded in 1873), who staffed the Massachusetts General Hospital, shows a marked difference.

In the records of the 181 candidates admitted to the Boston Training School in the decade of the 1870s, birthplaces were recorded in 119 cases. Only 14 of the candidates were natives of Boston; most of the others came from rural Massachusetts and other New England states (53), or from the Maritime Provinces of Canada (28). Of the 120 whose religion was recorded, 109 were Protestants. Previous occupations were noted, but only the paid ones. Eight pupils had been teachers, ten domestics, one a hospital attendant (hired nurse), five seamstresses, two machine operators, and one a clerk; the others must have been accustomed to hard work in small town or rural households.[32]

Fifteen years later, in 1889, the year the Johns Hopkins Hospital opened, the committee managing the Boston Training School assured the public that "the quality of the nurses" had improved, with "every effort" being made "to maintain and elevate the standard of teaching and requirements." Applicants now filled out a form with personal information and were required to furnish a reference from "some responsible person as to their moral character."[33] Between 1888 and 1891, 125 women entered training at the Massachusetts General. In some cases brief notes on education, intelligence, and "refinement" were entered in the ledgers that came to be known as enrollment books. In the 96 instances where previous education was evaluated, 50 were "poor" or "fair" and 46 "good." Judgments on intelligence, not surprisingly, corresponded with the educational ratings. Thirty-four women were considered "refined," 8 were judged to be lacking in refinement. Notes on the records of the latter make such comments as "liked by patients, good-natured, loud, flirtatious," "noisy, lacked attention to detail," and "talked too much."

The Boston Training School records show that the school in the years between 1888 and 1891 was drawing from the same largely rural and northern areas; only four pupils were from Boston. Twenty-eight had come from elsewhere in Massachusetts; twenty-five from Maine, New Hampshire, and Vermont; and thirty-four from Canada (almost all from the Maritimes). Southern New England contributed four, New York and New Jersey, twelve, and the Midwest, five.

At Johns Hopkins, Isabel Hampton began by setting up a records system later described as "the most perfect of its kind in any school" of the day;[34] this included complete duty records for both pupils and head nurses as well as correspondence with those applicants whom she accepted.[35] She herself made the admissions decisions; her authority in training school affairs is indicated by the reported experience of Dr. Hurd, who in her absence once wished to admit a Baltimore girl whom he knew, but with some irritation had to accept the reminder of associate superintendent Lavinia Dock that the decision must await Miss Hampton's return.[36] She based her judgments on a letter from the candidate, including specified information about education, health, and freedom from home responsibility, plus recommendations from a physician and a clergyman. The level of personal cultivation revealed in the candidate's letter weighed heavily.

The application records reveal a great deal about the candidates' backgrounds and motivations. The records of 105 pupils admitted in the school's first four years (September, 1889 through August, 1893) show that the would-be Hopkins nurses, like those at the Boston Training School, came mainly from regions close to the school and from Canada: 24 from Baltimore and elsewhere in Maryland, 12 from other states in the upper South and the District of Columbia, 10 from Pennsylvania, 8 from New York and New England, and 23 from Canada, virtually all from the province of Ontario. The letters, however, portray a middle to upper-middle-class group, drawn from the larger towns and cities rather than from rural areas. A large majority of the young women, moreover, had completed a good secondary education at a local seminary. In church membership they were heavily Episcopalian (53) and Presbyterian (14). Their physicians and clergymen were family friends who had known "Bessie" or "Effie" from girlhood and usually emphasized the family's elite social standing, as well as, on occasion, the writer's bias regarding work for women. Thus Susie Carroll of Little Rock, Arkansas, age twenty-five, was "a lady by heredity, breeding and culture and qualified by education and natural endowment to learn any vocation appropriate for her sex." Agnes Lease, twenty-eight, of Mt. Pleasant, Maryland, would be leaving "a happy and comfortable home in order to engage in labor in a harder field, is educated and intelligent beyond the average of your applicants as you will find. She is perfectly proper and refined in all her tastes."

Only a few of the applicants to the Johns Hopkins Training School were dependent on themselves for support. Most were simply restless, tired of the domestic responsibilities of the unmarried daughter or sister in the family, and eager for an absorbing occupation out in the world. The price of separation was often a painful conflict with parents who felt that woman's place was in the home and also, in many cases, that nursing was too hard and socially demeaning. Mary Heriot of Charleston, South Carolina, having at age thirty won such a battle, wrote "I am single, and my life is my own, to do as I please with, from now on." Mary Collins, twenty-three, daughter of a Washington, D. C., physician, had studied abroad and was accomplished in organ, piano, French, and German but had "no special occupations except home duties." According to her pastor, "Maidie" waged her campaign with "great fortitude and patience"; her father finally took her side against her mother and wrote Miss Hampton himself: "As her desire, for years, has been to prepare herself for a career of usefulness as a trained nurse, she now leaves home with my full consent and blessing. Her mother very naturally, under the circumstances, raises some objections. . . ."

Those few who had been employed had worked mostly in such genteel occupations as teaching and giving lessons in music and languages, or serving as companions and housekeepers to the aged. Two who entered in 1892 had had business experience: Harriet Carr, educated at a Sacred Heart convent, who had connected herself with a new industry employing women and was assistant secretary at "the telephone company head office" in Hamilton, Ontario; and Julia Feeley of Pittsfield, Massachusetts, a graduate of Miss Salisbury's School for Young Ladies, who at thirty-three had been for six years "cashier in a large dry goods house in this city." Evvy Smith of St. Catharines, Ontario, had been keeping house for her father since her mother's death; with a second marriage he had acquired stepchildren to support, and her way was now clear to "earning an independent living."

Even after a student had arrived in Baltimore and was enrolled in the school, family claims had priority. The monthly reports of the training school record a number of incidents where students or even head nurses were called home by family illness. In September, 1896, Kate Calloway, a senior (second-year) student, had to give up training and go home at her sister's sudden death to take charge of the latter's small children. In March, 1892, two pupils were even "called home by the illness of friends." In 1891, one pupil's mother came and took her away after she had been in school for a month; "objected to her being a nurse" was Dock's note.

The large number of Canadian women in American nursing schools and leadership posts in these early generations has often been noted. The Canadians were breaking loose from a domestic setting which, because of class traditions, was even more strictly bounded than that of the American girl. In British Canadian families of the middle and upper-middle class, no occupation other than teaching was permissible; to be sure, few others were available. Better economic opportunities, moreover, were drawing many young men west to make their fortunes, creating a surplus of women with few alternatives to marriage. Isabel Hampton had been able to enroll at Bellevue (in 1881) only because teaching primary school had made her independent at twenty-one; a friend who had been admitted at the same time, but who was still living at home, was not permitted to go by her parents. Adelaide Nutting, a Canadian woman of strong intellect who was to follow Isabel Hampton as the preeminent leader in American nursing, was thirty when she joined the first class at Johns Hopkins; Adelaide and her mother, who came of a "good" family, had struggled for years, despite meager resources, to keep up appearances so that the girl could "circulate" on the fringes of Ottawa society; her mother was dead and hope of marriage gone before she left home.[37] Ida McArthur, twenty-five, of Bowmanville, Ontario, who had had three years of schooling in Toronto, finally won her parents' consent to apply at Hopkins when her father lost his money. ("Though not accustomed to very hard work," she wrote Hampton, "I feel sure I should be able to do all that you desire.")

The applicants showed a striking eagerness for new experience, making touching efforts to convince Hampton of their suitability for nursing. Alice Preston of Troy, New York, had helped with the nursing in two fatal illnesses in her family. ("The undertaker didn't have to do a thing except carry the casket downstairs the day of the funeral. The nurse and I did everything for Miss Mollie even to the measuring for the casket. . . . Words cannot express my longing to become a nurse as soon as possible.") Katharine Laing of Philadelphia, thirty-two, earnestly "hope[d] that you will be able to accept me and let me begin as soon as possible. I have been waiting for this day, so many years, that now I feel, I do not want to lose a moment." Applications came also from several upwardly mobile nurses trained at other schools. Hannah Neill, thirty-three, wished to have a better training "and nice associates at the same time. . . . I have a horror of entering some of the Schools here who admit any class of pupils. . . . I am perfectly willing to unlearn everything not approved and to begin as a new beginner."

Some of the young women persisted despite considerable anxiety over their physical capacity to endure the training, not surprising in a day when many doctors felt that women lacked the stamina even for college study. As Lucy Sharp, twenty-eight, of North Carolina wrote, "I know of no particular way to guage *[sic]* my strength don't think I can lift much more than fifty lbs. without feeling it"; furthermore, she was "liable to suffer a good deal of pain every month when unwell am often obliged to lay quiet one day and sometimes even two."

Though they may have known little of medical science, the successful candidates, each through her own break with the past and her venture into an unfamiliar world, had prepared themselves for membership in the Hopkins community; in the 1890s, women as well as medicine were exploring the unknown. The remarkable spirit of unity, almost comradeship, that was shared by the people working in the hospital grew, in part, at least, out of a common past experience.

For the members of the first pupil class, their initial months of training were both exhilarating and confusing. Miss Hampton gave all the nursing instruction. Only one text had been written, Clara S. Weeks's *A Text-book of Nursing* (1885), which the author herself described as a mere compendium; "all the rest of our study," one of the pupils recalled, "and all our materia medica we got from notes which Miss Hampton had written herself for us to copy and study." The methods Hampton taught, however, were often not followed by the head nurses on the wards, who came from a variety of different training schools in the United States and England: each thought "her own . . . the only correct way." For the moment, however, there was time to feel a sense of participating in an historic undertaking. Everything was new, and as Lavinia Dock remembered, "a fresh and inspiring atmosphere did indeed permeate the whole place. . . . When I think of the hospital now," she mused in 1910, "it is always this picture that I see:—the nurses in their blue dresses streaming down the corridor, the green lawn, and young trees outside in the sunshine . . .; and Miss Hampton's caryatid-like figure, clad either in white or black, [her eyes] . . . radiant with pride and joy in her flock."[38]

Determined to give the school a clear identity as an educational institution, Hampton began by assuming a new title, Principal of the Training School, in addition to the standard Superintendent of Nurses. Her innovations in Chicago furnished a starting point for arranging the instruction. The central problem was to manage admissions and graduations of students, and to maintain a regular schedule of graded classwork, without disrupting the nursing service at the hospital. Hampton compromised. New pupils at Hopkins entered the hospital during three-month periods in the spring and fall and began their classes with the next term.[39] The twelve-hour day on the wards was eased to permit two hours off duty in the afternoon and one free afternoon a week. This made time for a few regular weekly classes: two a week, in nursing, by Miss Hampton for first-year students, and one for seniors. The staff physicians gave a weekly lecture to each group in the evening.

An expert teacher, Hampton emphasized the use of visual aids (what she called "object-teaching"). She equipped the classroom with a skeleton, a mannikin to demonstrate "visceral anatomy," charts, specimens, and pictures, and enlisted the doctors' aid in securing other material for "demonstrations." A collection of about twenty medical texts and other works in medicine and nursing made up a good working library. As at most of the better training schools, notes taken in class had to be carefully written out in ink and handed in to be corrected and preserved for future reference. Hampton required written as well as oral examinations and gave the seniors extra practice in writing through dictation, quizzes corrected and criticized in class, and the preparation of short papers on such subjects as the more important drugs, observations of symptoms, and treatment in emergencies.[40]

She also set the pace in introducing new subject matter in nursing. Other training schools had given pupils lectures on, or lessons in cooking, but Hampton, aware of new research in foods and nutrition, secured a resident "Diet School Teacher," a graduate of the Boston Cooking School, who not only taught cooking for invalids but also gave some elementary instruction in food chemistry. A course in Swedish massage, eight demonstration lectures by Miss Hampton herself, also offered a precedent for other schools.[41]

Even thus augmented, formal instruction could hardly be more than incidental to the strenuous on-the-job vocational training. This, in turn, was outstanding at Hopkins, not only because of the special quality of the hospital and its medical staff but because of the supervision given the pupils as they rotated on a fairly regular schedule through the wards, the operating room, and the dispensary. Hopkins wards were headed by graduate nurses, rather than by the second-year pupils found in such positions at most nursing schools, and Miss Hampton herself spent much time in supervision and ward teaching. Pupils soon were impressed with her governing concepts: a humanitarian sympathy for all sufferers; the importance of "thoroughly clean surroundings and pure air" as "conditions absolutely necessary to the recovery of patients"; and her insistence that "system and method prevail throughout . . .; the work is not done haphazard."[42] One student retained a vivid memory of her "taking me, a raw probationer, into an isolation backroom to nurse a baby with virulent gonorrheal conjunctivitis. She did not need to touch it; in clear words she explained the technique minutely, the danger to be incurred, and my responsibility to myself as well as to the child, and after assuring herself that I understood the significance of each act she watched me do the first dressing. I listened to her talking to the baby's mother, and I realized for the first time I had seen the ideal of a trained nurse."[43]

With such inspiration, morale was high.[44] In February, 1891, Dr. Hurd, submitting his first report as hospital superintendent, listed the work of the training school at the head of the achievements that had already given the hospital "an acknowledged position in the medical work of the country as a growing center of instruction and usefulness." In Baltimore the school, the city's first, had become the object of considerable pride and interest. Young women of good family were entering this "new field of usefulness," and Miss Hampton, introduced to local society by Francis King, found time for an occasional luncheon, tea, or concert, joined the Women's Fund Committee for the medical school, and "became well known as a delightful representative of the great Hospital and of a new profession for women." President and Mrs. Gilman gave pictures to decorate the Nurses' Home, and Miss Mary Garrett, a leader and chief donor of the Women's Fund Committee, supplied books for its library. When the first class graduated in June, 1891, the occasion was made a special ceremony. Francis King and Miss Hampton spoke briefly; Dr. Osler gave the main address and provided bouquets of roses, which Mrs. Gilman presented as each of the eighteen young women received her diploma from Dr. Hurd.[45]

Osler's address, entitled "Doctor and Nurse," and the courtly gesture of the roses hinted at a certain ambivalence on the doctors' part toward the women who had been trained to be their skilled assistants. For the nurses, the physicians were their superiors, their judges within the hospital and before the public, and their professional role models; they were also men, whom most of the young women were conditioned to regard as authority figures. To a large extent dependent upon these men for their own image of themselves, they received mixed signals.

Each of the famed Hopkins doctors had his own dramatic personal style, but in their official pronouncements and perhaps also their conscious minds they were united in hailing the trained nurse as an ally (as Osler put it) in "lessening the sad sum of human misery and pain by spreading . . . knowledge of . . . [the] grand laws of health." The chiefs of services enjoyed their association with Miss Hampton and then with her successor Adelaide Nutting, a more reserved personality, but a woman of breeding and intellect. They were also greatly interested in all the teaching that went on in the hospital, including the training school. Dr. Osler and Dr. Howard A. Kelly, however, never allowed the nurses to forget their lowly professional origins and the weaknesses which they, as women, were heir to. Dr. Kelly, for instance, reminded the second graduating class of their "inestimable privilege to have elevated the class you represent, from that of self-taught, selfish hired attendants." Democracy and enlightenment had created "a new and beautiful ministry," physicians and nurses joining with pastors in devoted and self-abnegating service to humankind. "I need not add," he continued, "that nurses dominated by this spirit do not everywhere fill the rank and file of the profession." Osler, on his part, was addicted to stereotypes of garrulous nurses babbling of patients' private affairs and "things medical and gruesome."[46]

It is hard to believe that Isabel Hampton's carefully selected candidates stood in need of these admonitions, yet considering them as women fresh from a domestic world of close personal relationships and informal, spontaneous sociability, with an education that at best had provided more cultivation than intellectual discipline, one can conceive that they may have had some difficulty in adjusting to a more formal, institutional setting.

The problem of professional relationships prompted the writing of *Nursing Ethics* (1900), Hampton's second book, which created and named a subject that still lingers in nursing school curricula. Like much else, the concept was borrowed from the doctors and then devalued. "Ethics," for nurses, turned out to be essentially a code of etiquette. Like most etiquette books, it was designed to enable the reader to acquire the standards of a higher social class. The complex history of nursing, however, imparted to the code a distinctive emphasis on stringent discipline.

Historically, this element was in part a legacy from the military, religious, and nursing orders going back to the Middle Ages, with their traditions of obedience, subordination, and self-abnegation. Imbibing these through her training and experience, Florence Nightingale transmitted them to the secular, progress-minded nineteenth century. The standards of behavior they set were useful in the difficult task of upgrading the nursing service, and, fitting in with the British class structure, tolerable to English nurses of the new breed. The few American training schools of the first generation had not attempted this degree of control, but by the 1890s, circumstances were changing. One has only to read the directions, in Hampton's earlier textbook (*Nursing: Its Principles and Practice*, 1893), for cleaning the ward or preparing a patient for surgery to visualize the strenuous and unremitting activity of the daily twelve-hour war against germs, with no other weapons than cleanliness. To carry this enormous workload, pupil nurses, no matter what their standing in the loosely defined American middle class, had to be habituated to organization and discipline.

Few American girls had disciplined work habits, those from more affluent families being perhaps the least accustomed to constraint. And as was not the case in the other professions into which women above the working class were moving, such as teaching, librarianship, and social work, the pupil nurses were coming into contact, and working closely with not only other women, children, and families, but with men, ranging from the patients at the bottom of the social scale to the Johns Hopkins doctors at the top. Isabel Hampton, with her Canadian background and a mother who, as Adelaide Nutting remarked in several biographical reminiscences, was "a great believer in law and order and government, and a staunch upholder of British ideals in discipline,"[47] clearly found the old military tradition congenial. She also thought discipline essential, for if women were to win acceptance and status as nurses, to earn a good living, and, as she dreamed, to play their part in social reform, they must demonstrate their usefulness, and first of all convince their superior officers, the doctors.

Nursing ethics offered the key to success. Hampton and her successors in the genre identified three problem areas: manners, work habits, and sex, and laid down rules designed to transform the girlish chatterbox into a dignified and discreet nurse able to pick her way in a complex world of work where middle-class women were new and conspicuous.

In the early days at Hopkins, in the relatively relaxed atmosphere of the new hospital, Hampton, in her textbook, had attempted to define for her pupil nurses a manner both professional and womanly. On the ward, the nurse should "extend the same courtesy that she would show to visitors in her own home," rising to greet "the medical officers connected with the ward, the superintendent of the hospital, superintendent of nurses, and strangers." By 1900, working in the now renowned Hopkins or any other crowded, busy hospital, the gracious hostess had become a member of a platoon. "The head nurse and her staff should stand to receive the visiting physician, and from the moment of his entrance until his departure, the attending nurses should show themselves alert, attentive, courteous, like soldiers on duty."[48]

The proper attitude toward the patient underwent a similar change. According to the textbook of 1893, the nurse "should always make the patients feel that they are her first consideration, and that to do anything for their comfort is her greatest pleasure." She was adjured to be "particularly attentive and kind to a new patient: the dread of entering a hospital is bad enough, but much of the gloom can be removed by the bright, cheerful greeting of the nurse. . . ." The patient's friends, acknowledged to be "often the greatest trials that a nurse has to contend with," were likewise to be treated with patience. By 1900 this positive approach had given way to a warning that the pupil must be "very circumspect in her own language, and encourage nothing from patients, or their friends, that borders on familiarity, vulgarity, or frivolity."[49]

Home training, it appeared, was no longer sufficient. The ebullient young woman sometimes adjusted with difficulty to hospital routine. The probationer had to be warned that "unnecessary questions, talking and noise, are absolutely prohibited during the rounds of the medical staff," the junior pupil reminded that "the desire to talk incessantly, or to make unnecessary comments, should always be controlled," and the senior pupil admonished that "the operating room is no place for indulging in talking or frivolity of any kind." It was not permitted when off duty to "go into the hospital to visit"; similarly, having friends from outside the hospital "to visit one in the ward is quite out of place."[50]

Relationships with both sexes were hedged about with cautionary advice. Toward each other, pupils should show "nothing in the way of personal feeling," equally avoiding on the one hand "personal jealousy, discord, and faultfinding," and, on the other, "sentimental, intense personal friendships."[51]

Relationships with the opposite sex presented dangers which, though only obliquely referred to, had been, as we have seen, a source of serious concern since the beginning of hospital reform. Furthermore, the spinsterhood of nurses summoned up images of females desperate to secure a mate. Dr. Osler was prone to fantasies about the "gradually accumulating surplus of women who will not or cannot fulfil the highest duties for which nature designed them," whom he regarded as "a dangerous element."[52]

Since male folklore made woman the aggressor, nursing ethics, like the society at large, assigned her the responsibility for chastity, with careful explanations. "The ordinary little attentions and social privileges" that the pupil nurse "may have been accustomed to in the small social circle at home" could not be allowed in "the large wards of a hospital." Encounters with interns or resident physicians during the solitary hours of night duty were a subject of particular concern. The nurse must "emphatically" discourage "any disposition on the part of the doctor to stop for a friendly chat," or prolong his stay. ("If she is the only woman in a ward full of men," she risked losing their respect, thus lowering "the professional dignity of the entire nursing staff.") Should the doctor have to be called several times during the night, she must resist the temptation of giving him "any refreshment from provisions belonging to the ward."[53]

Other admonitions completed the restraint of impulse and the cultivation of caution: gossip was repeatedly condemned in every possible context; sympathy and sentiment were given limits; above all, the nurse must take care "not to make in any direction any unnecessary advances."[54] Middle-class habits of neatness, punctuality, truthfulness, study, method and order, personal hygiene, and table manners were inculcated as fundamentals. Finally, the military and religious traditions were explicitly invoked. "Above all, let her remember what she is told to do, and no more. . . ." And, amid injunctions to patience, gentleness, cheerfulness, and good temper, "the nurse's work is a ministry; it should represent a consecrated service, performed in the spirit of Christ, who made himself of no account but went about doing good."[55]

Isabel Hampton's working relationships with the Hopkins doctors were the subject of considerable gossip. At times, in the hospital, their interests clashed. Hampton's rotation of pupils from one service to another disrupted continuity in the wards, and her insistence on her authority to appoint head nurses, because of their teaching function, brought her to an impasse with surgeon William S. Halsted, who understandably wished to choose and retain his own operating team.[56] There was also some clash of wills with Dr. Hurd, a strong administrator, reserved, meticulous, and frugal; but though he does not seem to have been a popular figure with the nurses, he believed in the improvement of nursing, and not only because, as he said of Hampton after her death and his own retirement, he had "rarely, if ever, seen a woman with a more winning presence."[57]

The work of Dr. William H. Welch, the hospital's pathologist, did not bring him in contact with the nurses, but in after years he, too, faithfully seconded their efforts to improve their professional standing. Dr. Osler, Henry Hurd remarked tactfully after his death, "seemed always appreciative and helpful while at the same time he had an air of detachment as one who was endeavoring to see where the movement for the education of nurses would ultimately lead." Hampton, like Adelaide Nutting, was doubtless aware that Osler "liked certain nurses because he liked them as women."[58] The unfailing support of Francis T. King resolved many issues in Hampton's favor through the trustees' power of the purse. King's daughter recalled of Hampton that it was one of her father's "greatest pleasures to confer with her, and to listen to and encourage her admirable plans"; Miss Hampton nursed him herself in his last illness.[59]

The doctors' influence on the training school and the development of nursing went far beyond nursing ethics. Hampton worked with them at a time when the medical profession itself was reaching for a higher status in society, on the basis of its new powers of healing, and the men at Hopkins were in the forefront of this effort. As they built a new clinical base for medical education and research by redefining the functions of the hospital, they were also influencing the profession at large. Each in his own way, they cultivated a wide acquaintance, took an active part in professional associations, selected and trained younger men and placed them in important posts, conducted research and published it, founded new journals, and delved into medical history for past glories with which to identify. William Osler, the professor of medicine, gentleman scholar, embodiment of masculine charm and wit, served as a role model to a profession moving upward. Shining in medicine's reflected light, caught by the magnetism of the doctors' personalities and their confident sense of mission, the nurses imitated their professional structures.

Among the many ways in which the Hopkins doctors' example left its mark was the use of history to establish a sense of professionalism. One of the medical staff's Monday evening clubs devoted itself to historical studies; Osler and Kelly collected books on the history of medicine. Kelly, the leading gynecologist of his day, built up a library on the history of women, and his assistant, Dr. Hunter Robb, gave a series of papers at Historical Club meetings on noted French and German midwives of the past, whose work he extolled as professional in many respects.[60] It was during these years that Adelaide Nutting began her collection of books relating to the history of nursing, and she and Lavinia Dock conceived the idea of writing a book to celebrate the ancient antecedents of their profession and its progress to their own day. In the twentieth century, medical history was to thrive, as the prestige of the profession grew; attracting able, trained historians with or without medical degrees, it became a distinguished sub-field within the historical profession. Nursing history, lacking these vital transfusions, was kept alive in nursing school curricula by faithful followers of Lavinia Dock but finally fell into a state of inanition.

In June, 1894, Isabel Hampton resigned her post at the Johns Hopkins Hospital to marry Dr. Hunter Robb and move with him to Cleveland. In keeping with nursing ethics, their courtship had been discreetly conducted outside the hospital, causing no gossip except among the doctors.[61] She had organized the school and administered it for nearly five years, choosing as assistants two of the ablest women of her generation, Lavinia Dock and Adelaide Nutting. Within the hospital she had achieved the best training program of the day and a clearly defined professional standard of nursing service: by 1894, every nursing post on the staff was held by one of her graduates. She had written, in the late afternoons of those early years, in her office, after the day's work was over, *Nursing: Its Principles and Practice*, a detailed, 480-page text that would be standard in nursing courses for more than a generation.[62] Dr. Billings, in a review, remarked that the book was of interest to doctors as well as to nurses, "indicating what a trained nurse of the present day may be expected to know and to be able to do."[63]

Hampton had also readied a plan for a major new advance in the training of nurses that would shift the balance from service to education by extending the course to three years, reducing the workday to eight hours, and eliminating the money payment to pupils. In addition, she had laid the groundwork for the remainder of her career, which was to be devoted to organizing and upgrading the profession as a whole, and presenting to the nurses and to the public her conception of the nurse's role in the contemporary movement for social reform.

Her plans for a professional organization, specifically for a national association of nurses, and an advanced training course for teachers and admin-istrators, had been at least partly formulated by the time she came to Johns Hopkins. Lavinia Dock, who remembered enthusiastic conversa-tions about "nursing growth, organisation and activities" over leisurely Sunday morning breakfasts in the alcove of the nurses' dining room, had no doubt that these ideas had originated with Hampton.[64] The system-atized program of training and practice at Hopkins was intended to be an example that would inspire efforts for uniform standards everywhere; the group loyalty Hampton strove to instill was intended as a base for a larger "sisterhood."[65] Her efforts to extend the pupils' outlook beyond the confines of the hospital would build an awareness of social issues and thus provide worthy goals for united effort.

Some of the Hopkins pupils, before entering nursing, had been active in their churches, and hence may have had some experience in group work with other women, but there is no evidence of this in the applica-tion letters. The first step in building loyalty was to reconcile the pupils to working with others "with whom in every-day life one would have lit-tle in common." Nursing ethics, mindful of women's proverbial lack of loyalty to other women, next required them to refrain from disparag-ing other pupils "either to friends in the city or to doctors."[66] Graduates grew accustomed to working together, and strengthened their loyalty to the school in an alumnae association, founded in 1892, only the third to be organized in a nursing school (after Bellevue and the Illinois Training School), and the first to which all graduates of the school were admitted.[67]

Loyalty to the school, carried to an extreme, however, could be counter-productive. Pupils were admonished that "a nurse can give no stronger evidence of ignorance or narrow-mindedness than by behaving as if she considered herself, her school and her hospital better than any other."[68] From opening day, when nursing superintendents from Philadelphia were invited to the ceremony, Isabel Hampton's cordiality worked to break down the isolation of schools. Starting with her Canadian friends in nursing, a stream of training-school superintendents came to Baltimore to visit the hospital, the beginning of a communications network.[69] Lucy Walker, the English-trained superintendent of Philadelphia's Presbyterian Hospital school, timidly ventured to Baltimore in 1893, hoping to learn something about the new system which she had heard of for training nurses in the preparation of diets for the sick. Having no letter of intro-duction, she was amazed to be "at once received" by Hampton, who spent the day with her, invited her to lunch, and "explained her kitchen to the minutest detail."[70]

To open up some views of the world outside to pupils and nursing staff, Hampton took a leaf from the Journal Club which had been formed by the Hopkins doctors for discussion of current medical literature, and whose meetings she and Dock sometimes attended. A Nurses' Journal Club, founded in 1891, met for an hour every other Monday evening, officially "to keep in touch with what is being done in other schools and hospitals," but unofficially, also, to give the nurses practice in expressing themselves and to introduce them to important issues in nursing. Most of the participants read aloud from articles in medical or nursing journals; a few short original papers of a very informal sort were produced each year, on subjects like "Loyalty among Nurses," or "The Care of Children." Lavinia Dock may have been responsible for inserting in the program occasional articles from current magazines of opinion touching on subjects like capital punishment, the Negro nursing school at Hampton Institute, and Hull House (Jane Addams's first published account). In May, 1892, Father James O. S. Huntington, the reform-minded Episcopal priest, gave a short talk. A meeting in Miss Hampton's last year at Hopkins was devoted to "The Unregarded Causes of Ill Health in American Women."[71]

As she prepared her students and staff for participation in a profession, the growing reputation of the hospital and the training school brought Hampton opportunities to present her concepts of nursing and its goals to the public. She took full advantage of these, beginning with her address at the school's opening exercises.[72] On each occasion, varying the approach and emphasis with the audience, she pictured the new nurse, educated and idealistic, fitted to bring skilled care to all classes of society, whether in the hospital or at home. She then deplored the lack of uniform standards of training. A principal target was the small hospitals which conducted "schools" without the resources to offer a rounded nursing experience, throwing on the market poorly trained nurses who gave the profession a bad name.[73]

The new nurse described in these speeches tended to separate into two very different identities. In her hospital role, the nurse was the physician's obedient and loyal assistant, but the district nurse, bringing to the sick poor, in their homes, skilled care and instruction in the laws of sanitation, was an independent figure. In the latter role, the nurse occupies center stage, her medical supervisor somewhere in a shadowy background. She is an expert in household economy, versed in bacteriology, a woman of refinement and tact, who can convert her patients to "a healthier, better way of living" without arousing antagonism. The nurse could thus join the ranks of the progressive citizens of the day, bringing her own answer to the question, "What is to be done with the lower social conditions of life?"[74]

With her usual quickness and perceptiveness, Isabel Hampton had recognized the potentialities of a new kind of work which would both fulfill woman's mission of social uplift and enhance the status of nurses. District nursing, first developed in England, had been introduced in several American cities in the late 1880s by women who founded charitable associations to direct and finance the program. Chicago ladies had established such an organization during Isabel Hampton's last year at the Illinois Training School.[75]

Hampton carried with her to Baltimore the hope of introducing district nursing into the instruction and practice of the pupil nurses at Johns Hopkins, an advanced idea that was not to be realized to any extent in nursing education until the 1930s.[76] The Hopkins doctors were much attracted to this concept of social reform through the medium of medicine and hygiene.[77] But even the Johns Hopkins Hospital's funds were not bottomless, and as its work swiftly expanded, the pupil nurses could not be spared for an expensive experiment.

In interpreting nursing outside the hospital, however, Hampton continued to present the district nursing dimension. In May, 1890, when the National Conference of Charities and Correction held its annual meeting in Baltimore, in order to inspect the innovative facilities of the Johns Hopkins Hospital, she became the first nurse to address this influential group. Her report emphasized nursing's role in both scientific medicine and the contemporary vision of scientific charity, and the necessity of "exceptional women and training" to perform this work. She described the plight of a worthy profession without professional organization or any fixed standards of practice.[78]

That summer, on vacation in England, she visited one of the district nursing branches in London; the following spring, on a trip to Boston, she studied the operations of the Instructive District Nursing Association, considered the best in the United States. With this background she appealed to the Charity Organization Society of Baltimore later that year for a combined effort on the part of doctors, clergy, religious sisterhoods, nurses, and businessmen to establish district nursing in the city, pointing out that dispensaries could not reach "mothers of families, . . . chronic patients, and those who still retain their old prejudice against hospitals."[79] A few years later Lillian Wald, in New York, would invent the term *public health nurse* and capture nationwide interest by combining district nursing with a new kind of charitable institution called the *social settlement.* Isabel Hampton had done much to pave the way.

Hampton's efforts to define the status and role of nursing crystallized in the International Congress of Charities, Correction and Philanthropy that was held in Chicago as part of the Columbian Exposition of 1893. Hopkins-connected medical men dominated the Congress special section on hospitals; Hampton's Hopkins position gave her a leading role in planning the meetings devoted to nursing, and a platform for her views.

The range of papers showed not only Hampton's wide knowledge of the field and the people in it but also her excellent political sense.[80] Dock recalled later that "Miss Hampton really went through a mental process of construction of the entire subsequent evolution of the nursing profession. She placed the papers so that certain ideas should be worked out, and waited almost breathlessly for the results. . . ."[81] The most crucial, the papers on the history and organization of American training schools, the importance of training school alumnae groups, and the need for an all-inclusive nurses' association went to her fellow Canadians, the superintendents with whom she had often talked about their common problems.

Meanwhile Dr. Billings and Dr. Hurd had arranged for the superintendent and the assistant superintendent of the Johns Hopkins Hospital Training School to speak at the two most prominent meetings. The congress convened in mid-June. Early in the week, when one session considered major aspects of hospital administration, Lavinia Dock, appearing with Dr. Hurd, Dr. Edward Cowles of Boston, a German hospital director, and a Philadelphia hospital trustee, discussed "The Relation of Training Schools to Hospitals." In midweek came a presentation before the entire congress, when Isabel Hampton, sharing the platform with Dr. Billings and the English hospital authority Henry Burdett, delivered her carefully prepared paper on "Educational Standards for Nurses."

The two women knew hospital nursing in institutions ranging all the way from city or county hospitals, "where local politics grow at the expense of the neglected sick poor, . . . hating to be interfered with," to the munificently endowed Johns Hopkins, where hospital and school enjoyed "identity of interest and aims; a sense of mutual obligation; a reciprocal feeling of personal pride, admiration and attachment." Most hospital-school relationships, they knew, fell somewhere in between, characterized by "a formlessness, a lack of tradition, an adoption of hasty and tentative methods, and an acceptance of imperfect results." For all this the public blamed the nurses, "though much of the fault lies with the hospital."[82]

Dock reminded her audience of hospital leaders that trained nursing, interacting with "a dawning rationalism in medicine, antisepsis in surgery, [and] a growing intelligence of public opinion," had done much to bring hospitals into their present high esteem, and that it alone was responsible for the improved moral atmosphere of "the once foul old hospitals." Admittedly the new nursing system was more expensive than the old, yet the schools, by promising an education, insured "a steady supply of intelligent women," who, under school discipline, performed "an amount and quality of work which the hospitals could not possibly secure if they had to pay for it." In addition, many hospitals still made the pupil nurses support the school as well, by sending them outside on private duty.[83]

What the training offered by a hospital school should be was the topic of Hampton's paper, which she regarded as "the culmination of her teaching work."[84] In it she served notice that the achievements of the pioneer generation of schools were no longer good enough. Although virtually all hospital nursing was now done by training-school pupils, so widely did the schools vary in their requirements that the term "trained nurse" could mean "anything, everything, or next to nothing." She spoke plainly for the first time of the hospitals' responsibility to provide a real education in return for the nursing service, rendered for less than the pay of a ward maid. Hampton called for a spirit of unity and cooperation among the superintendents to determine upon a uniform system of instruction and work toward it, and proposed her plan of a three-year course with an eight-hour day of "practical work." In conclusion, she described the ideal background for a trained nurse: an education equal to that of the best high schools, and, to instill habits of throughness and system, home training in household economy, "a branch of woman's work . . . neglected or superficially understood by so many women in all ranks of life."[85]

In public meetings before an international audience of leaders in hospital work, Hampton and Dock had frankly discussed the basic, interlocking problems of nursing: the variability in training-school standards and hospital support. The dilemma, in somewhat altered form, would still be dogging the profession seventy-five years later.

There remained the question of what nurses themselves could do to raise their professional sights and standards. Hampton, in her address, had called for cooperation among the superintendents; Dock, in another portion of hers, although not mentioning Florence Nightingale by name, had advocated a return to the Nightingale system of a clear separation of the areas of medical and nursing authority. "The organization of a training school is and must be military," she declared, with "absolute and unquestioning obedience," and a chain of command leading to the head of the school. In the direct care of the sick the doctors gave the orders; in the internal affairs of the school, including teaching and discipline, the superintendent's authority should be absolute.[86] These themes would be picked up by the succeeding papers given before the nursing subsection,[87] whose meetings many of the hospital administrators also attended, since the schedules of the two subsections had been planned not to overlap.

Dock's paper provoked an interesting discussion from the audience. The speakers, nurses and hospital men, agreed on the necessity of full authority for the training-school superintendent, though Dr. Billings argued that women able to exercise such power were "extremely rare, just as men who are qualified to take charge of and command a big establishment are extremely rare." The real difficulty, he thought, would come over a question of disciplining "some nurse who is perhaps attractive in manner and ways," and "particularly satisfactory" to some trustee or member of the medical staff. But even in these cases, he concluded, "the rule of the superintendent of the training school goes with me." Dr. Hurd added his earnest conviction that there was a unity of interest between hospital and school.[88]

Hampton and Dock were disappointed at the timidity of the other nursing papers, especially that of Edith Draper, superintendent of the Illinois Training School, on "The Necessity for an American Nurses' Association."[89] The formidable presence of Henry Burdett, arch-foe of the British organization of a similar name, may have been intimidating, as was the paper sent to the congress by Florence Nightingale, who denounced the modern tendency to make nursing a profession, instead of a calling, and dismissed "examinations, public registration, graduation" as affording no proof of the dedicated character necessary for the true nurse. Miss Draper referred only vaguely to "a system of registering" to be administered by the association, without mentioning legislation, and Irene Sutliffe of the New York Hospital School, clinging to the Nightingale image, offered as justification for "a well-regulated association of nurses" its aid in the restoration of such ideals as "the beauty of self-sacrifice."[90]

The conflict in the nurses' minds between, on the one hand, the ideals according to which trained nursing had been founded and on which it had depended to create a new image, and, on the other, the realities of a modern profession, surfaced in a discussion following the paper by Louise Darche, superintendent of the New York City Training School at the pauper hospital on Blackwell's Island. Darche had described a school registry as one of the American alterations in the Nightingale plan. The nurses present seized upon this opportunity to discuss "prices," despite a clearly uneasy fear that such concern might be considered mercenary. The custom of having fees fixed by the registry was defended as preventing any unpleasantness with private employers, and the nurse's right to give her services for nothing was anxiously reserved. Lilla Lett, of St. Luke's Hospital in Chicago, offered as a possible model the plan in effect at her registry, where by agreement her graduate nurses worked without pay on cases in poor families for two weeks out of the year. But Lillian Wald, who had just begun her work among immigrant families in New York, struck a vigorous modern note: the nurse "should have the privilege of setting her own price. It is as much professional work as that of the physician."[91]

Hampton had known at least half of the superintendents attending the meetings for several years, through Canadian or Bellevue connections, but many of the other women later remembered that the chief event of the congress had been getting acquainted, and then suddenly realizing that "the deficiencies and difficulties of their work were peculiar to the whole nursing profession, and not to one school or hospital."[92] Hampton herself made essential contacts at the congress with the leaders from the Massachusetts General and Boston City hospital schools.

In one of the discussions about nurses' associations, she had laid down professional priorities. A national superintendents' association should come first; later the alumnae associations in the individual schools, of which only a few had yet been founded, could form the base for an association of all nurses. Following her suggestion that the superintendents should meet to discuss organizing, a few of the leaders conferred in Lilla Lett's sitting room at St. Luke's and determined to call a meeting after the session. "About eighteen" stayed to form the American Society of Superintendents of Training Schools in the United States and Canada. The name would carry no aggressive connotations or overtones of British militancy, and the election of officers brought into the movement the essential New England contingent. The two vice-presidents were veteran graduates of the Boston Training School, associated with the Massachusetts General Hospital: Mary E. P. Davis, superintendent of the University of Pennsylvania Hospital and its training school, and Sophia Palmer, founder and superintendent of the school at the Garfield Memorial Hospital in Washington, D.C. Lucy Drown, of the Boston City Hospital, was made treasurer. Anna Alston, of New York's Mount Sinai Hospital, became the first president; Isabel Hampton's old friend Louise Darche, secretary.

With the perspective of after years, Lavinia Dock could smile at the "awful solemnity" with which this nucleus of a profession took its first combined step. So conscious of standards was the new body that it excluded superintendents of small hospital training schools even when their own training had been unexceptionable, and she marveled that those present who fell under this decree made not a murmur of protest.[93]

It is worth noting that the members of the new society must have been aware of other women's recent activity in forming organizations. National women's suffrage and temperance organizations were now some twenty years old; the rising women's colleges had associations of alumnae, whose nomenclature the training schools borrowed for their own organizations of graduates; the proliferating women's clubs had recently founded a General Federation. A month earlier the fair had seen a much-publicized gathering of delegates from women's organizations, the World's Congress of Representative Women; daily, in the Woman's Building, a continuous Congress of Women was meeting with presentation of papers by or about women that eventually filled a thick volume.[94] A society of nurses would be something different, organized from the top down, because of the hospital authority structure, yet potentially more widely inclusive than any of the strongly middle-class women's organizations of that day. And, conscious of a history of their own whose great leaders were still alive, the founder generation of nurses had its special, if only partly conscious, feminism. As Louise Darche had said in ending her paper, "From its nature nursing is peculiarly a woman's work; a woman originated the training-school system in England, women started it in this country, women have brought it to its present stage of development, and it is to women we must look for its future advancement."[95]

Looking back at the congress after the passage of eighty-five years, one can see that in a sense the nursing papers which Isabel Hampton arranged constituted the first of a series of investigative reports which, once every generation, would diagnose and prescribe for the ills of this indispensable but floundering profession.[96] Like the later reports, the World's Fair program singled out nursing education as the key problem; like them, also, it estimated society's needs for nursing more accurately than society's readiness to pay the cost. In contrast to the others, the program was almost entirely the work of the nursing leadership, particularly Hampton and Dock, prepared for this role by their participation in the remarkably open community that launched the Johns Hopkins Hospital.

The Society of Superintendents proceeded briskly with its organization. With Dr. Billings's aid, Miss Darche rounded up the names of seventy-one superintendents to approach, and when the group met again in January, 1894, in New York, there were thirty new members. The forty-four superintendents present adopted a constitution defining the object of the society: "to further the best interests of the nursing profession by establishing and maintaining a universal standard of training and by promoting fellowship among its members. . . ."[97] Succeeding annual meetings debated the central concerns that had emerged at the World's Fair: the raising of standards of training along the lines Hampton had laid down; the operation of registries—bread and butter to the private duty nurse; the nurse's obligation of moral and social uplift; and the organization of an all-inclusive association.

In the society's discussions, hope mingled with hesitation and doubt. Hampton took a leading part in the proceedings and kept her key projects alive by securing the appointment of sympathetic committees. Lavinia Dock submitted comprehensive and astute reports on the registry problem, and explained the operations of other national professional associations, especially the American Medical Association. Everyone could agree that pupil nurses should not be sent out on private duty (a resolution to this effect was passed in 1896) and that training-school alumnae associations should be encouraged. The idea of a three-year course made headway, and by 1900 many schools were changing over. But the eight-hour day seemed only remotely possible; it would not become standard for nurses until the New Deal in the 1930s made it standard for everyone. The nonpayment plan, Hampton's idea for financing "a really liberal education as an equivalent for the three years' service,"[98] was adopted only by the few schools like Johns Hopkins that could attract young women of some means. Most superintendents were sure that without the cash allowance, worthy candidates would be unable to enter nursing, and the society finally refused even to endorse nonpayment.[99]

As Adelaide Nutting, who became head of the training school at Hopkins in 1894, took up the leadership of the superintendents' effort to raise standards of training, Hampton concentrated on the remaining goals of her long-cherished plan for the nursing profession. Lavinia Dock's study having prepared the way, a national organization of nurses came into being at a small meeting of superintendents and representatives of training-school alumnae associations at Manhattan Beach, New York, in September, 1896. Hampton, absent from meetings that year for the birth of her first child, returned, to be triumphantly elected the first president of the Nurses' Associated Alumnae of the United States and Canada.[100] Within three years a professional journal was in publication.

Hampton then found the capstone for her structure and set it in place. A debate at the Society of Superintendents' meeting in 1898 over qualifications for membership enabled her to initiate a discussion of training for superintendents, and to propose replacing the hard school of experience with a formal course such as normal schools provided for teachers. The duly appointed study committee returned the next year with a fait accompli. Proceeding alone, after the committee as a whole had been unable to settle on a common meeting date, Hampton and Nutting had arranged with Dean James E. Russell, of the newly founded Teachers College at Columbia University, for a year's course in "hospital economics" for graduate nurses, to begin that fall,[101] the origin of the department of nursing education which would train most of the leaders in the profession for the next forty years.

The decade of the 1890s had seen professionalization advance from little more than an idea in Isabel Hampton's head to seeming completion. And yet as the decade, and the century, ended, a feeling of frustration set in among the superintendents, as if their goal had somehow eluded their grasp. The Spanish-American War publicly demonstrated the lack of public influence of the Associated Alumnae, whose offer to recruit nurses was totally ignored by the government. Instead, women of social position and influence won the ear of the Surgeon-General, and volunteers were selected by Dr. Anita McGee, under the sponsorship of the Daughters of the American Revolution.[102]

By 1898, too, the superintendents were uncomfortably aware of widespread public criticism of trained nurses, particularly of that great majority of graduates who earned their living caring for cases in private homes. For the most part, it was not the nurse's skill or knowledge that was questioned, but her personal conduct: she was said to be too talkative or too arbitrary, she was wasteful of household supplies. One may surmise that families under strain of serious illness had difficulty adjusting to the constant presence of a stranger with ill-defined status and authority, a normal share of human failings, and usually some ignorance of upper class mores. The superintendents responded to this criticism with a stepped-up effort (reflected in Hampton's *Nursing Ethics of 1900*) to stiffen the morals and conduct of the pupil nurses. Superintendents' control of admission and expulsion must be absolute; candidates younger than twenty-five, not yet past the "silly age," should be rejected. As for carelessness and extravagance, the fault, of course, lay in the pupil's upbringing, but it was nevertheless the superintendent's duty "by precept and example and continued watchfulness during the two or three years we have them with us in training" to reform the character and send out "examples of economy as well as angels of mercy."[103]

Had they known it, the superintendents, in their renewed affirmation of Victorian middle class standards of female behavior, were binding nursing to a code that was obsolescent and already being challenged by a rising current of feminism. They were also flying in the face of demographic change. The last great wave of immigration was adding millions each year to the population, at the same time that city life and the prestige of modern medicine began to draw not only the ailing poor but the middle classes into the hospital. New institutions had to be built, and the small hospital (Hampton's bête noir) suddenly multiplied, as the upper levels of society, shrinking at first from the general hospital with its pauper associations, patronized proprietary institutions established by enterprising doctors. To assure themselves cheap labor, these proprietary hospitals opened so-called training schools, without assuming the obligations of such schools, as Hampton and the society conceived them.[104] After a decade of exciting challenge and dedicated work, Hampton and her small corps of superintendents, with their weak educational system and fledgling professional institutions, saw the private-duty market flooded with a new multitude of "trained nurses" from "schools" indifferent or oblivious to "professional" standards or refined demeanor. The employer, already disappointed in his expectations of gentle womanly nurture and economical use of linens, neither a virtue imparted in the rugged ordeal of hospital training, now was further put off by such poorly trained personnel.

Even in the 1890S, Hampton and the other superintendents of the best hospital schools had at times been forced to accept students whom they considered unqualified, simply to meet the needs for nursing service. From 1900 on, as hospitals multiplied and other occupations less demanding and isolating opened up to women, even the good schools had to dip down into the labor pool and admit ever more youthful and more poorly prepared students. By 1912, more than 55 per cent of pupil nurses were only twenty years old, or younger. The supply of middle and upper-middle-class girls with good educational backgrounds dwindled further, as many who might have entered nursing in the 1890s elected to go to college. Of the 303 students in seven New York City training schools in 1910 (most of the seven among the best in the country) more than half had had less than four years of high school.[105]

In 1890, with 35 training schools in operation, and something under 500 graduate nurses in the United States, Isabel Hampton's long-range plans had seemed practicable. But even in 1893 her new Society of Superintendents did not represent the majority of existing schools and nurses. By 1900 there were 432 schools; in 1909 they numbered 1096.[106] Only a minority of their superintendents belonged to the society, and only a minority of graduates joined their school alumnae associations (and through them, the Associated Alumnae), or subscribed to the struggling *American Journal of Nursing*, which for years lacked money for an office outside the editor's home. The Hospital Economics course at Teachers College attracted a bare handful of students in its first half-dozen years, and was kept alive only by contributions of money and teaching services from Hampton, Nutting, and a few others.[107]

Hampton's remedy for the dilution of standards by small training schools was still the idea of a central school offering a rounded experience in several small hospitals with different medical specialties. By 1905 she had broadened this concept to advocate a coordinating central institution in each state.[108] But the bigger version, like the smaller one, failed to come to grips with the basic problem of securing adequate financial support.

Of Hampton's proposed instructional reforms, the three-year course, by reducing turnover, worked to the hospitals' benefit and was generally adopted, but only a few institutions enriched the educational program as she had expected; elsewhere the old two-year curriculum was just spread thinner. She had triumphantly abolished the practice of sending senior students out to duty in private homes, but now some schools were making money by assigning seniors to special duty with private patients in the hospital for long periods. She had introduced graduate head nurses at Hopkins; now many hospitals put senior pupils back in charge, under the direction of a graduate nurse supervisor.[109]

As nurses actually lost ground in their efforts to establish standards, their counterparts, the doctors, were well on the way to bringing their sprawling profession under control. The American Medical Association was reorganized in 1901, and in 1904 it began the process of inspection and grading of medical schools which, culminating in the Flexner report of 1910, forced dozens of inadequate schools to close.

Within the profession which she loved with a possessive affection, Hampton's leadership was inevitably challenged. The two stalwart leaders of the Massachusetts General Hospital contingent, Sophia Palmer and Mary E. P. Davis, old friends and classmates and shrewd businesswomen, quickly made themselves felt in the Society of Superintendents. Palmer had taken the lead at the Manhattan Beach meeting which founded the Associated Alumnae, and in 1900, Palmer and Davis, to Hampton's exasperation, single-handedly launched the *American Journal of Nursing*, much in the fashion that Hampton and Nutting had produced the course at Teachers College. Relations were further strained when Palmer criticized the management of the course. With the Hopkins group, of course, Hampton's ties were strong, but even her long, affectionate friendship with Adelaide Nutting cooled as Nutting's strong intellect and will carried her to the forefront of organized nursing and, in 1907, to a professorship at Teachers College.[110]

Meanwhile Lavinia Dock moved into a different world, Lillian Wald's Nurses' Settlement on Henry Street in New York. Isabel Hampton had been the earliest public champion of district nursing, which she correctly perceived to be a field that nursing could develop for its own, a role that could attain a distinct social importance. Now, however, while private-duty nursing became the weary target of public criticism, the public lavished appreciation and support on Lillian Wald and her visiting nurses. The organizations which Hampton had brought into being struggled with internal problems, while more broadly based activity by women in movements for health, education, and recreation receded from their view. Miss Wald allied herself not with the medical profession but with the growing public health movement, secured the endowment which finally put the Teachers College course on its feet, and eventually took a leading part in forming a separate professional body, the National Organization for Public Health Nursing. And all the while, Henry Street was becoming the center of a circle of brilliant women social reformers and feminists in which Lavinia Dock found herself completely at home.[111]

To Isabel Hampton, life in Cleveland as Mrs. Hunter Robb also brought some measure of disappointment. True, she enjoyed the social prestige awarded the wife of one of the city's leading physicians, and found time for local nursing affairs, serving on the executive committee of the Visiting Nurse Association from its founding in 1901, and as chairman of the training-school committee of the Lakeside Hospital. Looking back on those years, Clevelanders felt that she had created a strongly supportive atmosphere for the profession there. Considerable evidence survives to indicate that her marriage was less than happy, however, though Dr. Robb does not seem to have interfered with his wife's professional work in any way. Household duties did sometimes interfere, and irked her generally. She loved her two sons, but reportedly overindulged them; after the birth of the second, in 1902, when she was forty-two, she became less active professionally. In June 1910, at the age of fifty, Isabel Hampton Robb was killed in a streetcar accident in Cleveland.[112]

As Adelaide Nutting reflected after Hampton's death, she had had, at Johns Hopkins, an opportunity to "create standard, precedent, and tradition at will, under conditions which were at that time little less than ideal."[113] Trained nursing was just emerging from its pioneer stage. At Johns Hopkins, thanks in part to Hampton's leadership and magnetism, it received recognition as an essential auxiliary of modern medicine, and a good measure of encouragement to keep pace with medicine and share in its rising status. The Hopkins experience encouraged Hampton's attempts to make nursing an organized, self-regulating profession for women; the World's Fair provided a highly visible public debut, and, under Hampton's spell, the impetus for the rapid formation of professional nursing organizations.

But the Hopkins experience of the early 1890s was a unique historical moment, and the Hopkins ambience did not prove reproducible elsewhere. Within the expanding hospital world of the new century, competition for funds intensified, and the nurses and their training schools inevitably emerged a poor second to the staff physicians. Caught in a vicious circle of public criticism, they clung to outworn notions of female gentility that frowned upon aggressiveness. Isolated and overworked in the hospital and on private duty, they were separated from the vital branch of their profession which engaged in active combat with social problems in the outer world, and sought to raise the status of women. The leadership at the top of what came to be the nursing establishment, encumbered by middle class prejudice (in the guise of idealism), continued to call for higher standards, with little response from the general public or a major part of their own constituency. The status quo would be accepted as woman's place for a generation or more to come.

NOTES

1. *Twenty Years at Hull-House* (New York: Macmillan, 1910), p. 61.

2. In their tentative acceptance of the women's committee's proposal, the trustees carefully defined the sphere of women doctors. "This board is satisfied that in hospital practice among women, in penal institutions in which women are cared for, and in private life where women are to be attended, there is a need and place for learned and capable women physicians." "Medical School Fund," *Johns Hopkins Hospital Bulletin* 1 (November 1890): 103.

3.   Ibid., p. 104.

4.   Ibid. Both the women's committee and the trustees prefaced their remarks on the admission of women as medical students by strong statements on the importance of training women as nurses.

5.   Ibid., 1 (December 1889): 6–8.

6.   "The Structure and Ideology of American Nursing," in *The Nursing Profession*, ed. Fred Davis (New York: John Wiley and Sons, 1966), p. 69.

7.   M. Adelaide Nutting and Lavinia L. Dock, *A History of Nursing*, vols. 1 and 2 (New York: G. P. Putnam's Sons, 1907); Dock, *A History of Nursing*, vols. 3 and 4 (New York: G. P. Putnam's Sons, 1912). Many times revised by Dock and Isabel M. Stewart, and finally by Stewart and Anne L. Austin, this classic work reached its 5th edition in 1962. Other authoritative surveys by nursing leaders are Mary M. Roberts, *American Nursing* (New York: Macmillan, 1954), and Isabel M. Stewart, *The Education of Nurses* (New York: Macmillan, 1943). Richard H. Shryock *The History of Nursing: An Interpretation of the Social and Medical Factors involved* (Philadelphia: W. B. Saunders, 1959), is an excellent survey by a distinguished historian of medicine; see also his "Nursing Emerges as a Profession: The American Experience," *Clio Medica 3* (1968): 131–47. For sociological treatments see Davis, *Nursing Profession*, and Amitai Etzioni, *The Semi-Professions and Their Organization: Teachers, Nurses, Social Workers* (New York: Free Press, 1969).

8.   Ada M. Carr, "The Early History of the Hospital and the Training School," *Johns Hopkins Nurses Alumnae Magazine* 8 (June 1909): 54–75; John S. Billings *et al., Hospital Plans* (New York: W. Wood, 1875); Donald Fleming, *William H. Welch and the Rise of Modern Medicine* (Boston: Little Brown, 1954). For the history of hospitals, see W. Gill Wylie, *Hospitals: Their History, Organization, and Construction* (New York: Appleton, 1877), Henry C. Burdett, *Hospitals and Asylums of the World*, 4 vols. (London: J. and A. Churchill, 1893), vol. 3; Commission on Hospital Care, *Hospital Care in the United States* (New York: Commonwealth Fund, 1947), chaps. 30–33; Morris J. Vogel, "Boston's Hospitals, 1870–1930: A Social History" (Ph.D. diss., University of Chicago, 1974); Charles E. Rosenberg, "And Heal the Sick: The Hospital and the Patient in the 19th Century America," *Journal of Social History* 10 (Summer 1977): 428–47.

9.   See Shryock, *History of Nursing*, pp. 278–81.

10.   Elizabeth King Ellicott, address to the Maryland State Association of Graduate Nurses in 1900, quoted in Ethel Johns and Blanche Pfefferkorn, *The Johns Hopkins Hospital School of Nursing, 1889–1949* (Baltimore: Johns Hopkins University Press, 1954), p. 22.

11.   Johns Hopkins Hospital, *Reports and Papers Relating to Construction and Organization*, no. 1 (1876), pp. 6–8.

12.   Ibid., no. 3 (1877), pp. 8–10.

13.   Ibid., p. 11.

14.   "The Plans and Purposes of the Johns Hopkins Hospital," *Addresses at the Opening of the Hospital, May 7, 1889* (Baltimore: J. Murphy and Co., 1889), p. 29.

15.   Johns Hopkins Hospital, *Reports and Papers*, no. 3, p. 11.

16.   Ibid.; Henry M. Hurd, address at 25th anniversary of the Johns Hopkins Hospital, 1914, typescript in William H. Welch Papers, Welch Medical Library, Johns Hopkins Medical School, Baltimore, Md.; Billings, "Plans and Purposes," p. 30.

17.   Billings *et al.*, *Hospital Plans*, p. 9; Billings, "Plans and Purposes," p. 19.

18.   Harvey Cushing, *The Life of Sir William Osler*, 2 vols. (Oxford: Clarendon Press, 1925), 1: 303.

19.   "Hospital Organization and Management" (1897), quoted in Thomas S. Cullen, *Henry Mills Hurd* (Baltimore: Johns Hopkins University Press, 1920), p. 76; "The Relation of the Training School for Nurses to the Johns Hopkins Hospital," *Johns Hopkins Hospital Bulletin* 1 (December 1889): 7. Mrs. Hurd was an active member of the Women's Fund Committee for the medical school.

20.   "Relation of Training School to Hospital," p. 8.

21.   Hurd to King, 4 Sept. 1889, typed copy in Nightingale Collection, Welch Medical Library, Johns Hopkins Medical School, Baltimore, Md.

22.   William Osler, "The Inner History of the Johns Hopkins Hospital," *Johns Hopkins Medical Journal* 125 (October 1969): 187; Dock, *History*, 3: 122; Carr, "Early History of the Hospital," p. 65.

23.   Osler, "Inner History," pp. 187–88.

24.   Among the many glowing descriptions of her, see Lavinia L. Dock and Henry M. Hurd in "The Isabel Hampton Robb Memorial Fund," *Johns Hopkins Nurses Alumnae Magazine* 11 (April 1912): 6, 16. Also Elizabeth King Ellicott, in "Memorial Services for Isabel Hampton Robb," *Johns Hopkins Hospital Bulletin* 21 (August 1910): 11. For her maternal sense see, for instance, Edith W. Ware interview with Grace Baxter, n.d., typed summary, Department of Nursing Education Archives, Teachers College, Columbia University (hereafter cited as Dept. Nurs. Ed. Archives, TC).

25.   M. E. Cameron, "Isabel Hampton—Pupil Nurse in the Bellevue Training School for Nurses, 1881–1883," *American Journal of Nursing* 11 (October 1910): 10–13; Lavinia L. Dock, in "Memorial Fund," p. 7; M. Adelaide Nutting, in "Memorial Services for Isabel Hampton Robb," *Johns Hopkins Hospital Bulletin* 21 (August 1910): 6.

26.   Hampton to Elizabeth Birdseye, 11 July 1886, Nightingale Collection; Edith A. Draper, "Isabel Hampton Robb," *American Journal of Nursing* 2 (January 1902): 244.

27.   Lavinia Dock in "Memorial Fund," p. 7, Isabel McIsaac, "Should Undergraduates Be Sent Out to Private Duty," Society of Superintendents, *Third Annual Report* (1896), p. 67.

28.   Cora Overholt as quoted in "Memorial Services," *American Journal of Nursing* 11 (October 1910): 32.

29.   Dock, *History*, 3: 124.

30.   "Isabel Hampton Robb—Her Work in Organization and Education," *American Journal of Nursing* 11 (October 1910): 19.

31.   Isabel Hampton Robb, "An International Educational Standard for Nursing," reprint from *New York Medical Journal*, 15 (January 1910), p. 7, in nursing history files, Office of Director, Massachusetts General Hospital School of Nursing (hereafter cited as MGHSN), Boston, Mass.

32.   These and the following data on pupils of the Boston Training School come from the manuscript enrollment books, Office of Director, MGHSN.

33.   *Report of the Directors of the Boston Training School for Nurses Attached to the Massachusetts General Hospital*, 1889, pp. 4, 6.

34.   Carr, "Early History," p. 70.

35.   The monthly records of the nursing department and the files of letters

from applicants accepted are preserved in the Welch Medical Library at the Johns Hopkins Medical School. Unless otherwise noted, they are the source for this and the next seven paragraphs.

36.   Lavinia Dock's note on the application of Wilhelmina Wade, September 1891, records that Dr. Hurd was "displeased."

37.   See family correspondence in Nutting Papers, Dept. Nurs. Ed. Archives, TC.

38.   Georgia Nevins and Adelaide Nutting in "Memorial Services," *American Journal of Nursing* 11 (October 1910): 39, 28; Nutting in "Memorial Services for Isabel Hampton Robb," *Johns Hopkins Hospital Bulletin* 21 (August 1910): 8; Carr, "Early History," p. 73, Dock, "Recollections of Miss Hampton at the Johns Hopkins," *American Journal of Nursing* 11 (October 1910): 16–17. Since in the first years there were no medical students at the hospital, the nurses, as the only young people, may have enjoyed a special place in the sun. This could (in part, at least) account for the idyllic memories of Carr, Dock, and others.

39.   Hampton described this solution in her textbook, *Nursing: Its Principles and Practice* (Philadelphia: W. B. Saunders, 1894). The admission records confirm that she used such a system at Hopkins.

40.   Hampton, *Nursing*, pp. 19–20, 33, 34.

41.   Hampton, "Practical and Scientific Instruction in Invalid Cooking," *Johns Hopkins Hospital Bulletin* 1 (December 1890): 108, Henry M. Hurd, in "Robb Memorial Fund," p. 18, Carr, "Early History," p. 71, Hampton, *Nursing*, p. 40.

42.   Hampton, *Nursing*, pp. 56, 42, 17. "'The comfort of the patient' was the keynote of all our practical instruction," an early pupil recalled. Georgia Nevins, in "Memorial Services," *American Journal of Nursing* 11 (October 1910): 29.

43.   Grace Baxter to Adelaide Nutting, n.d. [probably about 1940], incomplete typed copy, Dept. Nurs. Ed. Archives, TC.

44.   "She filled us with great pride in our work," Adelaide Nutting later wrote. "It seemed to us better worth doing than any other work in the world." "Memorial Services," *Johns Hopkins Hospital Bulletin* 21 (August 1910): 9.

45.   *Second Report of the Superintendent of the Johns Hopkins Hospital, January 31, 1891*, pp. 32–33; Edith Ware, typed notes on two interviews with Adelaide Nutting, one undated, the other 31 June 1939, Dept. Nurs. Ed. Archives, TC; Johns and Pfefferkorn, *Johns Hopkins Hospital School of Nursing*, pp. 80–83; *Johns Hopkins Hospital Bulletin* 2 (July 1891): 95.

46.   Osler, "Medicine and Nursing," in *Essays on Vocation* ed. Basil Mathews (London: Oxford University Press, 1919), p. 9; Kelly, *The Ministry of Nursing* (Baltimore: Griffen, Curley, 1892), pp. 5–8; C. N. B. Camac, comp., *Counsels and Ideals, from the Writings of William Osler* (Boston: Houghton Mifflin, 1905), pp. 94, 121.

47.   Nutting, "Isabel Hampton Robb," *American Journal of Nursing* 11 (October 1910): 19–20; *"Memorial Services," Johns Hopkins Hospital Bulletin* 21 (August 1910): 9.

48.   *Nursing*, p. 55; *Nursing Ethics* (Cleveland: E.C. Koeckert, 1900), p. 173.

49.   *Nursing*, pp. 56–57; *Nursing Ethics*, p. 79.

50.   *Nursing Ethics*, pp. 65, 78, 52, 61.

51.   *Nursing*, p. 57; *Nursing Ethics*, pp. 139–40.

52.   William Osler, "Nurse and Patient," in *Aequanimitas* (Philadelphia: P. Blakiston's Sons and Co., 1905), p. 164.

53. *Nursing Ethics*, pp. 64, 132, 85.

54. Ibid., p. 63.

55. Ibid., pp. 57, 38.

56. Edith Ware, interviews with Ida Carr, 13 June 1940; Dr. J. M. T. Finney, 10 June 1940; Adelaide Nutting, December 1940; Dr. William T. Howard, 13 June 1940; typed notes in Dept. Nurs. Ed. Archives, TC.

57. Hurd, "Robb Memorial Fund," p. 16. On Hurd and the nurses, see, e.g., Edith Ware interview with [Ruth B.?] Sherman, 8 June 1940, typed notes in Dept. Nurs. Ed. Archives, TC.

58. Hurd, in *Sir William Osler, Bart.: Brief Tributes to His Personality, Influence and Public Service* (Baltimore: Johns Hopkins University Press, 1920), pp. 105–6; Edith Ware, interview with Isabel M. Stewart (Nutting's friend and successor at Teachers College), November 1940, typed notes in Dept. Nurs. Ed. Archives, TC. The highly articulate Osler often expressed (sometimes under heavy veils of literary allusion) the medical profession's perception of nurses and nursing as a threat. See, for instance, "The Hospital as a College," an address given in 1903, arguing for increased clinical teaching of medical students: "I envy for our medical students the advantages enjoyed by the nurses, who live in daily contact with the sick, and who have, in this country at least, supplanted the former in the affections of the hospital trustees." *Aequanimitas*, p. 333.

59. Elizabeth King Ellicott, in *Johns Hopkins Hospital Bulletin* 21 (August 1910): 11–12; Carr, "Early History," p. 71.

60. William Sydney Thayer, "Reminiscences of Osler," *Osler and Other Papers* (Baltimore: Johns Hopkins University Press, 1931), pp. 30, 37; for Robb's papers, see the following issues of the *Johns Hopkins Hospital Bulletin*: 2 (December 1891); 4 (September 1893); and 5 (January–February 1894). See also Kelly's review of John A. Ouchterlony, *Pioneer Medical Men and Times in Kentucky*, in *Johns Hopkins Hospital Bulletin* 3 (April 1892), which lauds the work of Mrs. Frances Coomes, "a surgeon, physician and obstetrician." Kelly's library on women's history forms part of the Nightingale Collection at the Welch Medical Library.

61. Osler, "Inner History of the Hospital," p. 188.

62. Lavinia Dock, "Recollections," p. 18. "Her power of concentration," Dock said, "was admirable, and she had a tranquil poise, not easily disturbed even by interruption. After coming in from last rounds I would sit down and hear the newest pages. Dr. Robb used also to wander in and help with suggestions as to phrasing." On the longevity of the textbook see Dr. Hurd's comment in "Memorial Fund," p. 18.

63. *Johns Hopkins Hospital Bulletin* 5 (April 1894): 55.

64. "Recollections," p. 17; Dock, *History*, 3: 123–24; Isabel M. Stewart and Anne L. Austin, *A History of Nursing* (New York: G. P. Putnam's Sons, 1962), p. 199.

65. She used this term in *Nursing*, p. 58.

66. *Nursing*, p. 58, and *Nursing Ethics*, p. 139.

67. Dock, *History*, 3: 124–25.

68. Hampton, *Nursing Ethics*, pp. 258–59.

69. Adelaide Nutting later wrote that Hampton and Dock, at this time, also "studied progress made in other training schools and in other branches of edu-

cation." "The Work of the Johns Hopkins School for Nurses," *Johns Hopkins Hospital Bulletin* 25 (December 1914): 5.

70. Lucy Walker-Donnell to Nutting, 25 May 1940, Dept. Nurs. Ed. Archives, TC; Nutting, "Work of the Johns Hopkins School," p. 5.

71. A notice of the club's establishment was carried in the 23 May 1891 issue of *The Nightingale*, one of the short-lived nursing periodicals of the day. The *Johns Hopkins Hospital Bulletin* printed its annual reports; see 2 (April 1891): 65–66; 3 (June 1892): 79–80; 4 (October 1893): 100. The report for 1893–94, printed in leaflet form, is in the Nightingale Collection as are typed copies of some of the original papers.

72. The other addresses were "Training Schools for Nurses," at the National Conference of Charities and Correction in 1890, "District Nursing," at the annual meeting of Baltimore's Charity Organization Society in 1891, and "Educational Standards for Nurses," at the Chicago World's Fair in 1893; all are cited below.

73. As an alternative, she proposed a central school connected with a group of small institutions which could provide training comparable to that of a large general hospital. Stepping carefully, she did not emphasize the opportunities for self-determination which such a school would afford, run by nurses, and with nurses on its board together with representatives of the hospitals and the medical profession.

74. "Training Schools for Nurses," *Proceedings of the National Conference of Charities and Correction* (1890), pp. 145–46; "District Nursing," in Hampton, *Educational Standards for Nurses* (Cleveland: E. C. Koeckert, 1907), pp. 52–53.

75. District nursing had been pioneered in the United States in 1877, as a charitable effort, under the nonsectarian Protestant auspices of the New York City Mission and Tract Society, with Mrs. William H. Osborn, board chairman of the Bellevue Training School, paying for the services of a Bellevue graduate. For the historical background, see Annie M. Brainard, *The Evolution of Public Health Nursing* (Philadelphia: W. B. Saunders, 1922).

76. The Johns Hopkins School of Nursing added public health nursing to the curriculum in 1933, the Massachusetts General Hospital School in 1938. See Sylvia Perkins, *A Centennial Review: The Massachusetts General Hospital School of Nursing, 1873–1973* (n.p.: [Massachusetts General Hospital] School of Nursing, Nurses Alumnae Association, 1975).

77. Dr. Hurd, in his annual reports, repeatedly called attention to the need for a system of district nursing in Baltimore, to "lighten the heavy burden of poverty and preventable disease" (*Second Report of the Superintendent*, p. 31). Dr. Kelly, an exponent of the social gospel, who had begun his medical practice in a mill town outside of Philadelphia, pressed the trustees to introduce such a system, in his address to the training-school graduates in 1892 (*The Ministry of Nursing*, pp. 10–13). Dr. Osler, deeply interested in containing the spread of tuberculosis, is reported to have told Miss Nutting, in a burst of enthusiasm, that if he had not been a physician he would have wanted to be a district nurse. (Edith Ware interview with Isabel Stewart, November 1940, typed notes in Dept. Nurs. Ed. Archives, TC).

78. "Training Schools," p. 145 and passim.

79. "District Nursing," pp. 46ff.

80. The papers were originally published in John S. Billings and Henry M. Hurd, eds., *Hospitals, Dispensaries and Nursing: Papers and Discussions in the International Congress of Charities, Correction and Philanthropy, Section III, Chicago, June 12th to 17th, 1893* (Baltimore: 1894). The papers on nursing were reprinted in *Nursing of the Sick, 1893* (New York: McGraw-Hill, 1949).

81. Dock, "Recollections," p. 18.

82. Dock, "The Relation of Training Schools to Hospitals," in *Nursing of the Sick*, pp. 14, 13.

83. Ibid., pp. 18, 21, 19, 20.

84. Dock, *History*, 3: 126.

85. Hampton, "Educational Standards for Nurses," in *Nursing of the Sick*, pp. 5, 7, 8, 11.

86. Dock, "The Relation of Training Schools to Hospitals," pp. 16–17.

87. See especially Louise Darche, "Proper Organization of Training Schools in America," in *Nursing of the Sick*, pp. 101–3.

88. Dock, "The Relation of Training Schools to Hospitals," pp. 23–24.

89. Dock, *History*, 3: 126.

90. Nightingale, "Sick Nursing and Health Nursing," *Nursing of the Sick*, p. 36; Draper, "Necessity of an American Nurses' Association," idem., p. 151; Sutliffe, "History of American Training Schools," idem., p. 92.

91. Darche, "Proper Organization," pp. 104–6.

92. Isabel McIsaac, presidential address to International Council of Nurses, Buffalo, New York, September 1901, in *American Journal of Nursing* 2 (October 1901): 2.

93. Dock, *History*, 3: 127; Society of Superintendents, *First and Second Annual Reports*, 1895, p. 3 (hereafter SS, *First Report*, etc.).

94. May Wright Sewall, ea., *The World's Congress of Representative Women*, 2 vols. (Chicago: Rand McNally, 1894); Mary K. O. Eagle, ea., *The Congress of Women* (Chicago: International Publishing Co., 1894).

95. Darche, "Proper Organization," p. 103.

96. Later reports are: Committee for the Study of Nursing Education, *Nursing and Nursing Education in the United States* [the Goldmark Report] (New York: Macmillan, 1923); Esther Lucile Brown, *Nursing for the Future* (New York: Russell Sage Foundation, 1948); and Jerome P. Lysaught, *An Abstract for Action* (New York: McGraw-Hill, 1970).

97. SS, *First and Second Reports*, pp. 8, 10. (The third and subsequent *Annual Reports* were published individually.)

98. SS, *Second Report*, p. 37.

99. SS, *First Report*, p. 16; *Seventh Report*, p. 29.

100. Dock, *History*, 3: 128–29; *The Trained Nurse* 16 (October 1896): 534. A scattering of the early records of this organization, now the American Nurses Association, may be found in the Nursing History Archives, Boston University.

101. SS, *Fifth Report*, pp. 66–70; *Sixth Report*, pp. 61–64. On the germination of the idea, see Dock, *History*, 3: 131–33; Dock, in "Memorial Fund," pp. 9–10; Nurses' Alumnae Association, Proceedings of the 12th Convention, in *American Journal of Nursing* 9 (September 1909): 955.

102. Hampton, "Some of the Lessons of the Late War and Their Bearing upon Trained Nursing," in her *Educational Standards for Nurses*; Sophia Palmer, "Women in the War," SS, *Sixth Report*, p. 69.

. 103. For a sample of the criticisms of private duty nurses and the superintendents' reaction, see, in SS, *Fifth Report:* Mary Agnes Snively, presidential address, p. 8; Eva Allerton, "How Far Are Training Schools Responsible for Lack of Ethics among Nurses" (and discussion following), pp. 45ff.; Linda Richards, "The Superintendent of the Training School," p. 52; in SS, *Sixth Report*, Alice I. Twitchell, "The Tendency of Trained Nurses to Extravagance" and discussion, pp. 38ff.; editorial, *American Journal of Nursing*, 9 (October 1908): 5.

104. Isabel M. Stewart, *The Education of Nurses*, p. 140.

105. Ibid., p. 153.

106. Ibid., p. 128, 130, 139.

107. In 1910, for instance, the Society of Superintendents had 360 members. (Adelaide Nutting in "Memorial Services," *Johns Hopkins Hospital Bulletin* 21 [August 1910]: 10.) In the same period less than half the graduates of the Massachusetts General Hospital training school belonged to their alumnae association. (Perkins, *Centennial Review*, p. 67.) Nurse historians have understandably glossed over the low participation in professional organizations, though Mary Roberts refers to it (*American Nursing*, p. 46). The difficulties of the early years of the Teachers College course are documented in Teresa E. Christy, *Cornerstone for Nursing Education* (New York: Teachers College Press, 1969), chaps. 2 and 3.

108. Stewart, *Education of Nurses*, pp. 173–74.

109. Ibid., pp. 155–56.

110. On the Manhattan Beach meeting, see Dock, *History*, 3: 129. Hampton's reactions to Palmer and Davis's entrepreneurship with the *American Journal of Nursing* are evident in her letters to Nutting, in Dept. Nurs. Ed. Archives, TC. See also, on her relationship with Palmer, Edith Ware, notes on interview with Harriet Fulmer, 14 November 1940. The cooling of the Hampton-Nutting friendship can be inferred from such letters as Hampton to Nutting, 28 December [1907], and Ware, notes on interview with Mrs. Lord, 12 June 1940, all in Dept. Nurs. Ed. Archives. On Palmer's criticisms of the Teachers College course, see Christy, *Cornerstone for Nursing Education*, pp. 23ff.

111. Hampton must also have found disheartening the rise of medical social work in hospitals, its early divorce from nursing, and its quick professionalization on an independent basis.

112. This account of Hampton's life in Cleveland is based on a skeptical reading of Edith Ware's notes (Dept. Nurs. Ed. Archives, TC) on the gossipy reminiscences given her thirty years after Hampton's death. See, for instance, Dr. Lewellys F. Barker and Mrs. Lord (a former pupil), 12 June 1940; Dr. Howard A. Kelly and Dr. William T. Howard, 13 June 1940; Isabel Stewart, November 1940; Mrs. John H. Lowman, Annie Brainard, and Elizabeth M. Folchemer, 18 November 1940, Marian G. Howell and Mrs. Charles F. Hoover, 19 November 1940; Helena McMillan, 16 November 1940; Louise Muller and Mrs. A. R. Colvin [Sadie Tarleton], 15 November 1940.

113. "Isabel Hampton Robb," *American Journal of Nursing* 11 (October 1910): 22.

4

Discipline, Obedience, and Female Support Groups: Mona Wilson at the Johns Hopkins Hospital School of Nursing, 1915–1918

Douglas O. Baldwin

Nursing education in North America in the late nineteenth and early twentieth centuries was noted for its reliance upon strict discipline and hierarchical organization in training young women to be efficient nurses. Based largely upon the personal correspondence of Mona G. Wilson, this article examines how Mona Wilson coped with the exacting discipline and stern routine at the Johns Hopkins Hospital School of Nursing during the First World War, and discusses the importance of the student nurses' informal network of support groups in enabling the women to survive the Hopkins experience.

Mona Wilson, the third child of Harold and Elizabeth Wilson, was born in 1894 in the prestigious Rosedale area of Toronto, Ontario.[1] Her father owned the Harold A. Wilson Company, a popular sporting goods store in Toronto, and belonged to several of Toronto's exclusive organizations, including the National Club and the Royal Canadian Yacht Club, where the family mingled with the city's commercial, political, and social elites.

The Wilson children received the finest education obtainable in Toronto's private schools. At a time when few women attended university, two of Mona's sisters studied at the University of Toronto, and one graduated from the Margaret Eaton School of Dramatic Arts. Mona attended the Toronto Model School, which was reputed to be the best

Note: This chapter was originally published in the *Bulletin of the History of Medicine 69* (1995): 599–619. Reprinted with permission.

elementary school in the city, before enrolling at Havergal Ladies' College in 1909. Havergal, which served as a nursery for Canada's future female social and religious leaders, combined sound academic training in the liberal arts and sciences with an emphasis on hard work, self-denial, Christian values, and the importance of public service.[2] Mona graduated from Havergal in 1913 and the following year attended the Lillian Massey School of Household Science at the University of Toronto. At the conclusion of this one-year course, Mona registered at the Johns Hopkins Hospital School of Nursing in quest of a nursing diploma.

After graduating in 1918, Mona enlisted in the United States Army Nursing Corps, and she was in the last group to sail to France in December 1918. The following June, she joined the American Red Cross Society and departed for Siberia. Quartered in Vladivostok, Mona spent eight months working in a women's medical ward and training Russian nurses' aides in the principles of practical nursing. By the time Mona left Siberia at the end of February 1920, she had experienced a failed coup attempt and had watched helplessly as mounted Bolshevik soldiers rode into her hospital ward looking for deserters. In May 1920, Mona was posted in Tirana, the capital of Albania. Since Muslim women refused to be examined by male doctors, Mona and the other American Red Cross nurses conducted home visits in this war-ravaged country. Mona also accompanied the mobile clinic into the mountains to preach the benefits of toothbrushes and soap, and to conduct baby clinics. In Tirana, she helped establish a small school for training local nurses. Late in June 1920, Mona hurried by car to the Adriatic coast, amidst a barrage of shells, to assist the Red Cross medical unit located only about ten kilometers from the warring Albanian and Italian armies. When the fighting ceased, the Italian Red Cross decorated Mona for her efforts.

Following the Armistice in August, the American Red Cross dispatched Mona to Ragusa (now Dubrovnik) on the Dalmatian coast to care for 30,000 White Russian refugees who had escaped from the Bolsheviks in the Crimea. Here, she clothed, fed, and nursed the expatriates back to health so they could be relocated elsewhere in Europe. When Mona left Ragusa at the end of February 1921, the "Russian Government [in exile] in the Kingdom of the Serbs, Croatians and Slovenes" presented her with yet another award for her "kindness and tireless efforts to alleviate the sufferings of our Refugees."[3]

April found her in Vir Pazar, Montenegro. During the next nine months she organized Mothers' and Little Mothers' clubs to teach the benefits of fresh air, disease prevention, infant care, and personal hygiene; conducted home visits; accompanied mobile clinics into the mountains; initiated school inspections; trained young women in the principles of public health nursing; and was the resident nurse in the Danilovgrad orphanage. For these efforts, Mona received the Red Cross Certificate.

Mona returned to Toronto in January 1922 and earned her Public Health Nursing Diploma at the University of Toronto the following year. In 1923, she became Chief Red Cross Public Health Nurse in Prince Edward Island. In the absence of a provincial health department, Mona and her small staff served the Island's health needs for the next eight years. She initiated medical inspections in the schools; established dental clinics, Junior Red Cross clubs, tuberculosis chest clinics, and crippled children's camps and clinics; and organized province-wide programs of smallpox and diphtheria vaccinations. Touring the rural sections of the province, Mona preached the necessity of planting vegetable gardens, drinking milk, and eating wholesome food. When the provincial government established a department of health in 1931, it appointed Mona Wilson Provincial Director of Public Health Nursing. Except for the period of the Second World War, she held this position until her retirement in 1961. In October 1940, the Canadian Red Cross seconded her as Red Cross Associate Commissioner for Newfoundland. Here, she took charge of ministering to the needs of shipwrecked soldiers and sailors on the North Atlantic Run. For this work she earned the nickname "the Florence Nightingale of St. John's," and received the Order of the British Empire (OBE). Returning to Prince Edward Island, Mona was instrumental in acquiring dental hygienists to conduct educational programs in dental health—the first time such personnel had been used in a public health department in Canada. She also played a major role in the establishment of the Division of Nutrition for Prince Edward Island, and in the introduction of a child and maternal health program.

In addition to these accomplishments, this dynamic woman helped to establish the Girl Guides, the Zonta Club, the Business and Professional Women's Club, and several other Island associations that sought to broaden the people's vision and boost women's self-confidence. By the time she died in 1981, Mona had been awarded the highest honor in international nursing (she was the ninth Canadian to receive the Florence Nightingale Award in 1963), in Girl Guides (the Beaver in 1957), and in Prince Edward Island (Island Woman of the Century in 1967).

Nursing had become a popular occupation for middle-class women by the end of the nineteenth century. It is doubtful, however, whether Mona would have entered nursing had it not been for the outbreak of the First World War. When the conflict began, the entire Wilson family rushed to assist the British cause. Elizabeth Wilson joined the Women's Patriotic Association, Margaret rolled bandages and knitted socks at the nearest Red Cross office, Jack enlisted in the artillery, and Jane worked in the Active Service Canteens. Harold, the Wilsons' eldest son, who was among the first soldiers to enlist in the Canadian Overseas Expeditionary

Force, warned the women of the family not to "let wild-fangled ideas of nursing wounded soldiers rush through your heads, that's all poppy-cock."[4] Unconvinced, and just as eager to participate as the others, Mona volunteered to be an overseas nurses' aide in the Voluntary Aid Detachment organized by the St. John's Ambulance Corps. Brimming with excitement to tell the rest of the family her news, Mona returned home only to meet a friend of her older sister who had dropped by for lunch. This woman had just received her nursing diploma at the Johns Hopkins Hospital School of Nursing in Baltimore, and discouraged Mona from becoming a nurses' aide, because she felt the position offered no career possibilities once the war was over. Because trained nurses were needed overseas, and as nursing offered chances for a future career, she urged Mona to apply to Johns Hopkins.[5]

Nursing wages compared favorably with teaching, clerical, and factory salaries, and nursing was now second only to teaching as a career choice for American women.[6] Nursing offered the prestige of professional standing, a measure of independence, and a chance for adventure. For Mona, who had been raised on the ideal of service to others, nursing provided an opportunity to do something useful with her life. It opened doors to religious missions in faraway lands, to hospital and sanitarium work, to settlement and mission homes in the crowded slums, and to public health work in schools and rural areas.[7]

Mona had always claimed that nursing was one profession in which she had no interest. Nonetheless, she said, "I felt I must do my bit in the war effort and so succumbed to the urging,"[8] a decision that must have surprised the entire family. This rambunctious girl, a "chronic peeve" in her own words,[9] was about to become a quiet, obedient nurse. Her oldest brother responded to the news by noting that he had always believed Mona would "marry someone and be happy. Hope she doesn't grow up to be an old maid. They always go sour, lose their figure, looks, humour, and temper very easily."[10]

Once Mona had decided upon becoming a nurse, she had to select a school. There were more than 1,100 training schools in the United States, and almost 100 in Canada.[11] Like many other Canadians, Mona traveled to the United States, where the "better class" enrolled in the prestigious schools.[12] Although the Johns Hopkins Hospital was not completed until 1889, by 1900 its affiliated medical school was already considered one of the best medical schools in North America.[13] Hopkins's nursing school was equally prestigious, having been a leader in adopting the three-year course of study, the eight-hour day, student scholarships, and tuition fees, and in hiring full-time nursing instructors. Hopkins graduates and superintendents of nurses, such as Mary Adelaide Nutting, Lavinia Dock, and Isabel Hampton Robb, had published textbooks on nursing principles,

ethics, and history, and had initiated the first professional nursing organizations and journals in the United States.[14]

Canadian-born nurses held prominent administrative positions at
Hopkins. Isabel Hampton Robb, M. Adelaide Nutting, Georgina Ross,
and Elsie Lawler, for example, filled the post of Superintendent of Nurses
and Principal of the Training School from its inception in 1889 to 1940.
Each year from 1892 to 1919, at least one Canadian nursing student graduated from Hopkins, with a high of ten graduates in 1918. Canadians
also served as residence directors and head nurses at Hopkins. Prior to
the First World War, so many Hopkins graduates resided in and around
Toronto that Ethel Berwick, a Hopkins graduate and William Osler's god-
child, opened a tearoom in Toronto which periodically held Hopkins
get-togethers for these nurses.[15] One such graduate recommended Johns
Hopkins to Mona Wilson in 1914.

When Mona wrote to Johns Hopkins for an application, she discovered that applicants had to be at least twenty-two years old, of average
height and good physique, high school graduates, and of good breeding.[16] Since most women had completed their education by age eighteen,
the age restriction discouraged working-class women from applying and
favored those who did not need to work after graduating from secondary
school.[17] Married women and those over thirty-five years old were refused
admission because the schools believed they were too set in their ways to
be properly receptive to training.[18] In addition to demanding good health
and a high-school education, Johns Hopkins required prospective students to forward a letter from their clergyman "testifying to good, moral
character and qualifications for undertaking professional work."[19] Since
the school routinely received over one thousand requests for information each year, and had more than two hundred and fifty applications
annually,[20] the superintendent advised each applicant to "think the matter over very carefully" and asked for a personal note detailing the applicant's health, physique, religion, occupation, social background, reasons
for wishing to become a nurse, and family ties and freedom from responsibilities.[21] This last request reflected the large number of drop-outs due
to family problems.

Mona easily satisfied all the requirements but one: born on 11 August
1894, she would not be twenty-two for another year. Of course, Mona
would have been admitted immediately to almost any other training
school,[22] but the Wilsons wanted their children to attend the "best"
schools. Mona's solution was to lie, and on the medical certificate accompanying her application, the family physician recorded her birth date as
11 August 1893. This subterfuge helps to explain why Mona seldom
recorded the date of her birth in later years.[23] The rest was easy. At 5 feet
3 inches and 132 pounds she was of average build. Her educational back-

ground, especially with a year of household science at the University of Toronto, was excellent; and Archdeacon Cody's recommendation referred to her high school as "one of the best Ladies Schools in Canada."[24] Mona's own letter of application was most impressive. She had been a residence prefect at Havergal, had had administrative experience at Young Women's Christian Association summer camps, and had been engaged in volunteer social work the previous winter. In addition, her family physician wrote on the reverse side of his medical certificate that Mona "was a very superior young woman, well bred and well adapted mentally, physically and morally to excel as a nurse."[25] Mona was admitted to the program and left for Baltimore by train on 17 March 1915. Her studies commenced one day later.

The Johns Hopkins Hospital was situated in the older, poorer section of Baltimore. "It is a district," Mona wrote shortly after arriving in Baltimore,

> *of colored people and white ones together—living next door to each other, so you can imagine the class of whites they are—they all just camp on the streets, move all their chairs out and literally camp on the sidewalk, so that a pedestrian is forced to pick his way over the cobblestones in the center of the road. Really it's awful to see life like that . . . horrible back passages between houses possibly leading to hovels in the rear and doors opening from cellar ways that seem to lead into the very depths of the earth. . . . So you get some idea of the district in which the hospital is situated, but Johns Hopkins stands out noble and grand in the midst of all the filth and poverty.[26]*

The first few days, Mona was too concerned about finding her way to pay much attention to the scenery, although the beauty of the campus must have impressed her—as it was designed to do. Mona was directed to the nurses' home, which was close to the hospital wards for easy communication, but sufficiently removed so as not to disturb the patients. The Hopkins trustees had originally wanted to provide nursing accommodations equivalent to a first-class hotel, with single rooms and a common parlor and dining room, to attract a better class of young women. The exterior, with its austere Renaissance form, symmetry, and order, was meant to reassure the girls' parents of the school's professionalism and probity.[27] Recent hospital expansion, which had increased the number of patients from 71,000 in 1911 to 131,000 four years later, had necessitated a corresponding growth in the number of nurses. As the nursing superintendent reported in 1915, "from every single corner of the hospital have come insistent demands that it has not been possible to comply with. The operating room finds it impossible to do the work with the staff provided, though a maid has been added to perform certain duties formerly assigned to the nurses. . . . In every ward the work becomes more complicated and consequently more taxing and difficult for the nurses, graduates and pupils alike."[28] The nursing class of 1915, with eighty probationers, was the largest in the school's history.[29]

The morning following Mona's arrival the new students assembled downstairs in the reception room, where Elsie Mildred Lawler, the superintendent of nurses and principal of the school of nursing, addressed them. Most of the students were in awe of Lawler, whose reputation as a leader in the struggle for shorter hours, better working conditions, and more generalized training for nurses was well known. In addition, as the *Circular of Information* warned, she could "terminate the connection of a pupil with the school at any time in case of misconduct, disobedience, insubordination, inefficiency, or neglect of duty."[30] The superintendent welcomed the women into the Hopkins "family," read the morning prayer, and outlined the rules and regulations. Mona left no record of how she felt that day, but as a contemporary nursing manual noted, "the entrance of the nurse candidate into this new world is a rather bewildering experience, and the process of adjusting herself to these new conditions, laws, and customs is rarely easy."[31]

For the next six months, Mona was on probation and wore a home-made pink-and-white uniform to indicate her lowly status. "We pinkies are not nurses you understand," Mona informed her sister, "merely probationers—much scorn in the word probationers!!!!"[32] Mona learned to sit in the section of the dining room set aside for probationers, to stand in the presence of a superior, to obey orders immediately, to keep her room neat at all times and ready for inspection, to ask permission to leave the hospital grounds or to have visitors in the dormitory, to keep her hair in a bun and tucked under her cap, and when to rise, eat, study, and retire. She was expected to refrain from wearing her uniform off campus, to avoid boisterous laughter, "common" language, and frivolous activities, and to confine her conversation while on duty to professional matters. "Every nurse who indulges in habits or practices which are undignified or vulgar, or in remarks which are flippant, 'slangy' or coarse," wrote a popular nursing manual, "is helping to lower the moral tone of the school, and making it harder for younger nurses to live up to the best that they know."[33] Careless work was punishable by suspension, and dating a doctor could lead to dismissal. In Mona's graduating year, for example, a fellow nurse who attended a party that included several doctors immediately "fell into disgrace," and "there was a general calling down from Miss Lawler etc. and a beastly rumpus all round."[34]

Following the Nightingale model, and in accordance with nineteenth-century pedagogical ideas, Lawler stressed character training, strict discipline, and hierarchical lines of authority. Lower orders were not to fraternize with their superiors, nor were nurses to become friendly with the patients or the staff, lest such behavior jeopardize their authority. The line of command devolved from the superintendent to her assistants, to the head nurses, senior students, intermediate pupils, junior nurses, and finally to the probationers. This hierarchy was reinforced through separate entrances and dining facilities. Distinctive uniforms, pins, and caps served both to fortify hierarchical authority and to symbolize the nurse's function in society.[35]

Hospital administrators such as Elsie Lawler viewed the training school as an extended family, in which the chief surgeon was the father, the nursing school superintendent was the mother, and the students were the potentially unruly and willful children—whose hours, living quarters, demeanor, virtue, and social relationships all needed close observation and regulation. Being women, the students required careful supervision. Their punctuality, personal neatness, and morality were constantly evaluated.[36] Student residences, significantly termed "homes," enabled the matrons to keep a close motherly eye on the students, and to maintain a "dignified, orderly, attractive and homelike household."[37]

As a probationary student, Mona was constantly monitored for her physical strength and endurance, adaptability to hospital work, powers of observation, and judgment. Her instructors completed monthly reports that commented upon Mona's industry, reliability, conscientiousness, promptness, patience, and kindness, and her "general conduct and loyalty to the governing rules."[38] The comments noted on the records of several of Mona's friends indicate the bias of the instructors, and the characteristics the school encouraged. Kathleen Caulfield, for example, was described as "a nice woman, reliable worker"; Ruth Barton was "slow and lacking in confidence"; Phyllis Higinbotham was "quiet and dignified"; Marion Rossiter "worked neatly and accurately," and had a "pleasing manner," but revealed "a tendency to talk too much if working with somebody." Mona was "a thoroughly nice woman." A less favored pupil was described as a "rough and ready worker," and one student nurse was spoken to several times about her "self-satisfied manner and her noisy way of going about," as well as her careless work and popularity with the patients. Other students were characterized as "resentful of criticism" and "lacking in force."[39]

The first five months involved a daily combination of six hours of practical training, and two to three hours of classes, lectures, and demonstrations, followed by two weeks of hospital work, and concluding with final examinations. Elsie Lawler's ethics classes sought to inculcate self-control over "natural impulses," proper habits, good judgment, and unselfishness. She also reviewed the school's code of ethics, which emphasized the nurse's duty to the doctor (who was due proper respect according to "his" higher professional standing) and the nurse's loyalty to her school (whose management, the students were warned, should never be criticized).[40]

Most of Mona's time was occupied in taking classes, copying out lecture notes for inspection, and studying for tests. "Any free minute," Mona complained to her parents, "I flop on the bed and go to sleep, whether it is 10 am, or 12 noon . . . and we have to study and study hard—which is about the hardest thing for me to do, for I never was a student."[41] As a result, she found it difficult to escape "the hammer of my conscience which is loudly beating Study! Study!"[42] In the summer the pupils worked eight hours a day in the hospital. They managed the diet section, dispensary, and surgical supply room, which allowed Elsie Lawler to reduce the salaried staff.[43] During this period, Mona experienced Baltimore's hot summers, and received her first taste of ward work. In late July, Mona grumbled that "the heat is—to say the least, extremely trying, I haven't slept for a week on account of it but just flop on the bed and swat mosquitoes and toss from side to side until my poor mattress is about worn to a frazzle, and my hands bruised from continuous contact with the wall and flying insects."[44] Ice-water baths provided only temporary relief.

In the colored men's ward, Mona soon learned that hospital nurses "do not move around slowly and gracefully, but are usually in a whirl, here one moment there the next." "Picture me," she continued,

> *when the head nurse told me to do up the surgical side of the ward—my scariness turned to terror—whatever was I to do?—only to go ahead and do it, so I got linen from the linen cupboard, bath blankets and a nurse's basket and sallied forth. . . . I didn't dare let them see I was a green horn, so I tried to look very professional and businesslike, bustling about. . . . Then there was dusting (dusting is a part of each day's work throughout the whole 3 years) and the cleaning of the lavatory where solutions are made up and instruments boiled etc. Then I had to rush patients off to x-ray and the operating room, run all the errands, and do all the odds and ends.*[45]

The work was exhausting, and after laboring a long eight hours one day, Mona wondered how the nurses at the Toronto General Hospital endured twelve hours.

The worst experience was night duty—of which Mona served 176 nights. Sleep was particularly difficult, and studying was almost impossible. "Most of the lectures were given during my siege of night duty [six weeks of nine to ten hours daily] when I had to get up in the middle of the night as it were (1:30 P.M.) for a lecture at 2. You can imagine how much of these lectures I absorbed, when I couldn't take any notes because I had to prop my eyes open."[46]

Ward duty was exacting and tension-filled, and drained Mona of all her energy. One contemporary hospital investigator used pedometers to discover that an average nurse walked over five miles a day in the wards, carried fifteen-pound food trays a total of two miles daily, and moved bed screens weighing thirty-one pounds each time a patient had to be washed or had to use a bedpan.[47]

The schedule at Hopkins was so debilitating that after six months Mona's original class of forty-one had been reduced to thirty. One student quit after receiving a one-day suspension for carrying out orders improperly.[48] Other pupils resigned because they felt inadequate following unfavorable evaluations of their work, or because of problems at home, marriage, or loss of interest.[49] Mary Marsh, Mona's first roommate, inherited some money and returned to Virginia to study medicine. The cramped quarters and the mixture of backgrounds and temperaments created personality conflicts that drove some women from the profession. "Some of the girls," Mona informed her sister,

> *haven't been getting on very well with each other and there have been catty fights etc.—Miss Maguire [a fellow probationer] being mixed up in it . . . [she] is rather small minded not being able to take a jest. It all came to a final point one night in a Dietetics class when we generally kicked up a row. Our Janie Jones pinned a note on Miss Maguire's back and she being perfectly furious (lacking a sense of humour) took it to Miss Lawler, and as a result we all got the deuce, there was a big row—and Miss Maguire decided to leave—probably it was just as well because she was most unpopular and ignored, or at least nobody was friendly with her.*[50]

The end of August brought the panic of final examinations. Despite gloomy predictions of failure, Mona finished with an average of 86.7 percent, and her instructors commented on her eagerness to learn and her quick mind.[51] The next two and one-half years resembled the first six months, except that there seemed to be even less leisure time. The normal day began at 6:50 *A.M.*, when the pupils assembled in the Nurses' Home for nondenominational prayers, a hymn, announcements, and assignment changes. Hospital work took precedence over lectures and class work. Days lost to illness had to be made up at the end of the year.

Although the regulations and restrictions seem overly onerous by today's standards, they were easily accepted in a society that stressed the authority of ministers, teachers, and parents. In one of Mona's first letters home, she enthused that they were all treated as adults and given independence.[52] However, the monotony of routine and the machine-like existence soon took their toll, and Mona began to feel like nothing more than a well-trained maid.[53] Eight months after arriving in Baltimore, following a trip to New York with her parents, Mona wrote to her sister: "Here I am back in the Nurses' Home of J.H.H. vainly endeavoring to settle down once again to institutional routine after a peep into the gayety *[sic]* of life in New York. . . . I hope you will never feel this hateful feeling of kicking against the pricks—the bitterness of lack of freedom especially when one has had that freedom dangled before one in such a tempting way. . . . [I]t makes me so restless and discontented."[54] The following summer, Mona confided to Jane, "I pine for sweaters, rocks, wilderness, bracing air and wide open spaces—hang it all, I've just *got* to have it. You cannot imagine how it affects one, living shut up like this for a year and a half, wearing a hot, tight-fitting uniform and moving according to routine and a set of hours, rules and regulations."[55] Even in the euphoria of graduation ceremonies, Mona concluded that although she hated to leave "all the girls, the excitement of managing a big ward, the routine, even the continual complaining, on the other hand, it is so wonderful to be free once again, to get away from the eternal restraint."[56]

Unfortunately, some head nurses carried the emphasis on authority and obedience to an extreme and their dictatorial ways tended to undermine Mona's self-confidence. Mary Glazier, the night duty superintendent in Mona's junior year, was particularly hard on the students, and they referred to her as the "devil" for her quickness to scold and harangue the nurses when they could not answer her questions. Mona parodied Glazier's attitude to her sister: "'You don't know?' (Withering contempt) 'And why don't you know?' (in stern command). 'It is your *business* to know! Do you mean to tell me that you are the night nurse on this ward, responsible for the lives of the patients (etc.) and *do not know* why such and such a thing happened?' (with a particularly icy penetrating accent on each word.)"[57]

The head nurse in the private wards of the Marburg Building also aroused the students' ire. Here, Louisa Kolb "creeps along behind you and jumps on you—oh it's horrible being shadowed that way—she keeps tab on the smallest detail of everything the nurses do. Absolutely nothing escapes her, everyone talks in a whisper and keeps one eye on the watch over the shoulder to see if you are being followed."[58]

The constant surveillance and criticisms took their toll on the students. For a mid-term test during the probationary period, Mona had to give a bed bath to one of the ward patients. "Heaven forbid," Mona wailed to her sister, "I can plainly see myself drowning the poor woman by dumping the water on her—really I'm the clumsiest individual, and slow!!!"[59] The physicians' rounds were particularly nerve racking. As the physicians moved from bed to bed, the nurses scurried around at their bidding, recording the patients' prescribed treatments, boiling instruments, changing compresses, getting supplies, and so forth. One day, when one of the hospital's "big medical men" made the rounds, Mona felt particularly uncomfortable, "as if awkwardness and stupidity were written all over me in huge letters."[60] By the middle of her intermediate year, Mona longed for the "great outdoors"; was depressed; felt slow, awkward, and stupid in the wards; and considered herself ugly. By the end of that year, however, Mona had become more accustomed to life at Hopkins, and began to feel more competent. 'You have always considered me the slowest most stupid one of your flock, nevertheless mother dear, I'm progressing, though it's scarcely noticeable at times."[61]

In February 1918, Mona took the Maryland State Board Examinations. The practical test in this "chamber of horrors" lasted a mere five minutes, as Mona had only to apply a turpentine plaster in front of "five pairs of examining eyes."[62] This was followed by ten written examinations over three consecutive days that tested the students' memory.[63] While there is no record of how well Mona did on these examinations, she received the school's highest "Officer's Mark" with a 97 percent average, and her instructors wrote that she was "unusually capable and efficient. Marked executive ability. A thoroughly nice, quiet and dignified nurse, one of the best in the class."[64] Graduation day was held several weeks earlier than usual to allow Mona and the other nurses who had enrolled in the Red Cross to go overseas as soon as possible. This was the largest graduating class in the school's history, with 68 of the original 80 probationers in attendance. Graduation ceremonies were followed by the first dance Mona had attended at Hopkins, which left her sore and aching, feeling "like a decrepit old woman the next day."[65]

How did young women such as Mona Wilson cope with the constant surveillance and the physical and psychological stresses of nursing school? Twenty years ago, Carroll Smith-Rosenberg's path-breaking article "The Female World of Love and Ritual" revealed that a network of intimate supportive relationships existed among American women during much of the eighteenth and nineteenth centuries, which enabled them to function successfully in society.[66] Nancy F. Cott's subsequent examination of the diaries and letters of young women during approximately the same period illustrated that female friendships provided women with needed emotional security.[67] Carol Lasser demonstrated that traditions of solidarity based on common events in the female life cycle, and similar tasks and assignments on farms and in the home, created a profound sense of connectedness among women.[68] More recently, Blanche Wiesen Cook documented the importance of personal relationships and female support networks in providing support for women in their public and professional roles.[69] To these studies, anthropology has contributed the concepts of kinship ties and networking as crucial factors in shaping women's lives and providing emotional nurturing.[70]

According to Nancy Cott, academies for girls were the best institutions for propagating friendships. Boarding schools encouraged the girls to think of each other as sisters to whom they could turn for moral support.[71] Schoolgirls, according to Smith-Rosenberg, assumed an emotional centrality in each others' lives; they helped each other to overcome homesickness, they gossiped about beaux, and they incorporated each other into their own kinship systems.[72] College, concluded Martha Vicinus, created lifelong friendships and a community of united women.[73]

Since nursing schools shared many of the characteristics of colleges and girls' academies, it might be surmised that student nurses employed similar patterns of female networking to help them survive the more rigorous demands of professional training. Unfortunately, this aspect of nursing history has been generally ignored. Nancy Tomes is one of the few historians who have explored the impact of the training school on individual nurses.[74] Although she outlined how the training school integrated women of diverse origins and motivation into a working institution, and discussed how the nurses occasionally banded together in acts of rebellion, Tomes did not explain how the nurses coped with the stresses and strains of training school. The only study to explore the existence of female support groups among nurses is Martha Vicinus's *Independent Women: Work and Community of Single Women 1850–1920.* Although Vicinus acknowledged that homesickness and shared miseries united probationers and created a temporary corporate loyalty, she concluded that "the constant rotation of probationers from ward to ward, the class divisions in the training home, and the exploitative work all acted to inhibit a sense of community from developing among women nurses."[75]

These studies have failed to explain how young nursing students survived three years of what Vicinus described as a combination of boot camp and boarding school. Mona Wilson's correspondence indicates that she was able to persevere only because of the supportive peer friendships that the young women fashioned at Johns Hopkins.

In retrospect, it seems only natural that the student nurses would create what Nancy Tomes has termed "a little world of our own."[76] They were separated from their families for the first time and facing an often hostile environment; the fact that they shared their living arrangements with others in similar positions inevitably led to the blossoming of intense friendships. Although Mona's first roommate, for example, was not a person she "would write a book about," the two women discovered their mutual enjoyment of fresh air and early evenings and became good friends.[77] Mona and her second roommate, Marion Rossiter, became lifelong friends. At the conclusion of Mona's first year, a fellow nurse who was leaving Hopkins to get married implored Mona not to return home to Toronto, but to spend the holidays with her prior to her marriage.[78] Social scientists have shown that friendships are especially important at times of transition, and admittance to nursing school certainly qualifies as a transitional stage.[79]

Equally important was the students' shared common vision. They wanted to be nurses. As women and as students, and later as nurses, they had little status or power in the male-dominated hospitals, but they did possess importance among themselves. Women highly valued peer relationships among their own gender because they were not well regarded by men. As Nancy Cott has argued, "a woman discovered among her own sex a world of true peers, in valuing whom she confirmed her own value."[80] A student nurse could best appreciate another student's anxieties, joys, and aspirations.

Hospital authorities recognized the existence of such friendships and acknowledged their importance for the nurses' happiness. They did worry, however, that friendships formed too hastily might lead to a poor selection of friends, and warned against "allowing the feeling to develop that one's friend is an absolute necessity to one's happiness."[81] In Mona's case, Marion Rossiter became an inseparable friend. Mona and Marion had their own private and emotional world. They shared sorrows, joys, and anxieties, devised methods for sneaking food up to their rooms, talked about life into the early hours of the morning, visited each other's families, spent summers together, and refused to be separated when they worked for the Red Cross in Siberia and the Balkans. In letters home, and in her diary, Mona referred to Marion as "my Mary Anne," or "my dearest friend."[82] When Marion died of tuberculosis in 1925, Mona's older sister wrote sympathetically, "I am so sorry Mona, it will be dreadfully lonely for you without her. One grows so away from other people when one has a real friend—and then there is that hopeless gap in one's life— and it will seem almost impossible to bridge."[83] This was exactly how Mona felt. "The dear, dear girl," Mona noted sadly to her sister, "I feel unutterably lonely to know she is not anyplace to chat with through letters or have the hope of joining up and going off together—but am glad that her suffering is over at last . . . but I feel that there is nothing worthwhile ahead of one now."[84]

In discussing female friendships formed at women's colleges, Barbara Solomon noted that it was natural for a girl to have one intimate friend as well as to create a small group of peers "who knew each others' deepest thoughts and feelings . . . and gave each other respect and affection akin to love, as well as encouragement in their new adventure."[85] A similar sense of companionship at the Johns Hopkins Hospital School of Nursing provided Mona and her friends with the support group they needed for survival. Their shared experiences created a solidarity and bonding that led to lifelong friendships. In keeping with the school's family metaphor, Mona's little clique of six or seven student nurses referred to themselves as "our family," and adopted nicknames for each other.

According to Carol Lasser, by voluntarily creating such kinships the women softened the harsh realities of isolation in daily life and reinforced their shared gender.[86] Mona's Hopkins family included Marion Rossiter (MaryAnne), who had always wanted to be a nurse, and came to Hopkins from Worcester, Massachusetts; Phyllis Higinbotham (Phyl), who had attended high school in Guelph, Ontario, and was a graduate of the University of Toronto, where she had studied music and modern languages; and Ruth Barton (Rufus), who had planned to attend college, but whose father's death forced her to take up office work. As a result, Ruth was thirty-one years old when she entered Hopkins. Mona often referred to her as "mother," and she and Marion signed letters to her as "your children." Margaret Leigh, "another damned canuck,"[87] plus several other Hopkins student nurses, also provided the group with the necessary emotional and spiritual support to endure the trials of nursing school. When graduation day came, the thought that she might not see her friends again cast a dark pall over this otherwise joyful occasion: "I'm quite lost and forlorn these days. It's awful to be bereft of one's dearest friends."[88]

Although entertainment was limited by the scarcity of time and finances, Mona and her friends found time to attend an occasional movie, walk in the woods, or picnic in the park. Shopping and "decent eats" were on the other side of town, fifty minutes away. "We cannot walk to places like in Toronto," Mona explained, "for one reason we are usually too dog tired and another that the streets are mostly up and down hill and tedious climbing for the footsore and weary. But one can get on a car at the corner here and go for a nice hour's ride in the country for 5 cents."[89]

Youthful rebellion against the stringent rules included the occasional illegitimate party, pranks such as pinning notes on people's backs, and thinking up uncomplimentary nicknames for especially strict nurses. Food orgies became an escape and a ritual of female friendship.[90] At first, the probationers hid fruit and sweets in boxes and flower vases in their rooms. Later, Mona and her friends took the streetcar to a cake shop in the "respectable part of town," where they spent evenings sampling different kinds of ice cream and "a large sized cake with three layers and nice gooey white icing and coconut on the top."[91] Soon, eating evolved into a ritual occasion. Every holiday, whether American or Canadian, was an excuse for a party. The ten Canadian nurses celebrated Victoria Day in Phyllis Higinbotham's room, "each person having a quart of chocolate ice-cream with chocolate sauce. My capacity is tremendous! I can see Mother lifting her hands in holy horror at the thought of a whole quart disappearing down my throat without a thought of it being at all unusual."[92] Both the parties and the gorgers became more numerous—

and Mona ballooned to 140 pounds, "husky, eh what?"[93] The "family" eventually stopped the per person quart of ice cream, but every letter home contained at least some mention of food, and Mona enclosed a photograph of herself in one letter, stating "you see I am still fat and flourishing."[94] By Mona's graduating year, the cook in the Nurses' Home had become a devoted friend and a supplier of illegitimate snacks.

An additional bond for these women was the fact that they would soon be graduates of Johns Hopkins, one of America's most distinguished nursing schools. Upon graduation they would have a special professional identity. Like contemporary women college graduates who felt united by their education,[95] Mona felt strong ties with other Hopkins nurses. In her travels around the world, Mona kept up her subscription to the *Johns Hopkins Nurses Alumnae Magazine* and actively sought help, recommendations, employment, and support of her fellow Hopkins nurses—normally with great success.

Mona and her circle of friends were among the elite of their school. The training at the Johns Hopkins Hospital School of Nursing was intended to produce supervisors and administrators—women graduates who could manage a staff, discipline other nurses, plan programs, keep orderly records, and communicate effectively with physicians and hospital trustees.[96] During the last half of her senior year, the head nurses at Johns Hopkins singled out Mona and eleven other students for special executive and administrative training,[97] which provided these nurses with a special professional identity and ensured excellent future recommendations.[98]

In the years following graduation, Mona kept in touch with the "family" of friends she had made et Johns Hopkins. Although Mona joined another informal support network of female friends in Prince Edward Island, she remained close friends with her Hopkins confidantes until her death in 1981. They exchanged letters, visited each others' homes, and traveled on holidays together in retirement.

Judging from Mona Wilson's subsequent career, Hopkins's stress on hierarchy, discipline, obedience, order, and efficiency proved successful. However, without the support groups that the women formed at Johns Hopkins, few nurses could have endured the ordeal. The women who survived this three-year trial owed their sanity to the camaraderie that the strict conditions forged amongst them.

NOTES

1.   The Wilson children included Helen (born in 1890), followed by Harold MacKenzie (1892), Mona herself (1894), Jack (1896), twins Jane and Doris (1900), and Margaret (1905). Another child died in infancy, and Doris passed away in 1906.

2.   R. Jones, "Travellers' Joy," in *Ellen Mary Knox*, ed. George Wrong (Toronto, 1925), p. 66.

3.   Mona G. Wilson Collection, Acc. 3652, Public Archives of Prince Edward Island, Canada.

4.   Harold to sister Jane from Valcartier, Quebec, 14 September 1914. This letter, plus several hundred more, were originally stored in a box under Jane's bed in Toronto. Jane allowed me to read these letters in installments and gave me permission to quote from them freely. When Jane died in 1991, her son disposed of all the letters except those few that I had copied or that Jane had given to me. The Public Archives of Prince Edward Island possesses approximately one thousand additional letters written by and to Mona Wilson.

5.   In fact, the heavy recruitment of nurses' aides for the Voluntary Aid Detachment resulted in a shortage of trained nurses following the war. Veronica Jane Strong-Boag, *The Parliament of Women: The National Council of Women of Canada, 1893–1929* (Ottawa: National Museums of Canada, 1976), p. 313.

6.   Nancy Tomes, "'Little World of Our Own': The Pennsylvania Hospital Training School for Nurses, 1895–1907," reprinted in *Women and Health in America: Historical Readings*, ed. Judith Walzer Leavitt (Madison: University of Wisconsin Press, 1984), p. 74; Jane E. Mottus, *New York Nightingales: The Emergence of the Nursing Profession at Bellevue and New York Hospital, 1850–1920* (Ann Arbor: University of Michigan Press, 1981), p. 93

7.   Fred Davis, ed., *The Nursing Profession: Five Sociological Essays* (New York: John Wiley & Sons, 1966), p. 88; Vern Bullough and Bonnie Bullough, *The Care of the Sick: The Emergence of Modern Nursing* (New York: Prodist, 1978), p. 95; Karen Kingsley, "The Architecture of Nursing," in *Images of Nurses: Perspectives from History, Art, and Literature*, ed. Anne Hudson Jones (Philadelphia: University of Pennsylvania Press, 1988), p. 65; Philip Kalisch and Beatrice Kalisch, *The Changing Image of the Nurse* (Menlo Park, Calif.: Addison-Wesley, 1987), pp. 22–27.

8.   Mona to sister Jane, 13 November 1947 and 26 April 1980, author's collection.

9.   Mona to Jane, 18 January 1915, author's collection.

10.   Harold (overseas) to Jane, 17 January 1915, author's collection.

11.   Kalisch and Kalisch, *Changing Image* (n. 7), pp. 21–22.

12.   Susan Reverby, *Ordered to Care.: The Dilemma of American Nursing, 1850–1945* (Cambridge: Cambridge University Press, 1987), p. 81. Approximately one-third of the nurses at the nursing training schools in New York were Canadians, and 21 percent were from Ontario. Mottus, *New York Nightingales* (n. 6), pp. 96–102.

13.   Abraham Flexner, *Medical Education in the United States and Canada* (New York: Carnegie Foundation for the Advancement of Teaching, 1910; reprint, Boston: Merrymount Press, 1960), p. 235 (page citation is to the reprint edition).

14.   Ethel Johns and Blanche Pfefferkorn, *The Johns Hopkins Hospital School of Nursing, 1889–1949* (Baltimore: Johns Hopkins Press, 1954), pp. 29, 131.

15.   *The Johns Hopkins Nurses Alumnae Magazine*, February 1921, *20*; May 1926, *25*: 80–82 (henceforth *JHNAM*).

16.   "The Johns Hopkins Hospital School for Nurses, Circular of Information, 1914–1915," William Henry Welch Medical Library, Johns Hopkins Medical

Institutions, Baltimore.

17. Martha Vicinus, *Independent Women: Work and Community of Single Women 1850–1920* (Chicago: University of Chicago Press, 1985), p. 104.

18. Reverby, *Ordered to Care* (n. 12), p. 85. The typical nursing student was young, single, native-born, and from a rural background. Barbara Melosh, *"The Physician's Hand": Work Culture and Conflict in American Nursing* (Philadelphia: Temple University Press, 1982), pp. 30–31. At the Bellevue Training School in 1900, one-quarter of the students were college graduates, one-half had graduated from high school, and the rest had graduated from normal or private schools. Mottus, *New York Nightingales* (n. 6), p. 75.

19. "Johns Hopkins Hospital School for Nurses, Circular of Information" (n. 16). Also see the statement on "culture" by the Committee on Education of the National League of Nursing Education, *Standard Curriculum for Schools of Nursing Prepared by the Committee on Education of the National League of Nursing Education, 1915 to 1918*, p. 27.

20. Johns and Pfefferkorn, *Johns Hopkins* (n. 14), p. 189.

21. "Johns Hopkins Hospital School for Nurses, Circular of Information" (n. 16).

22. In 1912, over half of the American nursing schools accepted women under twenty years of age. Reverby, *Ordered to Care* (n. 12), p. 85.

23. Dr. John Hall's letter of reference for Mona Wilson, n.d., Mona Wilson File, Student Records, RG 3, Series B, Alan Mason Chesney Medical Archives of the Johns Hopkins Medical Institutions (henceforth JHA).

24. H. J. Cody, St. Paul's Church, Toronto, 24 November 1914, Mona Wilson File, Student Records, RG 3, Series B, JHA. Cody, who later became the minister of education for Ontario and president of the University of Toronto, was the governor of Havergal as well as the Wilsons' family minister.

25. Mona Wilson File, Student Records, RG 3, Series B, JHA.

26. Mona to family, n.d., 1915, author's collection.

27. Kingsley, "Architecture of Nursing" (n. 7), pp. 69–72; Edward Stevens, *The American Hospital of the Twentieth Century* (New York: Architectural Record Publishing, 1918).

28. E. M. Lawler, "Annual Report," *JHNAM*, 1915, 14:140–41.

29. The probationers were admitted in two groups, one in March and the other in September.

30. "The Johns Hopkins Hospital School for Nurses, Circular of Information" (n. 16), p. 7.

31. Charlotte A. Aikens, *Studies in Ethics for Nurses* (Philadelphia: W. B. Saunders, 1925), p. 18.

32. Mona to sister Jane, 25 April 1915, author's collection.

33. Aikens, *Studies in Ethics* (n. 31), p. 150.

34. Mona to Jane, 23 February 1918, Acc. 3652, Mona G. Wilson Collection, Public Archives, Prince Edward Island, Canada (henceforth PAPEI).

35. For a list of recommended rules and regulations see Charlotte A. Aikens, *Hospital Management* (Philadelphia: W. B. Saunders, 1911), pp. 330–77.

36. Reverby, *Ordered to Care* (n. 12), p. 53.

37. *Standard Curriculum* (n. 19), p. 21.

38. "Instructor's Monthly Report of Students," Box 14, Student Records, RG 3, Series B, JHA.

39. Ibid.

40. *The Code of Ethics of the Alumnae Association of the Johns Hopkins Hospital Training School for Nurses* (Baltimore, 1896).

41. Mona to parents, 25 April 1915, Acc. 3652, PAPEI.

42. Mona to Jane, 31 May 1915, author's collection.

43. E. Lawler to W. H. Smith, "Board of Trustees Minutes," 8 February 1916, Box 9, RG 2, Senes A, JHA.

44. Mona to Jane, late July 1915, author's collection.

45. Ibid.

46. Mona to Jane, 9 March 1916, author's collection.

47. Philip Kalisch and Beatrice Kalisch, *The Advance of American Nursing* (Boston: Little Brown, 1978), pp. 307–8.

48. Aikens apparently did not consider this repercussion when she wrote that "suspension for a few days or weeks will often teach a lesson that can be taught in no other way, and lessons taught in this way have a salutary effect on the whole school." Aikens, *Hospital Management* (n. 35), p. 344. According to Vicinus, the drop-out rate in nursing schools from the earliest days through the First World War was seldom less than 30 percent annually. Vicinus, *Independent Women* (n. 17), p. 112.

49. "Board of Trustees Monthly Minutes," April, June, October, November, December 1915, JHA; *Twenty-Seventh Report of the Johns Hopkins Hospital for Year Ending January 31, 1916* (Baltimore: Johns Hopkins Press, 1916).

50. Mona to Jane, 31 May 1915, author's collection.

51. Mona Wilson File, "Student Records," RG 3, Series B, JHA.

52. Mona to parents, 25 April 1915, Acc. 3652, PAPEI.

53. Mona to Jane, 10 June 1916, author's collection. Lawler wrote that it required "eternal vigilance" to ensure that the hospital maids performed only the duties assigned, since otherwise, she explained, the nurses would never learn how to protect furniture, floors, and rugs, and would be careless of linen, dishes, and utensils. Elsie Lawler, "How Much Time Should Be Allowed for Specialization During the Training School Course," *Amer. J. Nursing*, July 1916, 16: 843.

54. Mona to Jane, November 1915, author's collection.

55. Mona to Jane, 1 August 1916, author's collection.

56. Mona to Dad, 15 May 1918, Acc. 3652, PAPEI.

57. Mona to Jane, 25 January 1916, Acc. 3652, PAPEI.

58. Mona to Jane, 10 June 1916, author's collection.

59. Mona to Jane, 31 May 1915, author's collection.

60. Mona to family, 17 April 1916, Acc. 3652, PAPEI.

61. Mona to Mother, 25 January 1918; also see older sister Helen to Jane, 6 February 1917, author's collection.

62. Mona to family, 28 February 1918, author's collection.

63. "Examination Questions of the Maryland State Board of Examiners of Nurses, October, 1916," *JHNAM*, February 1917, 16: 32–38.

64. Mona Wilson File, Student Records, RG 3, Series B, Mona Wilson File,

JHA.

65. Mona to family, 6 May 1918, Acc. 3652, PAPEI.

66. Carroll Smith-Rosenberg's "The Female World of Love and Ritual" is reprinted in Leavitt, *Women and Health* (n. 6), pp. 70–89.

67. Nancy F. Cott, *The Bonds of Womanhood: "Woman's Sphere" in New England, 1780–1835* (New Haven: Yale University Press, 1977), p. 173.

68. Carol Lasser, "'Let Us Be Sisters Forever': The Sororal Model of Nineteenth-Century Female Friendship," *Sign*, 1988, 14: 160.

69. Blanche Wiesen Cook, "Female Support Networks and Political Activism: Lillian Wald, Crystal Eastman, Emma Goldman," in *A Heritage of Her Own: Toward a New Social History of American Women*, ed. Nancy F. Cott and Elizabeth H. Pleck (New York: Simon & Schuster, 1979), pp. 412–44.

70. Also see Leila J. Rupp, "'Imagine My Surprise': Women's Relationships in Historical Perspective," *Frontiers*. 1981, 5: 61–70; and Karin Schultz, "Women's Adult Development: The Importance of Friendship," *J. Indep. Soc. Work*, 1991, 5: 107–22.

71. Cott, *Bonds of Womanhood* (n. 67), pp. 176–77.

72. Smith-Rosenberg, "Female World" (n. 66), p. 77.

73. Vicinus, *Independent Women* (n. 17), p. 142. For similar conclusions see Barbara Miller Solomon, *In the Company of Educated Women: A History of Women and Higher Education in America* (New Haven: Yale University Press, 1985).

74. Tomes, "'Little World of Our Own'" (n. 6).

75. Vicinus, *Independent Women* (n. 17), p. 110.

76. Tomes, "'Little World of our Own'" (n. 6).

77. Mona to parents, 25 April 1915, Acc. 3652, PAPEI.

78. Mona to family, 29 May 1916, Acc. 3652, PAPEI.

79. Schultz, "Women's Adult Development" (n. 70).

80. Cott, *Bonds of Womanhood* (n. 67), p. 190.

81. Aikens, *Studies in Ethics* (n. 31), p. 208.

82. *Diary*, 13 March 1920, Acc. 3028, PAPEI.

83. Helen Lea to Mona, 2 October 1925, author's collection.

84. Mona to Jane, 9 October 1925, author's collection.

85. Solomon, *In the Company of Educated Women* (n. 73), p. 98.

86. Lasser, "'Let Us Be Sisters Forever'" (n. 68), p. 164.

87. Mona to family, 29 May 1916, Acc. 3652, PAPEI.

88. Mona to family, 6 May 1918, Acc. 3652, PAPEI; also see Mona's comment in her diary about "those very dark days" when she left Hopkins. *Diary* (n. 82), 13 March 1920.

89. Mona to family, late July 1915, author's collection.

90. For the concept of food as a female ritual see Solomon, *In the Company of Educated Women* (n. 73), p. 97.

91. Mona to Jane, 31 May 1915, author's collection.

92. Ibid.

93. Mona to family, 8 August 1915, PAPEI.

94. Ibid., 29 May 1916, PAPEI.

95. Solomon, *In the Company of Educated Women* (n. 73), p. 95.

96. A 1929 survey of Hopkins graduates revealed that almost twice as many

Hopkins-trained nurses were engaged in institutional work (45 percent) as in private duty nursing (23 percent); nationally, some 54 percent of nurses held private duty positions. "What Our Graduates Are Doing," *JHNAM*, May 1932, 31: 64–66.

97.   In Siberia and in the Balkans, Mona's supervisors praised her for her executive abilities.

98.   Tomes, "'Little World of Our Own'" (n. 6), p. 478.

My thanks to Thomas Spira, at the University of Prince Edward Island; Gerard Shorb, archivist at the Alan Mason Chesney Medical Archives, the Johns Hopkins University; and this journal's anonymous readers, for their insightful comments and assistance. The Hannah Institute for the History of Medicine funded the travel and research costs involved in this study.

5

To Cultivate a Feeling of Confidence: The Nursing of Obstetric Patients, 1890–1940

Sylvia Rinker

Mothers of infants born at the end of the 19th century in America were the first to receive the assistance of the "trained obstetrical nurse."[1] Throughout the first half of the 20th century the nurses who cared for obstetric patients were charged with managing patients, their families, and their surroundings to make possible the aseptic delivery required by a growing medical science. Caring for new mothers who gave birth at home and later in hospitals, the pragmatic nurses of the first half of the 20th century were actively involved in developing an obstetric nursing practice that espoused the traditional nursing values of caring and compassion but also bore clear marks of the growing medical and obstetric science of the time.[2] In 1915, nurse Sara Bower stated emphatically that it was a particular responsibility of the nurse to "cultivate at all times a feeling of confidence in the patient."[3] However, as historian Judith Leavitt argued, new mothers who were submitted to the rigid scientific care of the era reported feeling not confidence but rather a sense of being left "alone among strangers."[4] Leavitt has offered a thoughtful analysis of this discrepancy, but further exploration of the problem is needed.[5]

Historical investigation into the evolution of clinical practice offers insight into the conflict between science and nurturing that erupted as nursing ideals confronted the everyday experiences of the nurses and patients involved. Tensions between the nurse's role as a scientific manager and her expected function as a nurturing caregiver were evident at

Note: This chapter was originally published in *Nursing History Review* 8 (2000): 117–142. A publication of the American Association for the History of Nursing. Copyright © 2000 Springer Publishing Company.

the outset of professional nursing; a century later the dialectic tension between the scientific base of nursing and its moral base of care remains unresolved.[6] Nurses shaped their practice by choosing actions from those that were possible within the context of the time.[7] The clinical practice nurses developed, viewed as an outcome of choices made, provides evidence that offers insight into the continuing ambiguity of the historical role of nurses expected to function as both scientific and caring practitioners.[8]

"Filling the gap between home and hospital adequately," and "smoothing the path for the obstetric art" were duties that the nurse, as an early 19th-century woman, was peculiarly qualified to perform. Recruited because she was a woman, the newly emerging "trained nurse" was charged with the task of convincing women to abandon the familiar female-surrounded birth-at-home experience in favor of the rapidly growing scientific medical childbirth in the hospital.[9] Dr. Joseph B. DeLee, a dominant figure in American obstetrics at the turn of the 20th century, prescribed a specific role for the nurse explicitly designed to benefit the new obstetric "specialty" and its physician practitioners.[10] He said:

> *The nurse may do much to aid the physician in obtaining from the public that recognition for obstetrics that the specialty so justly deserves. Thus, the nurse may smooth the path for the advance of the obstetric art. She becomes really a missionary spreading the gospel of good obstetrics.*[11]

As defined by the influential DeLee, childbirth required that strict limits, imposed by scientific asepsis rules, be applied to nursing practice. Thus, from the outset the nurse's innate female attributes, governed by the scientific principles of obstetric medicine, constituted the foundations for both the power and the limits of obstetric nursing. Welcoming the status afforded by their association with the newly emerging specialist obstetricians, nurses readily accepted a role that they were only partially able to define. Charged with delivering scientific care, the nurse remained on the periphery in defining the dimensions of that care.[12]

SOCIETAL FORCES

Obstetric nursing grew out of social forces in America in the early 20th century that combined to define birth as a medical event and propelled its move into the hospital. Industrialization and urbanization promoted the growth of institutions for birth. While the Progressive Era gave rise to the expectation that better health and living conditions for women and infants were both necessary and possible, confounding high maternal and infant mortalities continued to defy medical science throughout the period. Childbirth killed five times as many women aged 15–44 as did typhoid fever, and only tuberculosis outranked parturition as a killer of women in 1917.[13] Maternal mortality rates averaged over 60 per 10,000 throughout the period of this study and did not begin a steady downward trend until 1934, when sulfonamides became available to treat deadly puerperal infections.[14] During this time a prenatal emphasis developed also, in an attempt to curb infant mortality, thus expanding the physician's domain to include the scientific management of the woman before birth as well as at the delivery and beyond.[15] Attempts to cope with the desperate conditions of the Great Depression brought radical changes in government support for healthcare, and insurance became available to pay hospital costs. All of these factors combined to propel birth into the hospital, creating the need for skilled nurses to care for obstetric patients.[16]

The belief in the power of science held by Progressive Era Americans to improve the lives of citizens and the growing power of the medical profession made the association of nursing with medicine an attractive alliance to nurse leaders.[17] Eager to promote nursing as a respectable profession, Isabel Hampton referred to the nurse as the "physician's lieutenant," who, by virtue of her training, was "allotted a part to perform in the progress of medical science."[18] Hampton's vision of the possibilities for nursing included a clear commitment to standards, precision, and method for the organization, teaching, and practice of nursing.[19] Speaking at the Chicago World's Fair in 1893, and demonstrating her understanding that working within the system could strengthen the position of the nursing profession, Hampton willingly accepted a limited role for nurses, as she said: "To be sure, the nurse is only the handmaid of that great and beautiful medical science in whose temple she may only serve in minor parts."[20]

The rapid growth of hospitals and the system that developed for the employment of nurses fostered both the educational and economic dependence of nurses on physicians. Initially taught by physicians, student nurses at the turn of the century were indoctrinated into a hierarchy that made the nurse responsible not to the patient but to the physician. Because hospitals used pupil nurses to care for patients and did not employ graduate nurses until the 1930s, nurses had to rely primarily on the referrals from physicians for their private duty nursing cases after graduation. Novice nurses who, until the 1930s, were primarily students in the hospitals had neither the knowledge nor the authority to question a nursing practice that accepted a subordinate role dictated by medicine.[21] Anxious to establish themselves as valuable associates to physicians, nurses developed a practice that gave priority to medical science and the needs of physicians over the needs of individual patients. Scientific principles provided the foundation for the beginning practice of obstetric nursing and directly affected the relationships nurses established with their patients. Georgina Pope, Superintendent of Nurses at the Columbia Hospital for Women in Washington, DC, underscored the central role of the nurse and her value as a scientific practitioner when she said, "It is through the nurse that the doctor expects to combat the frightful disease of puerperal fever . . . she can become of no less importance than the physician himself in guarding the health and preserving the lives of mothers and children."[22]

Certainly the life-threatening danger of puerperal sepsis colored the evolution of obstetric nursing. Oliver Wendell Holmes had published his classic article "On the Contagiousness of Puerperal Fever" in 1843, and by 1879, Louis Pasteur had demonstrated that the infectious streptococcus was responsible for puerperal fever.[23] Science had provided a way, through antiseptic and aseptic practices, to overcome the killer, and its principles must *not* be violated. In 1924, Dr. Charles Reed, speaking to the Illinois State Association of Graduate Nurses, identified the "foundational qualities" of the nurse to be courage, tenderness, and self-control. He continued:

> *and yet, though she have the courage of a lioness, the divine tenderness of a mother, and the self-control of a Capulet, and have not science, it shall profit her nothing. Her training in science, science clear, precise, inevitable, is the necessary medium through which her mind and emotions express themselves. It is the master tool of her profession.*[24]

The traditional nursing values of compassion, comfort, and support for the whole person clashed with the rigors of scientific asepsis that defined the medical practice of obstetrics; the nursing care that developed bore the marks of this conflict.

OBSTETRIC NURSING IN HOME DELIVERIES

Despite an active campaign conducted by physicians to promote hospital birth in the early decades of the 20th century, in 1940, half of all deliveries in the United States still occurred at home.[25] Once the pregnancy was confirmed, the mother-to-be usually initiated an employment interview with the prospective nurse.[26] While it was common for the physician to recommend private duty nurses for employment, in obstetric cases the situation was often reversed. The nurse was key to promoting medical care for childbirth at the turn of the century because, just as women had felt comfortable in approaching the female midwife in the past, many women contacted the nurse before selecting their physicians.[27] Katharine DeWitt urged the private duty nurse whose patient had not yet consulted with a physician to offer to go with the patient to the doctor's office or come to the house when the doctor was first summoned if "nervousness" were the reason that the woman had postponed her initial contact with a physician. DeWitt loyally followed DeLee's dictates that when available, specialist obstetricians be employed as birth attendants because "a nurse can never forget what complications may arise requiring the greatest skill obtainable."[28]

The nurse who assisted at an operative delivery in the home faced a task of daunting proportions.[29] A nurse's tactful ability to secure the patient's cooperation was as crucial as her scientific training because she was required to convert the patient's private home into an aseptic field for scientific birth.[30] Building a trusting relationship with her patient was an essential first step as the nurse was responsible for convincing the mother that it was necessary to scrub all floors, walls, and furniture and otherwise rearrange the family's furnishings for birth. She must ensure that all equipment was sterile and at hand. After the environment was cleansed the nurse was expected to wash thoroughly her patient also, both internally and externally.[31] A warm bath, soapsuds enema, and in the early years an antiseptic douche were followed by additional scrubbing of the skin from the breasts to the knees, including the perineum, the buttocks, and the thighs.[32] Perineal shaving, begun in the early decades of the 20th century, continued, despite its demonstrated futility, well into the 1980s.[33] Following the cleansing, the mother-to-be was placed in an elaborately prepared bed for her labor. The nurse's responsibility then was to remain with her patient and send for the doctor when delivery was imminent.[34]

Considerable skill was required to comfort and reassure women who were normally frightened and anxious at the onset of labor. Graduate nurses who were experienced in the care of childbearing women recognized the value of the personal relationship with their patients. Nurse Louella Adkins wrote in 1903: "A thorough acquaintance of the peculiarities of each patient is a wonderful help, and should be sought in all ways short of inquisitiveness before the confinement."[35] She believed that the "well-bred observance of the patient is the guide to the *unobtrusive control* which the successful nurse must exercise."[36] The nurse who functioned autonomously to help her patient accept medical interventions for birth and maintain self-control throughout the ordeal of labor not only facilitated aseptic deliveries, she also made the entire experience much more pleasant for the physician and the family.

As nurses soon learned, developing good relationships with physicians was also essential for a pleasant birthing experience. According to Nurse Mary Keith the "wise" nurse had consulted with the physician before labor to find out when he wished to be notified.[37] Central to ensuring a safe delivery, the nurse must use her scientific knowledge to judge when to send for the physician. At the same time that such clinical judgments were expected of the nurse, she was cautioned repeatedly not to diagnose because diagnosing was considered exclusive medical territory.[38] The nurse was to inform the physician of the condition of his patient,

> *without giving her opinions. It is the duty of the nurse to inform the doctor that there is some antepartum flowing, for instance, or that the uterine tumor bulges sideways . . . but it is not her business to suspect aloud that it is a case of placenta previa, or a transverse position of the child.*[39]

The nurse's tact and flexibility were essential to provide safe care to the patient while maintaining the appropriate medical hierarchy. A certain amount of finesse was also required for the procedure of notifying the physician to come for the delivery: "The nurse should know enough never to send peremptorily for the doctor when there is no immediate necessity."[40]

A very common occurrence in home births was the arrival of the infant before the physician. Distances between patients' homes, difficulty in delivering messages, and their other patient responsibilities all prevented the physician's presence at the moment of birth. This was especially true in rural areas. Studies by the Children's Bureau reported repeatedly that even in the rare event when a physician had been engaged to attend births, he usually did not arrive in time.[41] The competent, adaptable nurse functioned in the doctor's presence as his "assistant;" in his absence, she functioned as the previously noted "lieutenant."[42] In recognition of this fact, nursing textbooks of the period gave instructions to the nurse first on her delivery duties in the physician's absence and then on her tasks in his presence.

Inherent in the nurse's role was preventing the unwarranted disturbance of the physician. The doctor's role was to manage the birth, not the labor leading up to the birth.[43] Dr. Stanley Warren saw "no intrinsic fitness in the obstetrician serving as a watchful nurse at the bedside forty-eight hours before he is wanted."[44] Clara Weeks-Shaw, author of an early nursing textbook, gave fair warning: "Perhaps more often in obstetric cases than in any others, the nurse is called upon to assume, in his absence, responsibilities properly belonging to the physician."[45] Some private duty nurses refused to take obstetric patients for this very reason.[46] Although uncomfortable with the responsibility for managing birth, the nurses who took obstetric cases did accept the delivery as part of their role as valuable helpers to the physician.[47] According to A. Worcester the "best assistants are those who themselves are able to take charge."[48] By limiting the types of cases she took, a nurse developed her expertise and could claim to be a "specialist" in obstetric nursing just as the physician had become a specialist by limiting his practice to obstetrics. A major reason obstetric nurses were embraced by scientific medicine while lay midwives were not is that nurses were always careful to recognize and protect the physician's authority even when fulfilling duties that were properly defined as medical obligations. The obstetric nurse accepted a dependent role, sanctioned by the authority of scientific medicine, that midwives refused. By assuming the delivery duty without the decision-making power to determine how the birth should be managed, nurses became firmly entrenched as subordinates in the medical sphere.[49] By accepting responsibility for managing the delivery, defined by medical science as strictly within the medical domain, nurses made themselves central to a process they had little authority to define or control.

Nurses quickly became indispensable assistants in providing the scientific medical advantage of anesthesia to women at birth.[50] Hampton encouraged nurses to use every opportunity while in training in the hospital to prepare themselves for giving anesthetics when they became private duty nurses in homes.[51] DeLee wrote in 1907 that since the doctor frequently prescribed chloroform the nurse should know the procedure well because "when the child is coming through the vulva, the nurse may have to administer the chloroform."[52] The nurse's duties while giving anesthesia included protecting the patient's face from the irritating vapors by smearing vaseline around the patient's mouth and nostrils, dripping the anesthetic on a handkerchief or an ether cone held over her face, and watching the patient's pulse and facial appearance very carefully for untoward signs.[53] The nurse was to give her full attention to this responsibility as the life of mother and infant were literally in her hands.[54]

Following delivery of the infant and the placenta, the responsibility for preserving the newly delivered mother's life landed squarely on the nurse's shoulders. In the first hours after delivery the nurse's "vigilant watchfulness offered the only security."[55] The nurse's observation of signs and symptoms were pivotal for safe medical care, and there was no question that the nurse was held responsible for the accurate interpretation of signs and the ultimate fate of her patient. In 1916, Nurse A. Young literally saved her newly delivered patient's life by her alert assessment of the deteriorating vital signs that followed the high forceps delivery of her patient.[56] Left alone to monitor her patient's recovery following delivery, she called the physician back to the home when it became clear to her that the patient must be transferred to the hospital for a life-saving blood transfusion and surgical repair of a hemorrhaging cervical tear. Young continued to care for the patient, carefully recording her vital signs, during the course of her hospitalization. At the end of 3 weeks, Young reported that "in spite of all Mrs. A. had gone through, there was no infection, and mother and baby left the hospital in good condition." Young demonstrated a sophisticated understanding of the pathophysiology involved in the medical treatment of postpartum hemorrhage. Scientific medical care, though admittedly the probable cause of the cervical tear that led to the hemorrhage in the first place, eventually saved this mother's life. Because of the nurse's intelligent, rapid response to her patient's deteriorating condition, the medical care she desperately needed had the opportunity to be successful.

The medical treatment receives center stage in Young's account of her experience, while the nursing care that made it possible is not recorded. Any emotional support and care given as nurse and family faced the trauma of an emergency transfer from the home to the hospital and the potentially imminent death of the mother were not part of the record she published in the professional journal. Instead, the authoritative knowledge of scientific medicine was the knowledge this nurse deemed important to document. The clinical judgments nurses made on the basis of their scientific observations clearly differentiated professional nurses from untrained attendants. In the developing profession of nursing, documenting the contributions of nurses to medical practice was a first step necessary for the acknowledgment of nurses as skilled professionals. In the evolution of nursing, expertise in the application of scientific medical knowledge was foundational for the future acceptance of the profession as a legitimate partner with medicine.

Nurses learned their lessons well; gaining scientific knowledge and experience, they began to evaluate the performance of physicians. When necessary, well-trained scientific nurses took the responsibility to ensure safe medical practice. Bower described a home delivery in 1915 at which it was her "painful duty and professional privilege" to protect her patient from a lax physician.[57] She reported that when he arrived, the physician had, "incredible as it may seem, fingernails that were black, absolutely filthy." By providing scrub brushes, pouring water, placing solutions where he could hardly avoid them, and using "mental suggestion" with all her force, Bower successfully protected her patient against infection. Proud of her practice, she said: "I came out victorious, a clean baby, and a complete and happy recovery." In 1915, with a maternal mortality rate of over 60 per 10,000 and an infant mortality rate of over 100 per 1,000, a safe recovery from childbirth was no mean accomplishment.

In addition to interpreting strictly scientific principles, graduate nurses proved to be very capable of actively translating their scientific knowledge into actions that could be safely adapted to the individual situations of their patients. Adkins was convinced, in 1903, that "Good antiseptic technique could be carried out in a barnyard, if the brain that directs it is trained in principles and details."[58] On the subject of care of the newborn's cord she said:

> *If we know we want to desiccate the cord as quickly as possible, and remember that any liquid put upon it will delay that result, we will be rewarded by a clean little pink dimple, whether we keep the stump clean and dry with the daintiest absorbent cotton, or with the scorched, and therefor sterile rag of the old-time nurse.*[58]

The nurse's ability to individualize the scientific care prescribed by medicine was important to the development of nursing as a profession with its own approach to patient care.

The patient record of a mother who did not survive her birth experience offers an example of nursing practice that combined the best available scientific medical care with the nurturing new mothers expected from their nurses. Susan Moore's pregnancy ended abruptly on June 4, 1908, when she suddenly began having the first of a series of convulsions that eventually required her admission to Columbia Hospital for Women in Washington, DC.[59] The best medical care and medications were unable to stop the convulsions, and Moore's infant was delivered, via high forceps, stillborn.[60] Within the nurse's postpartum notes are many medical assessments, including frequent recordings of the patient's temperature that spiked to 105° 5 days after delivery. Repeated doses of strychnine, laxatives, and whiskey were given, along with oxygen, in desperate attempts to save the patient's life. Nurses' observations, "respirations very rapid and painful; complaining of pain in left side; sighing a good deal in sleep; quite restless, seems very uncomfortable; very bad wheezing in chest; talked irrationally greater part of night; seems brighter this morning" documented in the nurses' notes, indicate the close attention her nurses paid to caring for this mother.[61] On the night before Moore died the nurse on duty wrote: "Does not want to be alone." One of the last nursing actions recorded, in the face of imminent death, was the placement of a hot water bottle on to the patient's left side. Nearly comatose, she could not have directed this action. No doubt the nurse had remembered Moore's earlier complaints of pain in her left side. Within an hour the patient's respirations had ceased. The scientific observations documented by Moore's nurses were important for helping physicians decide on the medical treatment she would receive. The nurses' recordings of Moore's responses to various medicines and treatments give evidence that nurses' actions were based not only on physicians' orders, but also on their own interpretations of the comforting measures Moore needed.

OBSTETRIC NURSING IN HOSPITAL BIRTHS

The gradual movement of birth from the home to the hospital gained momentum as the 20th century progressed. Mothers who delivered in hospitals before 1920 were primarily single or indigent women; however, by the mid-1920s, Americans had begun to see hospitalized birth, as well as hospitalization for other conditions, as symbolic of economic and social status.[62] Nationwide the 37% of hospital births that occurred in 1936 had grown to 55% in 1940 and by 1951 had reached 90%.[63] By the 1930s a growing number of middle-class women, whose healthcare expenses were occasionally subsidized by insurance, began to choose hospitals for birth.[64] The hospital nursing staff also changed; beginning in the 1930s, student nurses were replaced by graduates employed as staff nurses.[65]

The hospitalization of birth facilitated a greater number and frequency of procedures that greatly increased nurses' duties. From 1890 to 1940 a dramatic increase in the "operative interventions" used for childbirth in hospitals is clearly evident. The use of forceps, induction via inflatable balloons, versions, episiotomies, and cesarean sections had all been available since the mid-19th century but were not widely used until the 20th century.[66] The overall operative intervention rate for deliveries at Columbia Hospital in Washington, DC, more than tripled from 20% in 1892 to 66% in 1920.[67] Sixty-five percent of the women who delivered at the Chicago Lying-In Hospital between 1918 and 1925 had operative deliveries; by 1931, 80% of women received some type of intervention for birth.[68]

The strict asepsis that nurses and physicians tried to uphold in home births was even more rigorously pursued in hospitals. Rigid routines were developed to streamline the extra care required by the growing population of patients who were receiving increasing numbers of interventions for their births. Physicians lent their authority, and nurses used it willingly to promote scientific birth restrictions. Asepsis rules required banning family and friends from the laboring rooms in the hospitals.[69] Dr. Anna Fullerton noted that the nurse "succeeds best" in this process by telling the friends that it is the doctor's wish that she exclude them.[70] Nurses willingly supported policies that separated a woman from her family on her admission to the hospital, stripped her of her clothes, shaved and purged her, and sometimes restrained her, all in the pursuit of asepsis.[71] Individualized care suffered under this regime and certainly contributed to the dissatisfaction among mothers that Leavitt documented.[72] The nurses who participated in such actions believed the scientific training they had received; they were convinced that such policies were justified to save mothers and infants from death. One 1937 graduate nurse reported: "Infection didn't stand a chance. We used Lysol solutions for perineal care and sprayed merthiolate on the perineum every time we could!"[73]

Second only to the fear of death in childbirth among women at the end of the 19th century was a nearly universal dread of pain.[74] American women actively sought anesthesia, offered as one of the chief advantages of scientific birth.[75] Mary Blackwell, R.N., understood the challenge and the prestige of nursing the medicated woman in labor when she observed in 1931, "the nursing care of obstetric patients having analgesia and anesthesia is a difficult, though interesting duty."[76] The nurse administered the medication and applied the restraints, changing in the process, as historian Margrete Sandelowski has noted, "from a sisterly companion to an unfeeling robot."[77] Birth became an event not to be accepted and celebrated but to be managed and controlled. Because the anesthetized, restless patient could give no warning of an impending birth, making precipitous delivery very likely, the nurse who managed such a process successfully was obviously an accomplished partner in scientific birth.

As at-home births, the good nurse in the hospital saved the physician's time by calling him at just the right moment for the delivery. She became skillful at preserving the peace by giving careful attention to maintaining the established hierarchy. One nurse who began her practice in the 1930s reported that she was always careful, in reporting her laboring patient's condition, not to make a medical diagnosis.[78] "I'd call the intern and tell him 'I think' the patient is ready for delivery," she said. The intern came, examined the patient, and "informed" the nurse of the patient's progress. The intern notified the resident, who appeared on the labor unit in time to tell the nurse to call the attending physician; then he gave the order to move the patient "immediately" to the delivery room. Within the hospital system the nurse's knowledge was validated only when confirmed by the physician's authority. Experienced nurses knew, however, how to manage the system so that inexperienced interns and residents made the right decisions. While the intern and resident were busy confirming what this nurse already knew, she had already notified the anesthetist, the scrub nurse, and the circulating nurse so that all could be "in the delivery room, lined up and ready to go" before the attending physician arrived. That she managed, repeatedly, to get all of the personnel in their proper places at the right time, without ruffling feathers, was an accomplishment that this nurse reported with obvious pride, 50 years after the fact! Central to the action that facilitated a smooth delivery, the nurse kept her "place" by allowing the interns and residents to pronounce the medical judgments she had already made and acted upon. The mother was safely delivered, and the nurse's position as a valuable assistant within the system was maintained.

By giving priority to science and the physician over individual attention to the patient the nurse compromised the traditional woman-to-woman connection that had made her so valuable a missionary of the gospel of good obstetrics. Once the public had been convinced to accept medical attendance at birth, the womanly attributes of the nurse were redirected to support physicians and medical procedures rather than the patient who was giving birth. As good missionaries, obstetric nurses believed the gospel that strict adherence to asepsis principles was requisite to saving the lives of mothers and babies. As there could be no tolerance for breaks in aseptic technique, there could be no deviation in the hospital routine that might permit the introduction of the infectious germ. The hard-fought battle against maternal mortality was just beginning to lower the death rates of mothers in the late 1930s, and despite patients' complaints, nurses were convinced that the rigid policies were justified to protect their patients.

CONFLICT: MANAGING THE SYSTEM AND SUSTAINING THE PATIENT

Charged with spreading the gospel of good obstetrics, nurses discovered that their management skills were necessary to keep the household functioning during the disruption caused by scientific birth. As domestic managers in the hospitals, nurses were also responsible for promoting the smooth, efficient running of the institution. Nurses became adept at the scientific management of equipment, patients, and personnel in the hospitals. The priority for nursing care remained, throughout the time period of this study, to "smooth the path" for the physician and to ensure the economic efficiency of the hospital.

As hospitals changed from charity institutions to business enterprises, efficiency was prized for its economic value as well as for its influence on the happiness of physicians.[79] Beginning in the 1920s, caught in an ever greater push for hospital efficiency and economy, nurses participated in time-motion studies of nursing procedures and divided nursing care into component parts.[80] In the process the sympathetic, womanly qualities, so crucial for the acceptance of medical birth, were submerged under a scientific mold that required conformity and a standardized approach to patient care. Nurses developed and published clearly delineated standards and procedures in professional journals that reflected the values of the developing profession. The "Stewart Standards," used for evaluating nursing techniques in the 1930s included safety for patient and nurse; therapeutic effect; comfort and happiness of the patient; economy of energy, time, and materials; adaptability of the procedure to new situations; and the artistic, finished appearance of the work.[81] Detailed drawings in texts and journals showed *the* correct way to bind the abdomen and breasts following birth and *the* correct way to place instruments on a perineal care tray, and outlined strict schedules for maternal and infant elimination and feeding.[82] As they developed nursing procedures, questions about the relative merits of various solutions used for perineal care, about the most efficient breast care, and about what was the quickest way, compatible with safety and comfort, of getting twenty bedpans to twenty patients were all of concern to the developing professional nurses in the 1930s.[83] Articles published in journals of the time show that nurses were beginning to follow the medical model of scientific research to validate nursing interventions. Documenting the contributions of nurses to medical practice was a first step, necessary for the acknowledgment of nurses as skilled professionals. In the evolution of nursing, expertise in the application of scientific medical knowledge was foundational for the future recognition of nursing as a legitimate profession.

Permeating the asepsis and efficiency emphases, however, is evidence that nurses valued comforting, compassionate nursing actions that paid attention to their patients' human needs. Their scientific training provided nurses the building blocks for their practice, but as Carolyn Van Blarcom, one of the first nurses to write an obstetric nursing text in the 1920s noted, "No matter how well-trained or how complete the routines may be, the quality of the nurse's mind and the spirit that pervades her work are the determining factors in the effectiveness or futility of her endeavor."[84] The stereotypical approach required by medical asepsis created discomfort for mothers and conflict for nurses who were taught: "Sustaining the patient is the heart of the matter so far as nursing is concerned: the individual patient is the point. We see the problem from the patient's point of view so far as is humanly possible."[85] In the midst of burgeoning science and expanding technology, nurses recognized that comforting the patient was an appropriate, even expected, realm for nursing. The nurse's expertise in developing relationships with female patients was an important reason physicians enlisted nurses to promote medical care for childbirth in the first place. Speaking at the 1893 Chicago World's Congress, Pope said: "The mind of the pregnant woman is very susceptible to disturbing impressions, and the influence of a good nurse at such a time is immeasurable."[86] Although scientific efficiency and technical procedures clearly impinged on those relationships, nurses continued to recognize their interactions with patients as important for the delivery of effective nursing care. Practicing nurses clearly recognized that attention to patients' needs for emotional support was a crucial component of effective nursing practice. One wrote, "the nurse has not done well if she neglects to pay particular attention to the mental condition of the patient."[87]

Sustaining the patient required responding to patients' expressed needs. As time passed, new mothers became more vocal, clearly shaping the nursing care they received. Obstetric patients eventually changed the practice of the time that restricted newly delivered mothers to bedrest during the 10–14 days after their deliveries.[88] Initially, nurses tried to make new mothers follow the rules. However, nurses who were constantly with their patients during this long bedrest noted that the longer the patients stayed in bed, "the weaker they got."[89] One nurse noted that despite nurses' attempts to enforce doctors' orders, "you couldn't *keep* mothers in bed when they wanted to get up."[90] She reported that nurses just pretended not to see when patients got out of bed earlier than they were supposed to. Although physicians gave the orders, nurses decided when and where to enforce them, and the patients ultimately obeyed or not. Despite their position as dispensers of powerful medical science, doctors did not have total control. While physicians dictated what was to be done, nurses and patients began to define the manner in which medical treatments were accomplished, signaling an emerging sphere of nursing practice that emanated from a response to patient needs.

NURSE'S POINT OF VIEW

As nurses became more proficient in managing the details of aseptic delivery, they also promoted education that focused more specifically on nursing responsibilities. Physicians had been the first teachers in nursing schools, but by 1928, Jane McLaughlin wrote that nursing students needed instructors who could teach obstetrics "from the nurse's point of view."[91] This "nurse's point of view" included proficiency in medical assessments as well as a cognitive identification of the "art of nursing" or the manner in which skills were performed. Van Blarcom was particularly sensitive to the effect of the nurse as an empathetic supporter to the woman in labor: "this kind of assistance is indeed a comfort to the patient who appears to derive from it both a moral and physical sense of being helped in her struggle."[92] Not all nurses adopted the nurturing approach promoted by the leaders of the profession, but nurses were encouraged to "adopt a warm and sympathetic attitude" toward their patients.[93] Practicing obstetric nurses recognized that their ability to affect the mother's experience fell within the nurse's sphere of action. One nurse wrote, "I have found that if the mother is relaxed, contented, and happy, the baby will be a sleepy, contented baby awakening only long enough to take nourishment. I bend all my efforts in this direction."[94] Another noted, "The details of care, of course, are specified by the physician, but the effectiveness of the planning is largely dependent on the nurse's intelligence, interest, and conscientiousness."[95]

By 1940, nurses who worked in specific labor and delivery, postpartum, and nursery units began to develop a clinical expertise and familiarity with the routine that freed them to pay attention to patients' needs for comfort beyond the strict scientific application of medical treatments. In the process of smoothing the path for the advance of obstetrics, nurses had begun to develop a vision no longer confined to the field of medicine. While cooperative with medicine, nursing was moving beyond a physician definition of the function of nurses. Nurses lent their energy, intelligence, and abilities to promoting medical care for childbirth, but because of their relationships with patients, nurses were privileged to a particular kind of knowledge that while derived from and complementary to medical knowledge, was different. As the profession developed, nurses used their insights to shape nursing practice; the missionary began to craft her own message. Van Blarcom clearly stated: "Asepsis must come first and foremost, but the nurse's attitude and care of her patient must be mellowed by an always deepening sympathy and understanding." She continued:

> *Good nursing implies more than the giving of bed baths and medicines, boiling instruments and serving meals. It is more than going on duty at a certain time, carrying out orders for a certain number of hours and going off duty again. It implies care and consideration of the patient as a human being and a determination to nurse her well and happily, no matter what this demands.*[96]

While clearly acknowledging the physician as the authority, trained nurses began to identify specific areas that were the nurse's responsibility. In the process they also established nursing as a reputable profession with a sphere of practice that was complementary to, but separate from, that of physicians. In a subtle shift from the silent subservience of early practice, nurses began to participate in patient care discussions with physicians, in some instances presenting case studies at regularly scheduled conferences with physicians.[97] Using their knowledge and experience to discuss patient care, nurses began, formally, to define and develop nursing procedures. Navigating the shifting boundaries of science and nurture and struggling to meet the diverse expectations of patients, physicians, and hospital administrators, practicing nurses between 1890 and 1940 established the clinical practice of obstetric nursing as an integral component of medical care for birth.

CONCLUSION

The obstetric nurses of the first half of the 20th century fulfilled their mission to convince women of the need for medical attendance at birth. From a historical perspective the rigid scientific nursing of obstetric patients that developed by 1940 was a logical consequence of the circumstances within which it developed. The efficiency and efficacy that were the primary goals of obstetric nursing care in the 1920s and 1930s clearly conflicted with delivery of the individualized nursing care mothers needed and eventually demanded. Initially sought for their domestic abilities, nurses soon learned that scientific expertise gave them welcomed authority and prestige in the medical environment where they practiced.[98] Scientific expertise was the focus for the newly emerging profession of nursing, while the "deep sympathy of a woman" was an expected attribute, seen as a naturally occurring, particularly desirable characteristic of an obstetric nurse.[99] Nurses of the era would not have conceived there to be an incompatibility between science and nurturing. One was learned, and the other was expected. Both were requisite for the practice of professional nursing, but the history of clinical practice indicates that the prestigious scientific approach did take priority in the early years of nursing.

Convincing women to accept scientific birth and transforming homes and hospitals into aseptic environments required expert managerial abilities. The "tactful" nurse who could manage growing numbers of patients and physicians as well as the equipment for birth was valued as an accomplished professional. Nurses' skillful movement between their essential and ancillary positions smoothed the path for obstetrics, but also contributed to their invisibility within the early healthcare system. As a result, the nurturing relationship requisite for effective nursing and satisfied patients was also hidden, overlooked, and devalued. Historian Thomas Olson has documented that the "handling, managing, and controlling" abilities of students were the attributes praised by nursing superintendents between 1915 and 1937, while the "language of caring" was absent.[100] Historical investigation of the clinical outcome as real nurses translated ideal practices into the confines of everyday nursing, however, indicates that a fundamental source of nurses' power, knowledge, and influence was found in the relationships they established with their patients. Nearly a century ago, Bower recognized the significance of nurse-patient relationships when she identified that the nurses' primary duty was "to cultivate at all times a feeling of confidence in the patient." Her insight remains relevant today.

Across the ages (and across cultures), new mothers and their families have consistently identified nursing support as a primary ingredient for their satisfaction with childbirth care.[101] The human person-to-person connection, so easily taken for granted, was at the core of effective nursing in the first half of this century. Today, as burgeoning technology continues to require ever more technically proficient scientific practitioners, the problem of humanizing scientific care surfaces again and again.[102] Historical investigation of clinical practice indicates that nurses who would provide effective nursing care must temper needed scientific interventions with a compassionate approach that also nurtures patients' individual, human needs. At the outset of the new millennium, patients continue to need competent nurses who know how to give the best of scientific care by developing relationships that recognize and support the individual needs of patients.

Historical studies of the evolution of clinical practice have just begun. Examining the everyday practices of nurses in contact with patients has the potential to illuminate both productive strategies and limiting compromises nurses have made as practice has evolved. Over time, nurses' knowledge and expertise remained perversely hidden in the rush to meet the rapidly changing needs of an ever-evolving healthcare system. Exploration of the historical record can correct this picture by making explicit the distinct impact of nursing. What better source for evidence-based practice than the insights available from studying the documented outcomes of historical clinical practice? The history of developing nursing practice in all clinical areas offers a rich source of data that has barely been tapped. Such research holds the potential to offer a deeper understanding of the ongoing paradoxes of the nursing profession—enduring dilemmas such as the tensions between nurture and science—that continue to confound questions about the nurse's proper function and role.[103] How nursing ideals were transmitted into everyday practice and the results of nurses' alliances with patients, families, and physicians are other areas that need to be explored. Investigation of the history of clinical practice, where nurses meet patients, warrants serious efforts from historians who wish to explore the complex history of nursing.

NOTES

1.   Herbert Stowe, "The Specially Trained Obstetric Nurse—Her Advantages and Field," *American Journal of Nursing* (hereafter cited as *AJN*) 10(1910): 550–554.

2.   Diane Hamilton, "Constructing the Mind of Nursing," *Nursing History Review* 2 (1994): 3–28.

3.   Sara Bower, "The Obstetrical Nurse," *AJN* 15 (June 1915): 734–5.

4.   Judith Leavitt, Chapter 7, "'Alone Among Strangers': Birth Moves to the Hospital," in *Brought to Bed: Childbearing in America 1750–1950* (New York: Oxford University Press, 1986);

5.   Judith Leavitt, "'Strange Young Women on Errands': Obstetric Nursing Between Two Worlds," *Nursing History Review* 6 (1998): 3–24.

6.   Alison Kitson, "Does Nursing Have a Future?" *Image* 29 (Second Quarter 1997): 111–15.

7.   Judith Leavitt, "'Science' Enters the Birthing Room: Obstetrics in America since the Eighteenth Century," *The Journal of American History* 70 (September 1983): 281–304.

8.   Charles Rosenberg, "Clio and Caring: An Agenda for American Historians and Nursing," *Nursing Research* 26 (January/February 1987): 67–68.

9.   Richard Wertz and Dorothy Wertz, *Lying-In*, expanded ed.(New Haven: Yale University Press, 1989); Judith Leavitt, *Brought to Bed: Childbearing in America 1750–1950* (New York: Oxford University Press, 1986); Nancy Dye, "Modern Obstetrics and Working-Class Women: The New York Midwifery Dispensary, 1890–1920," *Journal of Social History* 20 (1987): 549–564.

10.   Charlotte Borst, "The Professionalization of Obstetrics," in Rima Apple, Ed. *Women, Health, and Medicine in America* (New Brunswick, NJ: Rutgers University Press, 1992), 197–216.

11.   Joseph B. DeLee, *Obstetrics for Nurses,* 2nd ed. (Philadelphia: Saunders, 1907), 18; DeLee, "The Prophylactic Forceps Operation," *American Journal of Obstetrics and Gynecology* 1 (1920):34–44.

12.   DeLee, *Obstetrics for Nurses;* Stowe "The Specially Trained Obstetric Nurse," 550.

13.   U. S. Children's Bureau, *Save the Youngest: Seven Charts on Maternal and Infant Mortality, with Explanatory Comment* (Washington: Government Printing Office, 1923), 2.

14.   Nancy Dye, "The Medicalization of Birth," in Pamela Eakins, Ed., *The American Way of Birth* (Philadelphia: Temple University Press, 1986), 42. Irvine Loudon, "Maternal Mortality: 1880–1950. Some Regional and International Comparisons," *The Society for the Social History of Medicine* 1 (1988): 183–228, Footnote 6, p. 188.

15.   The infant mortality rate, at a staggering 100 deaths per 1,000 live births in 1915, began a slow but steady decline to the 47 per 1,000 rate of 1940. Federal Security Agency, National Office of Vital Statistics. "Table 3: Trend of Infant Mortality in the United States Expanding Birth-Registration Area by States, 1915–1948." In Louise Zabriskie, *Nurses Handbook of Obstetrics,* 9th ed. (Philadelphia: J.B. Lippincott, 1952), bound between pages 608 and 609; Richard Meckel, *Save the Babies: American Public Health Reform and the Prevention of Infant Mortality, 1850–1929* (Baltimore: Johns Hopkins University Press, 1990); Elizabeth Enochs, "Maternal Mortality: The Situation in Fifteen States," *The Trained Nurse and Hospital Review* (September 1934): 211–215.

16.   Beth Rodgers, "The Great Depression, 1929–1940: An Era of Reform," *Virginia Nurse* (Spring 1984): 12–13; Ronald Numbers, "The Third Party: Health Insurance in America," in *Sickness and Health in America,* eds. Judith Leavitt and Ronald Numbers (Madison: University of Wisconsin Press, 1978), 142.

17.   Robert Wiebe, *The Search for Order: 1877–1920* (New York: Hill and Wang, 1967); Leavitt, " 'Science' Enters the Birthing Room," 303.

18.   Isabel Hampton, "Educational Standards for Nurses," in *Nursing of the Sick 1893: Papers and Discussions from the International Congress of Charities, Corrections, and Philanthropy, Chicago 1893* (New York: National League of Nursing Education, 1949), 2.

19.   Ellen Baer, "Nursing's Divided House—an Historical View," *Nursing Research* 34 (January/February 1985): 32–38.

20.   Hampton, "Educational Standards," 2.

21.   Patricia Benner, *From Novice to Expert* (Menlo Park, California : Addison-Wesley, 1984).

22.   Georgina Pope, "Obstetric Nursing," in *Nursing of the Sick 1893: Papers and Discussions from the International Congress of Charities, Corrections, and Philanthropy, Chicago 1893* (New York: National League of Nursing Education, 1949), 166.

23.   Oliver Wendell Holmes, "On the Contagiousness of Puerperal Fever," *The New England Quarterly Journal of Medicine and Surgery* VI (1842–1843): 503–530;

Elaine Larson, "Innovations in Health Care: Antisepsis as a Case Study," *The American Journal of Public Health* 79 (January 1989): 92–99.

24. Charles Reed, "Teaching Obstetrics to Student Nurses," *AJN* 24 (December 1924): 1210–11. Quote is on p. 1211.

25. Neal Devitt, "The Transition from Home to Hospital Birth in the United States, 1930–1960," *Birth and the Family Journal* 4 (Summer 1977): 47–58.

26. Katharine DeWitt, *Private Duty Nursing*, 2nd ed. (Philadelphia: Lippincott, 1917), 143.

27. In 1902, an obstetrician in Maine noted that only half of patients in his experience had selected a physician before the delivery, while all of the women had chosen their nurses. Stanley Warren, "Technique of Labor in Private Practice," *American Journal of Obstetrics and Diseases of Women and Children* XLV (January 1902):26–39.

28. DeWitt, 144.

29. Trained as generalists, graduate nurses, like medical students, often graduated with little practical experience in caring for maternity patients. May Burgess, *Nurses, Patients, and Pocketbooks* (New York: Committee on the Grading of Nursing Schools, 1928).

30. See Pope, "Obstetrical Nursing;" Henry Fry, "Obstetrical Emergencies," *AJN* 1 (November 1900): 107–111; Mary Keith, "Preliminaries of Obstetric Nursing," *AJN* 1 (January 1901): 257–9; Louella Adkins, "The Care of an Obstetrical Patient," *AJN* 3 (June 1903): 709–11; Jennie Putnam, "An Obstetrical Case at Home," *AJN* 10 (April 1910): 469–71; Elizabeth Burttle, "Obstetrical Nursing," *AJN* 16 (October 1915): 195–7; Louise Zabriskie, "Maternity Nursing in Hospital and Home," *AJN* 29 (October 1929):1157–64; and Florina Carbone, "Obstetrics in the Home," *Trained Nurse and Hospital Review*, 95 (September 1935): 228–31.

31. Pope, 587; Keith, 258; Putnam, 469; Hampton, 368; and Weeks-Shaw, 275.

32. At the Cook County hospital, in 1906, the vaginal douche was used before delivery. Henry Lewis, "Obstetrical Technique in the Cook County Hospital," *Surgery, Gynecology, and Obstetrics* 2 (January/June 1906): 81–82. See Pope, "Obstetrical Nursing," 542; Anna Fullerton, *Handbook of Obstetrical Nursing* 3rd revised ed. (Philadelphia: P. Blakeston, Son, & Co., 1893), 70; Weeks-Shaw, *Textbook of Nursing*, 275.

33. R. Johnston and R. Siddall, "Is the Usual Method of Preparing Patients for Delivery Beneficial or Necessary?" *American Journal of Obstetrics and Gynecology* 4 (December 1922): 509–12; Mallie Montgomery, "An Obstetrical Case Study," *Trained Nurse and Hospital Review* 91 (September 1933): 245–51; Catherine Betz, "A Study of an Obstetrical Patient," *AJN* 34 (November 1934): 1109–1116; Margaret Martin, "A Normal Mother and Baby," *AJN* 39 (October 1939): 1144–49; Karen Landry and Darla Kilpatrick, "Why Shave a Mother Before She Gives Birth?" *Maternal Child Nursing* 2 (May/June 1977): 189–190.

34. A. Worcester, "Obstetrical Nursing, *Boston Medical and Surgical Journal* CL (1904): 1–5; Pope, "Obstetrical Nursing;" Fry, "Obstetrical Emergencies."

35. Adkins, "The Care of an Obstetrical Patient," 711.

36. Ibid.

37. Keith, "Preliminaries of Obstetric Nursing," 258.

38.   Anne B., R.N., 1931 graduate of Youngstown Hospital School of Nursing, interview with author, Lynchburg, Virginia, 25 July 1994.

39.   A. Worcester, *Monthly Nursing*, 2nd ed. (New York: Appleton, 1890), 46. The placenta previa is an implantation of the placenta low in the uterus that may cause bleeding, or "antepartum flowing" in labor. A transverse position of the child in labor occurs when the presenting part is an arm or a shoulder.

40.   Worcester, *Monthly Nursing*, 46.

41.   See Frances Bradley and Margretta Williamson, *Rural Children in Selected Counties of North Carolina*, Publication No. 33 (Washington: Government Printing Office, 1918); Elizabeth Moore, *Maternity and Infant Care in a Rural County in Kansas*, Publication No. 26 (Washington: Government Printing Office, 1917); Florence Serbon and Elizabeth Moore, *Maternity and Infant Care in Two Rural Counties in Wisconsin*, Publication No. 46 (Washington: Government Printing Office, 1919); Viola Paradise, *Maternity Care and the Welfare of Young Children in a Homesteading County in Montana*, Publication No. 34, 1919.

42.   A. Worcester, "District-Visiting Nursing in Obstetric Practice," *Boston Medical and Surgical Journal* 89 (December 1898): 539.

43.   Fry, "Obstetrical Emergencies," 109.

44.   Stanley Warren, "Technique of Labor in Private Practice," *American Journal of Obstetrics and Diseases of Women and Children* XLV (January 1902):26–39. Quote is on p. 30.

45.   Weeks-Shaw, *A Textbook of Nursing*, 268.

46.   Ninety-four percent of four thousand physicians in 1928 reported that they often needed a nurse for their obstetric cases. May Burgess, *Nurses, Patients, and Pocketbooks* (New York City: Committee on the Grading of Nursing Schools, 1928); Of fifty graduate nurses surveyed in Kentucky in 1923, only twelve percent accepted obstetric cases. William McConnell, "The Trained Nurse in Obstetrics," *Southern Medical Journal* 16 (October 1923): 792–799. Quote is on p. 797.

47.   One elderly nurse reported that she took a private duty case in a rural community, and while she knew what to do for a delivery, she reported that she was "praying hard" for the doctor to arrive before the baby. "He showed up," she said, "just as the head was born." Of course, the nurse had already made all the preparations needed, and while the delivery was completed smoothly and quickly, it was not without distress and anxiety for the nurse. Immediately following this experience, the nurse refused two other obstetrical cases, even though she knew that to do so might place her on a "black list" and compromise her future earnings. Bland R., R.N., 1937 graduate Virginia Baptist Hospital, interview with author, Lynchburg, Virginia, 20 March 1994.

48.   Worcester, *Monthly Nursing*, 65. Nurse authors Elizabeth Fishback, "Obstetrical Nursing as a Specialty," *AJN* 14 (July 1914): 806–811; Bower; Elizabeth Burttle, "Obstetrical Nursing," *AJN* 16 (October 1915): 195–197; Mary Keith, "Preliminaries of Obstetric Nursing," *AJN* 1 (January 1901): 257; Pope, and Adkins, all addressed "obstetric nursing" as a specialty.

49.   Margrete Sandelowski, *Pain, Pleasure, and American Childbirth* (Westport: Greenwood Press,1984), 70.

50.   Cynthia Pitcock and Richard Clark, "From Fanny to Fernand: The Development of Consumerism in Pain Control During the Birth Process," *American*

Journal of Obstetrics and Gynecology 167 (September 1992): 581–587; Leavitt, *Brought to Bed*; and Sandelowski, *Pain, Pleasure, and American Childbirth*, document the process of women demanding pain relief for childbirth in the early decades of the twentieth century.

51.   Hampton, *Nursing: Its Principles and Practice*, 331.

52.   DeLee, *Obstetrics for Nurses*, 2nd ed., 1907, 119.

53.   Untoward signs included "the breathing or the pulse may suddenly cease and the face take on a livid hue or become ghastly pale." Hampton, *Nursing: Its Principles and Practice*, 338.

54.   Nurses were instructed in 1912 to "Devote your sole attention to the anesthesia. Do not try to do or see anything else at the same time," Weeks-Shaw, *Textbook of Nursing*, 251.

55.   Worcester, *Monthly Nursing*, 92.

56.   A. Young, "Transfusion of Blood in an Obstetrical Case," *AJN* 17 (November 1916): 128–129.

57.   Bower, "The Obstetrical Nurse," 735.

58.   Adkins, "The Care of an Obstetrical Patient," 710.

59.   Birth Record #416, *Patient Records, April-June 1908*, Columbia Hospital for Women. The name of the patient has been changed. Patient records are located in the administrator's office, Columbia Hospital for Women, Washington, D.C.

60.   Chloral Hydrate, Veratrum Viride, a spinal and arterial depressant, and Strychnine Sulfate, a tonic, affecting especially the nervous system, were all tried in futile attempts to stop the convulsions. Weeks-Shaw provides a useful list of "Drugs in Common Use," in Clara Weeks-Shaw, *Textbook of Nursing*, 139–153.

61.   Although the notes are not signed, the changing handwriting in the medical record indicates nurses' shifts that varied in length from seven and a half hours to fourteen hours.

62.   Sixty percent of births occurred in hospitals in Washington, D.C., 63% in Chicago, 65% in St. Paul, and 77% in Minneapolis by the mid 1920s. Dorothy Mendenhall, *What is Happening to Mothers and Babies in the District of Columbia?* (Washington: Government Printing Office, 1928), 24; Editor, "Maternity, Child-Welfare and Social Service (in Chicago)," *Transactions of the American Hospital Association* 31 (1929):31; Robert Woodbury, *Maternal Mortality: The Risk of Death in Childbirth from all Diseases Caused by Pregnancy and Confinement*, Children's Bureau Publication No. 158 (Washington: Government Printing Office, 1926), 87; and Fred Adair, *Prevention of Neonatal Mortality from the Obstetrician's Point of View*, (Washington: Government Printing Office, 1929), 2.

63.   Neal Devitt, "The Transition from Home to Hospital Birth in the United States, 1930–1960," *Birth and the Family Journal* 4 (Summer 1977): 47–58.

64.   See Molly Ladd-Taylor, "'Grannies' and 'Spinsters': Midwife Education Under the Sheppard-Towner Act," *Journal of Social History* 22 (Winter 1988): 255–75; and Rosemary Stevens, *In Sickness and in Wealth: American Hospitals in the Twentieth Century* (New York: Basic Books, 1989).

65.   Marilyn Flood, "The Troubling Expedient: General Staff Nursing in United States Hospitals in the 1930s," (Ph.D. diss., University of California, Berkeley, 1981).

66.   Mechanical induction involved the use of inflatable balloons pushed

through the cervix or other instruments to forcibly dilate the cervix. Janet Ashford, "A History of Accouchement Force," *Birth* 13 (December 1986):241–249. Version was a method of turning the infant in the uterus for a more favorable presentation for birth. Stephen Thacker and David Banta, "Benefits and Risks of Episiotomy: An Interpretive Review of the English Language Literature, 1860–1980," *Obstetrical and Gynecological Survey* 38 (1983): 322–338; Jane Sewell, *Cesarean Section—A Brief History* (Washington: American College of Obstetricians and Gynecologists, 1993); and Speert, *Obstetrics and Gynecology: A History*.

67.   *Annual Reports of the Columbia Hospital for Women: 1800–1920*, located in the hospital administrator's office, Columbia Hospital for Women and Medical Center, Washington, D.C.

68.   *Statistical Report of the Chicago Lying-In Hospital and Dispensary, 1918–1925; 1925–1927; and 1928–1931*, Lying-In Hospital Records Collection, University of Chicago Library, Chicago, Illinois.

69.   Interviews by the author with six nurses who practiced in the 1930s and 1940s and six mothers whose deliveries occurred by the 1940s reveal a consistent pattern in hospital births. All felt that families mainly "got in the way" during labor.

70.   Fullerton, *Handbook of Obstetric Nursing*, 110.

71.   Bernice Gardner, "Nursing Care During the Administration of Rectal Anesthesia," *AJN* 31 (July 1921): 794–8; Anne Yelton and Marie Hilgediek, "Rectal Ether Analgesia from the Nurse's Standpoint," *AJN* 33 (May 1933): 420–2; Harold Rosenfield, "Analgesia in Obstetrics," *AJN* 35 (May 1935): 437–40; Catherine Yeo, "Technic of Administration [Analgesia in Obstetrics] and Nursing Care," *AJN* 35 (May 1935): 440–42.

72.   Judith Leavitt, "Strange Young Women on Errands."

73.   Bland R., R.N., 1937 graduate of Virginia Baptist Hospital, interview with author, Lynchburg, Virginia, 20 March 1994.

74.   Wertz and Wertz, *Lying-In*; Sandelowski, *Pain, Pleasure and American Childbirth*; and Sylvia Hoffert, *Private Matters: American Attitudes Toward Childbearing and Infant Nurture in the Urban North, 1800–1860* (Urbana: University of Illinois Press, 1989).

75.   Leavitt, *Brought to Bed*. See especially Chapter 5: "'The Greatest Blessing of This Age:' Pain Relief in Obstetrics."

76.   Mary Blackwell, "The Nursing Care of Obstetric Patients Having Analgesia and Anesthesia," *AJN* 33 (May 1933): 425–7; Pierce Rucker, "Obstetric Analgesia and Anesthesia," *AJN* 33 (May 1933): 423–5.

77.   Sandelowski, *Pain, Pleasure, and American Childbirth*, 68.

78.   Anne B., R.N., 1931 graduate of Youngstown Hospital in Youngstown, Ohio, interview by the author, 25 July 1994, Lynchburg, Virginia.

79.   Charles Rosenberg, *The Care of Strangers* (New York: Basic Books, 1987) and Stevens, *In Sickness and In Wealth*.

80.   Wasserberg, Chelly, and Northam, Ethel, "Some Time Studies in Obstetrical Nursing," *AJN* 27 (July 1927): 543–4; Clayton, S. Lillian, "Standardizing Nursing Technic: Its Advantages and Disadvantages," *AJN* 27 (November 1927): 939–943.

81.   Quoted in Mary Louise Habel and Hazel Milton, *The Graduate Nurse in the Home* (Philadelphia: J.B. Lippincott, 1939), 6.

82.   Nellie Brown, "A Movable Perineal Dressing Tray," *AJN* 24 (November 1924): 875–6; Mildred Newton, "The Noiseless Perineal Dressing Cart," *AJN* 28 (July 1928): 667–8; M. Cordelia Cowen, "A Study of Breast Care: Part I," *AJN* 29 (October 1929): 1165–70; and Cowen, "A Study of Breast Care: Part II," *AJN* 29 (November 1929): 1299–1306; DeLee, *Obstetrics for Nurses;* Weeks-Shaw, *Textbook of Nursing;* Louise Zabriskie, *Nurses Handbook of Obstetrics,* 1st through 6th eds. (Philadelphia: J.B. Lippincott, 1929, 1931, 1933, 1934, 1937, and 1940); Van Blarcom, *Obstetrical Nursing.*

83.   Emily Shaffer, "Perineal Technic," *AJN* 34 (January 1934): 26–28; "A Survey of Methods Used in Four Hospitals," *AJN* 31 (March 1931): 313–17; Joyce Roberts, "Maternal Positions for Childbirth: A Historical Review of Nursing Care Practices," *Journal of Obstetric, Gynecologic, and Neonatal Nursing* 8 (January/February 1979): 24–32.

84.   Carolyn VanBlarcom, *Obstetrical Nursing,* 2nd ed. (New York: Macmillan, 1932), 433.

85.   Ibid., 439.

86.   Pope, "Obstetric Nursing," 166.

87.   Keith, "Preliminaries of Obstetric Nursing," 259.

88.   Hampton, *Nursing: Its Principles and Practice,* 379; Worcester, *Monthly Nursing,* 110.

89.   Lillian M., R.N., 1948 graduate Virginia Baptist Hospital, Lynchburg, Virginia, interview by the author, Lynchburg, Virginia, 24 March 1994.

90.   Carolyn L., R.N., 1933 graduate of Riverside Hospital, Newport News, VA, interview by the author, Richmond, Virginia, 10 March 1993.

91.   Jane McLaughlin, "Teaching Obstetrics to Nurses," *AJN* 28 (June 1928): 605–607. Quote is on p. 607.

92.   VanBlarcom, *Obstetrical Nursing,* 255.

93.   Ibid., 9.

94.   Eva Renwick, "Why I Prefer Obstetrics in Private Nursing," *AJN* 17 (October 1916): 42–44. Quote is on p. 43.

95.   Van Blarcom, *Obstetrical Nursing,* 11.

96.   Ibid., 5.

97.   Mary H., 1930 graduate of Stuart Circle Hospital, Richmond, VA, interview by the author, Lynchburg, Virginia, 27 April 1994.

98.   Patricia O'Brien D'Antonio, "The Legacy of Domesticity: Nursing in Nineteenth Century America," *Nursing History Review* 1 (1993): 229–246.

99.   Obstetric nurses listed as valuable attributes that were also associated with womanhood: adaptability, tact, sense of humor, virtue, conscience, courage, alertness of mind, deftness of hand, and "the love of a baby in her heart." Burttle, 196. The public press also praised the womanly qualities of nurses. Sarah Constock, "Your Daughter's Career," *Good Housekeeping* 61 (December 1915): 728–36.

100.   Thomas Olson, "Laying Claim to Caring: Nursing and the Language of Training," *Nursing Outlook* 41 (March/April 1993): 68–72.

101.   A. Wilcox, L. Kobayashi, and I. Murray, "Twenty-five years of obstetric patient satisfaction in North America: A Review of the Literature," *Journal of Perinatal and Neonatal Nursing* 10 (March 1997): 361–78; Brigitte Jordan, *Birth in Four Cultures,* 4th ed. (Prospect Heights: Waveland Press, 1993); Davis-Floyd, *Birth*

as an American Rite of Passage (Berkley: University of California Press, 1992); Eakins, *The American Way of Birth.*

102. Linda Kobert, "Are Universal Precautions Changing the 'Nurture' of Obstetric Nursing?", *AJN* 89 (December 1989): 1609. See Sandelowski, "(Ir)Reconcilable Differences? The Debate Concerning Nursing and Technology," *Image* 29 (Second Quarter 1997): 169–174; and Sandelowski, "Making the Best of Things": Technology in American Nursing, 1870–1940," *Nursing History Review* 5 (1997): 3–22.

103. Joan Lynaugh and Claire Fagin, "Nursing Comes of Age," *Image* 20 (Winter 1988): 184–190.

6

Midwives as Wives and Mothers: Urban Midwives in the Early Twentieth Century

Linda V. Walsh

Midwifery has been described as an occupation, a spiritual calling, and a profession. Any description of the practice has been influenced by the scholar's beliefs about health and illness, sources of knowledge, the role of the health care provider during childbirth, and the sociocultural role of women. Few historians have used feminist methods to provide new ways of seeing, and thus interpreting, midwives' lives and practices. Not until we analyze midwifery in the context of women's life experiences will we better understand the actions and influences of midwives in the changing American health care system of the early twentieth century.

Historian Elizabeth Pleck has noted that in analyzing the behaviors of family members in the home and workplace, scholars must address the question, "How did the physical and emotional demands of work alter family life?"[1] Few unskilled occupations generate demands on family outside the actual work hours that the mother is absent from the home. Professional careers, on the other hand, often place demands of time and energy on the life of family members. In this context, midwifery fits more in the category of profession or career, rather than occupation. Indeed, the European model of care to childbearing women that evolved in the twentieth century maintained the centrality of the professional midwife in the health care delivery system. However, those shaping the American system for obstetrical care excluded midwifery as an outdated and unscientific approach to childbearing women. Until recently, there

Note: This chapter was originally published in *Nursing History Review* 2 (1994): 51–65. Copyright (c) 1994 by The American Association for the History of Nursing. Reprinted with permission

has been little investigation of the midwives' actions during this dramatic change in the care available to women during their birthing experiences.

In order to better understand midwifery practice in the first three decades of this century, this research uses the "voices" of midwives, their family members, and women who hired them to identify previously overlooked sources. Interview data was supplemented by written public records such as birth certificate data, midwife registries, and church records. Anna Carastro, a midwife in practice in Philadelphia from 1923 to 1940, provided the central voice for this article. While she speaks as an individual, additional data support her experiences and beliefs as representative of other formally urban immigrant midwives.

ECONOMIC STATUS OF MIDWIVES' FAMILIES

Most previous studies of immigrant working women have analyzed the work and family experiences of women in unskilled or semiskilled employment.[2] The fact that midwifery was perceived by women and communities as professional work suggests that midwives' experiences may have been different from those of women working in factories, stores, offices, or in homes. Midwives occupied positions of social status similar to that of physicians, teachers, or other professionals within the immigrant communities. One well-known, busy Philadelphia midwife, Maria Straka, saw herself professionally "like a doctor," and perceived herself as more socially privileged than other families in the neighborhood.[3] Another midwife, Salie Mackiewicz, was "like a doctor [or] nurse."[4] Anna Carastro and Rebecca Gorodetzer, both educated in university-level midwifery programs, were respected in their communities as professional practitioners.[5]

Income is often used as an indirect indicator of professional or social status. Midwives with active practices were able to attain a comfortable income from practice earnings. When a midwife maintained an active practice among the working-class families in her community, she had the ability to generate practice revenue that usually surpassed the family incomes of her patients. As one neighborhood woman recalls, "The midwives, they always had the nicest homes and their children had the best clothes."[6]

The median working woman's income in Philadelphia in 1923 was $13–$15 per week, or about $750 annually if she was able to work steadily throughout the year.[7] Full-time work throughout the year was not the norm, however, and it was not unusual for married women workers to be laid off during slow seasons.[8] In that same year, Maria Straka attended ninety-eight births and collected $1,569 in fees. A midwife who maintained a practice that averaged eight to ten births per month generated income comparable to female clerical workers, teachers, librarians, and social workers in the mid-1920s.[9] Even when a midwife with an active practice did not have additional wage earners in the household, she was able to maintain a respectable standard of living.

When a midwife maintained a fairly small practice, she usually supplemented family income in a way that facilitated attainment of the growing middle-class standard of living. Anna Carastro averaged three to four births per month in the late 1920s and early 1930s. The $750–$1,000 per year collected in fees allowed her and her husband to buy real estate and to send their children to college; eventually, Anna was able to open a licensed day nursery.

Many midwives resided in households where there were other adult wage earners. Review of the Philadelphia City Directories for the years 1915–1936 identifies numerous workers in midwife households. No doubt, most were husbands and adult children of the midwives. Occupations noted for householders indicate that the wage earners were skilled, semiprofessional, and professional workers. This finding, when compared to the occupations listed for the fathers of babies delivered by Anna Carastro and Maria Straka, suggests that the midwife households had a stronger financial base than those households of the women hiring the midwives.

In general, when householders in midwife families were identified, they occupied positions of regular, full-time employment. This was in contrast to the fathers of the infants in the birth records of Anna Carastro and Maria Straka, who typically were day laborers. Anna Carastro recalls that her husband, Mario, an ornamental ironworker, "was never a day without work. His work was in demand."[10] Rebecca Gorodetzer's husband, Meyer, made a "good living" prior to 1932 as a violinist in an orchestra and as a music teacher. The family was financially secure enough that there was always household help until the Depression.[11]

Caroline Manning, in her study of working immigrant women in Philadelphia in the 1920s, found that working mothers continued to do most of the household work necessary to maintain the family. However, she also found that it was not unusual for husbands to contribute to the efforts of housework.[12]

PRACTICAL SUPPORT IN MIDWIFE HOUSEHOLDS

Although they tended to occupy a different socioeconomic class than the working wives in Manning's study, midwives also maintained primary responsibility for the daily needs of meal preparation and child care, with husbands participating in many chores. It was not unusual for couples in working class, immigrant, and rural families to share household work while supporting each partner's outside work.[13] The concept of "separate spheres" developed by earlier historians described the development of upper-middle-class family division of labor and responsibilities, but data from other population groups suggest that the concept was not universal.[14]

Husbands of midwives often shopped, prepared meals, and provided child care to ensure that household responsibilities were assumed when midwives were called away for a case. Many Italian husbands were known for their culinary skills, particularly in the preparation of traditional pasta and "gravy."

> *[My husband taught me to cook] I didn't know how to cook. My mother did everything. . . . But he learned in the service. In fact, I never did go to the butcher to buy meat. Whatever we need, he'd buy enough that during the week I didn't need to go to the store. Except for special things sometimes. But he liked to do that. I don't think it was unusual. I don't know what other people do. My mind, I'm telling you what my husband did.[15]*

Other husbands completed the preparation of meals that had been planned and initiated by their wives. Maria Straka's husband, Edward, was crippled by a stroke early in his adult life but was able to get around enough to complete meals if his wife was called away. Mrs. Straka prepared food in large quantities and stored prepared dishes that needed only to be warmed in the oven. Her daughter remembers that they always had "lots of food," and that between her father and herself, complete meals were always ready at traditional mealtimes.[16]

In addition to their contributions to household help, midwives' husbands' childcare activities were essential to the smooth functioning of the family. Obviously, for those midwives whose husbands were disabled and/or not working outside the home, the constant presence of an adult family member provided stability to the children's lives. Although Maria Straka's husband could not ambulate outside the home, he was able to move around inside enough to watch the children. The children were instructed not to go outside as long as their mother was away so that they would be strictly supervised.

Able-bodied employed husbands often shifted their working schedules to accommodate their wives' work hours. Anna Carastro recalls that if she had been called away during the night, her husband would stay home from work until she returned or until he was able to find someone else to watch the children. Occasionally, their schedules did not function as smoothly as planned, and Mrs. Carastro had to take her children with her when called to a birth.

> *Sometimes if there was a case, my husband was home. Sometimes I used to take the baby with me. I remember I delivered this case. I delivered the child, and this lady was from our home town. They had a fire-place in the big room*

upstairs. So I took the baby with me. People understood, you know. Especially because they were Italian people and they knew of me from home. The name. I didn't have any trouble.[17]

Mario Carastro sometimes took the children to the seashore for holiday while Anna Carastro stayed home because of commitments to women in the neighborhood. "And when my husband and the children went to the seashore—to Atlantic City or Wildwood—I couldn't leave because I expected some confinements. But my husband went there with the children."[18]

Older children and other relatives often helped with childcare too. With eight surviving children, there were young children who needed care in the Gorodetzer household until the late 1920s. Older siblings frequently watched Rebecca Gorodetzer's youngsters when she w as called to a birth. Occasionally, relatives in the neighborhood would watch her children for short periods of time. But Mrs. Gorodetzer also had to bring one or more of her children with her on occasion when she left the house on professional business. Millie, her youngest child, remembers being taken to Polyclinic Hospital when her mother went for bag checks and renewal of her midwifery certificate. She also recalls being taken to at least one house and being watched downstairs by householders while her mother attended a laboring woman upstairs.[19]

Almarinda Cimini's household consisted of her husband and children, as well as her husband's brother, his wife, and their children. Almarinda developed a busy midwifery practice while raising three children. Her sister-in-law provided the necessary childcare for both families and assumed many of the household responsibilities while Mrs. Cimini and the two husbands worked outside the home. In this way, the families could save money while they planned the purchase of a second home.

When married, separated, or widowed working-class or poor mothers entered the workforce, they often did so only until children could begin to supplement the family income with their own wages. Studies in the 1920s indicated that once children in poor working class families were of working age, they quit school to pursue paid work.[20] The education and work history of the children of midwife mothers, however, suggests that wages of children did not become a substitute for midwife earnings. Midwives' children staved in school and often pursued higher education. Anna Carastro's two children both went to college.

My husband said, "My children will never go to factory work. I am the working man. My children will go to school until they have a good education." I had education myself and so I wanted our children and my husband wanted our children to go as long as they wanted to go. Nancy went to Penn State College. She graduated in journalism. Joe went to Drexel Institute.[21]

Rebecca Gorodetzer's children all pursued careers, with four of the eight becoming musicians and the others entering the business professions. Maria Straka's children graduated from high school, and her son attended Pierce Business College. He pursued a career in accounting with an international oil company, while her daughter went into retail sales.

Adult children often provided continued support to their midwife mothers, even after they married and settled in their own households. Midwives who did not write in English usually had their husbands or children complete the birth registrations and reports of births that needed to be turned in to the Midwife Inspectors. Michelina Tiano's and Anna Dlugosz's grown sons completed all of their records. Even when the midwives were skilled in completing the records in English, the children often completed them because their mothers were busy. The Gorodetzer children often completed their mother's records in order to help her finish her work.[22]

Adult sons also drove their mothers to births at night. If the adult sons did not drive or have access to a vehicle, they walked with their mothers when the midwives were called out at night.[23] Adult children of midwives also acted as interpreters for their mothers when meetings with state and city officials were necessary.[24]

In addition to support from immediate family members, midwives received practical and emotional support from relatives and friends in the neighborhood. The support of women neighbors was especially important for immigrant women who had no close female relatives in this country. Anna Carastro points out:

Believe it or not, I never had any relatives, any blood relatives whatsoever, that came to this country. No one. I know those that were my husband's. But on my own line, there was nobody.[25]

Mrs. Carastro's transition to American life was assisted first by her husband's brothers' families in Tampa, Florida, and then by his aunt in Philadelphia. However, her relationship with his aunt never developed into one that offered support through her years as a mother and a working wife. And, although her husband felt strongly about not becoming close to neighbors, a special family-type relationship developed between the Carastros and the Scotts next door.

We never had a close [relationship] with the other neighbors. My husband didn't like the idea of being close with the neighbors. Stayed away from everybody. [We'd] be nice, but never get chummy with the neighbors. If you get chummy with the neighbors, trouble will come. They like to know everybody else's business. We were friendly, said "Hello" day or night—but not chummy. But next door, Mrs. Scott. She was like a mother to me. She had two children—Emma and Johnny. She had married late in life and had two children and her hus-band died. She remained a widow.[26]

Mrs. Scott's children frequently provided childcare for Mrs. Carastro's small children.

I remember when Nancy was a little girl, when our children were young, Johnny and Emma, brother and sister, said, "Do you have to go out so we can take care of Nancy. Joe and Nancy?" They loved the children. They would remain in their care. It pays to have good neighbors. There are peo-ple . . . who make nice things happen. Never any trouble. They were nice neighbors. And my husband was not so keen to be goody-goody with every-body. Mrs. Scott was to us like a mother and father.[27]

COMMUNITY RESPECT FOR MIDWIVES

The respect held for midwives by the women and families in their com-munities further facilitated practice in the early decades of the century. Women recognized those midwives with skills necessary for managing problems during labor and those midwives who maintained sterile and aseptic techniques in caring for mothers and infants. Members of the community also were aware of midwives whose techniques were poor.

Of the 959 families cared for by Maria Straka during her years of prac-tice, half hired her for at least two births, and ninety-seven hired her for three or more births. Eighteen of those families hired Mrs. Straka for five or more births.[28] Certainly, if women did not have faith in a midwife's knowledge and skills, they would not continue to hire her to attend births.

Anna Carastro also attended births for women who had hired her pre-viously. Generally, the families for whom she offered care had lower par-ities than those cared for by Maria Straka, but her birth registrations document eight families who hired her for three or more births.[29]

Addresses of families hiring both Anna Carastro and Maria Straka doc-ument that popular midwives often attended most births on neighbor-hood blocks. Within one small four-block area in the Gray's Ferry area, Maria Straka attended 172 births between 1919 and 1933. This was dur-ing the time that two other midwives—Maggie Scarcutty and Eva Grzybowska—lived on those blocks. Mrs. Grzybowska, a Polish midwife who advertised in the City Directory in 1910, was licensed by the state in 1914 and registered with the Philadelphia Health Department in 1930. Mrs. Scarcutty may have begun practice as Mrs. Straka's practice was declining, since she was licensed and registered in January 1931.[30]

The financial support of both Maria Straka's and Anna Carastro's prac-tices indicates that their services were respected by their clients as professional services worthy of payment, even when the client was experiencing financial burdens. Maria Straka's financial records from 1923 to 1927 document that many families paid in installments—often in increments of $2.00 per week. The total amount in fees collected through those years indicates that families paid their bills in full, accepting their obligation to Mrs. Straka.[31] Additionally, many families continued to repay Straka for her services with gifts of fruits and vegetables, meats and poultry, wines, and money.

Midwives often received gifts from family members during religious celebrations following the births. Polish and Hungarian families supported the custom of the midwife preparing the infant for baptism or berith. During the bathing of the infant, the midwife was allowed to keep the gold pieces that relatives and friends threw into the bath water.[32]

Anna Carastro's patients usually paid for her services, although not always in cash. She recalls:

Some people, I knew who could afford and who could not. Those who couldn't afford, what could we do? But then during August time they bring the grace of God to your house—fruits and everything that the soil produces. . . . They were honest people. They pay what they could.[33]

During the Depression, she found that people could not pay her.

Some people did not pay. They did not have money. They were starving. [During the Depression] the midwifery—there was nothing to do. The people had no money to call the midwife.[34]

Mrs. Carastro's perception of why women who had previously hired midwives gradually moved to going to the hospital for births provides further support of the pride those women felt in hiring a midwife. The immigrant women (primarily Italian) for whom she provided care did not believe in going to doctors for their care. "They didn't go to doctors at the time. They didn't call the doctors. If I need the doctor [because of a problem with the pregnancy or labor] then I said, 'Get the doctor.'"[35] Her explanation of why women who preferred midwives to doctors reversed their position reflects her observation of the economic effect on choices made for health care. "They didn't go to the *doctor* at the time. They went to the *hospital*—for nothing! They went to hospital, and they paid nothing. Or a few dollars."[36] Other neighborhood residents and institutional reports also suggest that it was the Depression that forced women who believed in midwifery care into the hospitals. When they couldn't afford the twenty to twenty-five dollars charged by the midwife, women would attend the hospital dispensaries, where they paid only twenty-five cents per visit. They could then enter the hospital when they were in labor and pay nothing for their care if they were truly destitute.[37]

Midwives also were respected as community members who contributed to assorted community organizations and causes. Rebecca Gorodetzer was active in a variety of charitable causes. She was instrumental in coordinating efforts to care for the terminally ill during the flu epidemic of 1918 when there was no room in area hospitals for admissions. She worked closely with the staff in her children's schools and would often bring knishes or strudel to the teachers and principals. Her baking skills were renowned throughout South Philadelphia, as were her nursing and midwifery skills.

The Catholic midwives were active members of their parishes and seemed to be recognized as important members of the church community. The Diamond Jubilee Parish Souvenir Book of St. Ladislaus Church notes:

> *Perhaps the best known ladies in the early period of the parish were the Polish mid-wives of Nicetown. They were Mrs. Veronika Szablewska of Rowan Street, Mrs. Anna Dlugosz of Hunting Park Avenue, and Mrs. Kazmierska of Juniata Street. They assisted at a large majority of about 5,000 births that were registered at our rectory to 1942, when the last of these mid-wives stopped her practice. Mrs. Szablewska's records show that she alone accounted for about 1,200 births up to 1930, when she retired. Mrs. Anna Dlugosz participated in even more births.*[38]

In many ways, the midwife served similar functions to the parish priest. She was involved with family members through birth and death. When infants were stillborn or in danger of dying in the immediate neonatal period, she baptized them to save their souls. To a certain extent, she even heard confessions regarding issues surrounding a woman's sexuality. Midwives were given the religious and civil authority to determine paternity, and in that role, had to be highly trusted members of the community. Occasionally, the question of paternity would be investigated by the civil courts, and it appears that midwives would answer inquiries truthfully but in a way that was also protective of the women for whom they cared.

> *I had a case once that went to court and I had to testify in court. I can tell you because you don't know the person and you don't know where I come from. Two ladies came to call me—was winter time. And they told me that so-and-so was in labor. So I went. She was big, sitting, but she didn't have a contraction. Well, I was supposed to go visit two patients, so I said, "I'll come back if you have contractions." She said, "Please don't leave me alone." All they knew, not to make a long story, was that the husband was in service. Therefore the pregnancy was not her husband's. She didn't want people to know. She, I presume, wanted to have some confidence with me, but there was those people. So I then understood. I said, "Look, I'm coming back.*

I have another one that is giving birth." That was not the truth. That was a lie. That was to get out so that the ladies would leave. Anyhow, she gave birth when I came back and the two neighbors were there. They knew her husband was in service and she gave birth. And I didn't know all this [at the time]. Somebody must have called—I don't know. But he came a day later. He came to my house. I said, "What can I tell you? I don't know anything about [the father of the baby]." . . . When I was called to testify in court, what did I have to testify? I said, "I was called. She said she was pregnant. It was not time. I went home. Was called again. I delivered the child. I don't know any secrets."[39]

CONCLUSION

The demands on the midwife's time, as well as the professional energy and attention she retained when at home, certainly intruded on family members' lives. When Anna Dlugosz moved in with the laboring woman's family to provide consistent care throughout the immediate postpartum period, other family members had to absorb those responsibilities that she ordinarily assumed. When Maria Straka went from one birth to another, in addition to completing her postpartum rounds, and was away from the home for more than twenty-four hours at a time, her husband and children had to adjust their usual routines to continue the daily household rituals. And, when Anna Carastro returned home after finding a woman in the very early stage of labor, she deferred any planning for family activities, knowing she would be called out again as soon as the woman's labor progressed to a more active phase.

Because of the irregular and unpredictable hours encountered in midwifery practice, householders needed to go beyond the expected chores and responsibilities shared by many families with working mothers. Unpredictability was (and continues to be) one of the most difficult factors encountered in midwifery practice. The positive effects of personal satisfaction, personal support from loved ones, and professional support from the community and colleagues in the medical field must be strong enough in a midwife's life to balance the unpredictability of her practice. For most Philadelphia midwives with successful practices that spanned the first three decades of this century, there was support sufficient to facilitate careers that continued into their older years.

Studies of working women in the early twentieth century document that on marriage, and certainly by the birth of the first child, most women left the paid workforce and committed all their time to the roles of wife and mother. Midwives, however, followed the pattern of professional women. Midwives who had successful practices or who had invested time and finances in higher education rarely left their professions altogether. Anna Carastro never considered giving up her career when she married. She was well aware of the demands of her busy practice in Sicily, yet when asked whether her husband expected her to leave her profession and remain at home with children, she was adamant. "No. I said I would never leave my profession."[40] Rebecca Gorodetzer, too, never considered leaving her profession when she married and had children. Those midwives who trained for their practices after having children also maintained their practices, even when their social and financial status changed. Michelina Tiano, Anna Nicklas Lange, and Annie Papciak Mielinichek remarried after widowhood or divorce, and stayed in practice following the subsequent marriage. Michelina Tiano chose to keep her first married name as her professional name, rather than adopt her second husband's surname.

Evidence suggests that four factors were instrumental in facilitating ongoing midwifery practice that spanned decades. Perhaps most important was the strong personal and professional support of the spouse and/or other family members. Midwives who maintained practice while married had husbands who respected their professional role enough to balance the inconveniences of work demand and unscheduled unavailability to the family. Those husbands tended to truly accept the marriage as a partnership, perhaps believing that the social position and financial remuneration rewarded the whole family, not just the individual midwife. Older and adult children and other extended family members also needed to support the midwife's efforts in order to facilitate smooth functioning of the household.

Second, any midwife with young children required reliable childcare. Whether that care was provided by the midwife's husband, older children, mother or mother-in-law, cousin, other relative, or friend, an individual who could take care of young children—often with no notice—was necessary to allow the midwife to respond to calls at all hours of the day.

A third factor that influenced the success of ongoing practice was respect among the women in the community. The midwife depended on referrals from women for whom she had provided care. Without recognition for the knowledge and skills necessary for safe practice, in addition to the strong moral values necessary for the trust inherent in the nature of the work, midwives would not be able to maintain a practice.

Finally, successful practice depended on sufficient financial remuneration to balance the demands of the position of midwife. Many women who practiced midwifery did so because their families needed the income. If the income generated by midwifery practice was not sufficient to maintain a satisfactory status of living, an assertive, intelligent woman would seek other employment. Anna Carastro, when faced with a practice that no longer was active enough to support her professionally and financially, explored further career options and opened a licensed day nursery.

Historian Alice Kessler-Harris has noted that almost all American women have been wives at some point in their lives.[41] In this respect, the midwives practicing in urban America in the early twentieth century were no different from other American women. The sociocultural roles of wife, mother, health care practitioner, and neighbor have implied work roles that have varied in demand and effort as the views of gender roles have evolved. The balancing of multiple roles was sometimes difficult, but women committed to both career and family responsibilities were able to find that balance. Anna Carastro reflects:

If she has that ambition [to be a wife, mother, and career woman] it's not going to be hard. Anything you do with all your heart, you don't think of the hardship. You enjoy every moment. You are thirsty or going forward for what is in your own mind. No trouble. I loved the profession, but I loved children. For, what is life without children?[42]

The Philadelphia midwives represented in this sample matured in their professional roles through the maintenance of relationships that validated them as strong, intelligent, resourceful career women. Those same relationships validated the midwives' roles in the family systems of their communities. Further analysis of the life experiences of professional women will increase our understanding of the influence of family and work culture on women's experiences in the workforce.

NOTES

1. Elizabeth H. Pleck, "Two World's in One: Work and Family," *Journal of Social History* 10 (1976–1977): 187 (hereafter cited as *JSH*).

2. For analysis of immigrant women's experiences in the United States, see Carol Groneman, "Working-Class Immigrant Women in Mid-Nineteenth Century New York: The Irish Women's Experience," *Journal of Urban History* 4 (1978): 255 (hereafter cited as *JUH*); Tamara K. Hareven, "The Laborers of Manchester, NH, 1912–1922: The Role of Family and Ethnicity in Adjustment to Industrial Life," *Labor History* 16 (1975): 249; Corinne Azen Krause, "Urbanization without Breakdown: Italian, Jewish and Slavic Immigrant Women in Pittsburgh, 1900–1945," *JUH* 4 (1978): 291; Elizabeth H. Pleck, "Two Worlds in One," 178; Elizabeth H. Pleck, "A Mother's Wages: Income Earning Among Married Italian and Black Women, 1896–1911," in *The American Family in Social-Historical Perspective*, 2nd ed., ed. Michael Gordon (New York: St. Martin's Press, 1978); Diane C. Vecchio, "Italian Women in Industry: The Shoe Workers of Endicott, NY 1914–1935," *Journal of American Ethnic History* 8 (1989): 60; Janice Reit Webster, "Domestication and Americanization: Scandinavian Women in Seattle, 1888–1900," *JUH* 4 (1978): 275.

3.   Interview with Mary Harvey, 30 January 1989.

4.   Interview with Edward Wojcik, 31 October 1989.

5.   Millie Imber-Rutko, personal letter; phone interview with Harry Gorodetzer, 4 October 1988; phone interview with Michael Gorodetzer, 3 November 1988; interview with Anna Carastro, 7 April 1989.

6.   Interview with Frances Suder, 6 January 1989.

7.   Caroline Manning, *The Immigrant Woman and Her Job*, United States Department of Labor, Women's Bureau Bulletin No. 74 (Washington, D.C.: Government Printing Office, 1930).

8.   See Louise Odencrantz, Italian Women in Industry (New York: ARNO Press, 1977).

9.   G. E. Manson, "Occupational Interests and Personality Requirements of Women in Business and the Professions," *Michigan Business Studies* III (April 1931).

10. Interview with Anna Carastro, 9 October 1989.

11. Millie Imber-Rutko, personal letter.

12. Manning, *The Immigrant Woman.*

13. For discussion of shared household responsibilities, see Pleck, "Two Worlds in One."

14. For example, see Nancy Cott, *The Bonds of Womanhood: Women's Sphere in New England, 1780–1835* (New Haven: Yale University Press, 1977).

15. Interview with Anna Carastro, 9 October 1989.

16. Interview with Mary Harvey, 29 January 1989.

17. Interview with Anna Carastro, 7 April 1989.

18. Ibid.

19. Millie Imber-Rutko, personal letter.

20. See U.S. Congress, *Report on Condition of Woman and Child Wage Earners in the United States*, Vol 2 (Washington, D.C.: Government Printing Office, 1910); Elyce J. Rotella, *From Home to Office: U.S. Women at Work, 1870–1930* (Ann Arbor, Mich.: UMI Research Press, 1981); Gwendolyn S. Hughes, *Mothers in Industry: Wage-Earning by Mothers in Philadelphia* (New York: New Republic, Inc., 1925); Manning, *Immigrant Women.*

21. Interview with Anna Carastro, 9 October 1989.

22. Interviews with Charles Carpino, 12 October 1988; Ann Rakszawski, 21 August 1989; Elizabeth Wolf, 9 January 1989.

23. Interviews with Charles Carpino, 12 October 1988; Harry Gorodetzer, 4 October 1988.

24. Minutes, Bureau of Medical Education and Licensure, Pennsylvania State Archives, 4 February 1921.

25. Interview with Anna Carasrro, 9 October 1989.

26. Ibid., 10 October 1989.

27. Ibid.

28. Maria Straka, Birth Records.

29. Anna Carastro, Birth Records.

30. Maria Straka, Birth Records; Midwife Register, Philadelphia Department of Health, Philadelphia City Archives.

31. Maria Straka, Family Papers.

32.   This custom was discussed in interviews with Anna Carastro, 7 April 1989; Mary Harvey, 30 January 1989; Harry Gorodetzer, 4 October 1988; Millie ImberRutko, personal letter.

33.   Interview with Anna Carastro, 7 April 1989.

34.   Ibid.

35.   Ibid., 8 April 1989.

36.   Ibid.

37.   The Annual Report of Pennsylvania Hospital, 1935, addresses the fact that the institution provided free care to increasing numbers of individuals during the first five years of the Depression. Also, interviews with Ella Ruggerio, 9 November 1988, and Edward Wojcik, 31 October 1989, identified the belief that women no longer were able to pay a midwife and so sought cheaper or free care through the dispensaries and lying-in wards of the city hospitals.

38.   Diamond Jubilee Parish Souvenir Book, St. Ladislaus Roman Catholic Church, Philadelphia, Pa., p. 75.

39.   Interview with Anna Carastro, 7 April 1989.

40.   Interview with Anna Carastro, 8 October 1989.

41.   Alice Kessler-Harris, *Women Have Always Worked: A Historical Overview* (Old Westbury, N.Y.: Feminist Press, 1981).

42.   Interview with Anna Carastro, 8 October 1989.

SECTION 3

THE NATURE OF POWER AND AUTHORITY IN NURSING

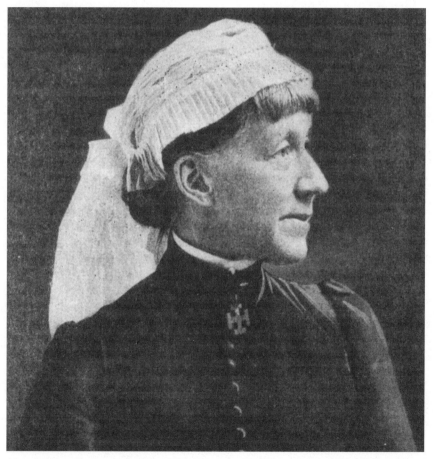

Alice Fisher, circa 1885. Courtesy of the Center for the Study of the History of Nursing, University of Pennsylvania.

Introduction

Patricia O. D'Antonio

From the moment Florence Nightingale set foot in the Crimea in 1854, nursing has struggled to gain for itself both the power to shape its own destiny and the cultural authority to match its critical clinical responsibilities. It has been a battle fought, as we well know, amid profound social ambivalence about the nature and the economic value of nursing. And it has been a battle whose success has been compromised by deep divisions within the discipline's own ranks about the very definition of, and standards for, professional nursing practice.

Such an explanation does construct a shared framework within which nurses might understand the dilemmas surrounding the issues of power and authority in the discipline. But it still neglects the ways that the dimensions of the particular social context within which the struggle is waged structures ideas about what the battle is about, how it can be fought, and if it will withstand the press of change and competing constituencies. As Ellen Baer argues in her analysis of why the University of Chicago failed to honor its early twentieth century contractual agreement with the Illinois Training School (ITS) to establish a baccalaureate nursing program, "timing is everything." Then, the longstanding (and carefully financed) dream of some lay supporters and nursing leaders went up in the smoke of contentious debates about the necessity of "book learning;" conflicting loyalties to old and new orders; the decimation of the ITS endowment in the wake of the Great Depression; that era's passing of a sense of responsibility for the health needs of the poor from the private to the public domains; and the dearth of assertive advocates.

Baer's study, however, and those of the other historians presented in this section, should not be read as one about dismal blunders in the quest for disciplinary power and authority. Rather, given historians' assumption that as much can be learned from what failed as from what succeeded, these studies should be read as ones about contextual limits. Karen Buhler-Wilkerson, in fact, joins the constraints of time to that of place and social custom. Full of confidence (and armed with the considerable power and social legitimacy they earned by decreasing the mortality and morbidity rates of the urban north), northern public health nursing leaders sought to bring to the seemingly more backward rural and Southern Red Cross chapters the same professionalizing agenda that had worked so well for them in the past. They failed. In Charleston, South Carolina, the venerable Ladies Benevolent Society chose to remain purely local and increasingly insignificant rather than submit to the judgement and vision of a "stranger" unfamiliar with southern mores.

Judith Walker Leavitt's portrait of mid-century obstetrical nurses, an admittedly bleak picture painted by the birthing women who were their patients, adds gender to the contextual mix. Her historical nurses did seem cold, callous and more concerned with counting than with comforting. Yet, Leavitt's analysis suggests sympathy for the predicament of these women. Caught between the simultaneous and conflicting demands of two entirely differently gendered systems, these nurses simply asserted the priority of their own needs. Moreover, they blunted, for a time, both their sense of bewilderment about the social experience wanted by birthing women (with whom they had little in common), and their feeling of powerlessness in the face of the demands made by the male-dominated hospital environment (to which they were bound by explicit nursing codes).

Finally, Margarete Sandelowski delves deeply and carefully into the relationship between nursing and the technology that has given medicine and hospitals their mantles of cultural authority. Her study suggests just how much contemporary clinicians might be empowered if they could understand the complicated, nuanced, sometimes unsuccessful but always exciting negotiations between nurses and their times, their places of practice, their particular patients, and the social mores they both reflected and worked to change. For if the theme of this section emphasizes the multi-dimensional social context within which nurses seek disciplinary power and cultural authority, then the arguments of Sandelowski, in particular, and the studies in this section, in general, suggest the quintessentially social agenda of this quest. We have wanted (and still do want) control. Historically, as Sandelowski points out, we have been extraordinarily ambivalent about challenging the social mores that deny us the right to make this seemingly self-evident claim. And even today, we continue to cloak our demands in language highlighting our altruistic commitment to our patients and our communities. We are certainly nothing if not altruistic. But we are also social actors with needs and wishes that may not always match those of our identified constituents. Acknowledging this, and then working to resolve the inevitable tension, might, finally, set us free to pursue the clinical power and cultural authority we want and we need to legitimate our ownership of our work.

7

Aspirations Unattained: The Story of the Illinois Training School's Search for University Status

Ellen D. Baer

In the last quarter of the nineteenth century, sparked by reaction to the Civil War and the growing blight of industrialization, some Americans became personally involved in helping others. Focusing on needy people in prisons, schools, almshouses, and hospitals, these wealthy, benevolent citizens tried to help those who could not meet their own obligations. But, by the second decade of the twentieth century, people came to regard care of the needy as a governmental responsibility and personal benevolence declined. This shift in responsibility forced nursing and other social institutions founded in that period to seek new sponsors for their activities.

One example of this phenomenon was the Illinois Training School for Nurses (ITS), founded in 1880 by philanthropic women of vision on the edge of the United States frontier. The school trained nurses to care for the sick in Chicago, primarily at Cook County Hospital. In 1926 the ITS Board contracted with the University of Chicago to contribute ITS's assets to the university in exchange for the creation of a school of nursing "of the same rank and standing as the other Schools of the University."[1]

But the University of Chicago did not start the school the bargain called for, and those aspirations of the Illinois Training School were not attained. Against a backdrop of one century turning into another, with attendant changes in the garb of charity and the power of medicine, the ITS story illustrates how nursing got caught between shifting social pri-

Note: This chapter was originally published in *Nursing Research 41* (1992): 43–48. Reprinted with permission.

orities. The events center in Chicago as its population grew from 100,000 to over two million in the years between the Civil War and the Great Depression.[2]

Chicago: America's Heartland

When a canal linked Lake Michigan to the Illinois River in 1848, the connections among the Great Lakes and Mississippi River shipping networks were completed. Chicago became the busiest port in America, shipping midwestern grain, meat, and minerals to the East. In 1856, the Chicago Theological Seminary, the Academy of Sciences, Hahnemann College, and the Chicago Historical Society organized. The first city high school and the first University of Chicago opened in the same year; Northwestern University had already been founded.[3] With the beginning of these institutions, the initiation of its cattle stockyards, the completion of the transcontinental railroad, and its position at the center of the grain-producing prairie, Chicago became the heart of the nation. But the growing action in Chicago created other, less fortunate consequences. Untended injuries in the stockyards and on the rails, illnesses of lone travelers in town on business, the terrible fire of 1871, and the general rootlessness of society on the move caused concerned Chicago citizens to act.

First Nursing School West of Buffalo

In 1880 "sixteen ladies met at the Palmer House, for the purpose of organizing a Training School for Nurses, for the benefit of the sick, [and] . . . to furnish to those women who desire to become skilled nurses, such facilities as would open to them a self-supporting and honorable profession."[4] As the movement to systematize care of the sick extended westward, similar events took place among civic or religious-minded benefactors in Kansas City, St. Louis, Cincinnati, and Detroit.

The Illinois Training School, like the first American Nightingale-type training schools for nurses in the East, owed its birth to the efforts of public-spirited, philanthropic women who wished to add nursing to ". . . institutions for the relief of suffering humanity. . . ."[5] Women who observed hospital care in the East or studied Nightingale's work in England became convinced that nursing schools associated with hospitals were needed to replace the "unkempt, untrained and politically chosen attendants then employed."[6] The Cook County Hospital, opened in 1866, "needs but the school in connection with it to become perfect."[7] Such a school would offer women a chaperoned, protected life while delivering nursing care as pupils. After graduation, they could seek respectable, paid work in private duty or visiting nursing. The school would become the nursing service department of its affiliated hospital, and the pupil-nurses would deliver all of the care under the supervision of a few instructors and the superintendent, the only graduate nurses employed by most hospitals prior to the 1930s.

Allied with the cream of Chicago society, the women persuaded husbands, physicians, and friends to join them in convincing a reluctant Board of County Commissioners to allow pupils of the proposed school to take over nursing in the County Hospital. As the school's first Board of Managers' President, Mrs. Charles B. Lawrence explained:

> . . . *It was not understood in the beginning that county hospitals are under the control of politicians, and that a committee of women without votes could bring no influence to bear upon a board composed almost entirely of office-seekers. But a majority of the Board of Cook County Commissioners were indifferent alike to the needs of the sick and the importance to the public of the proposed scheme. For a long time they ignored all petitions and communications addressed to their body. They would answer no notes, and observe no appointments. At last came a change; an election carried off some of the objectors, and the new members who took their place were more amenable to humane considerations. The ladies, too, armed themselves with a new weapon. Realizing their disability of sex, and their old-time privilege of gaining their end by indirect means, they deliberately married their board to another, of masculine power and proclivities, and renewed their attack upon the fortress they were determined to possess. . . .*[8]

Chartered on September 15, 1880, as a not-for-profit corporation, the Illinois Training School had 25 women corporate directors, 23 women managers (with approximately half serving in both capacities), and 4 men on a finance committee. Of the 53 men appointed to an Advisory Board, four were county commissioners, three were county hospital physicians, and the remainder community members with social influence and general commercial interests. Bellevue Training School's associate superintendent, Mary E. Brown, became the first superintendent at a salary of $800 per year. The county commissioners bowed to the pressure from citizens and allowed the school to become the nursing service agency for at least some wards in the hospital.[9]

Nursing by Contract

Incorporated independently, the school's finances were kept separate from the hospital. Unlike other hospital training schools, County Hospital accepted no responsibility for providing room or board for the pupils, wages for the instructors/head nurses, or wages for the superintendent. As a fortuitous consequence of the county commissioners' lack of cooperation, various citizen support groups embarked on fund-raising campaigns in the name of the Illinois Training School Corporation. Public meetings drew impressive turnouts and garnered substantial contributions. Newspaper accounts kept people advised of progress and within three months of County Hospital's acceptance of the school, the board raised over $14,000 to secure living accommodations for the pupil-nurses. The board purchased the school's first building lot in May 1882.[10]

The County Hospital paid untrained nurses prior to the school's inception and the school's managers continued that fee structure. Whatever had previously been paid to untrained nurses on specific wards was transferred to pay the training school. The school and its budget grew by replacing untrained nurses ward by ward with pupil-nurses. As other hospitals developed in Chicago, such as Presbyterian Hospital in 1885, they looked to ITS for nursing services. The school kept careful budget analyses and billed hospitals accordingly for the Illinois Training School nursing services. A similar system dictated fees paid to the school when pupil-nurses "specialled" private patients in-hospital or did private duty in patients' homes. Profit was not the intent or the result. The school's managers needed to pay wages and purchase necessities such as living space, furnishings, and school equipment. The county government's erratic financial and political practices kept ITS continually on the financial brink, even as the school's nonliquid assets increased in value.

The yearly budget system started in 1881 before the school opened. Worried that misunderstandings would occur with the county commissioners, the school's board submitted a list to the commissioners documenting expenses and payments. In 1891 the yearly budget became a signed contract, with provisions enabling the school to obtain reimbursement for the many unexpected County Hospital expenses that the commissioners were so reluctant to pay. Often the city paid in scrip, requiring the school to borrow from a bank until the scrip could be redeemed.[11] Even with a contract, money remained exceedingly tight and the school developed other means to earn income. Most of those were consistent with practices in other training schools. The difference lay in the larger scope of the Chicago enterprise and the fact that ITS kept the funds it earned.

The school earned additional income by charging a $5 fee per private duty nurse to list graduate nurses in the formerly free directory. The year after Isabel Hampton became superintendent (1886), the school discontinued the pupil-nurses' monthly allowance. By running a small model hospital developed by state benefactors in the Women's Building of the 1893 Chicago World's Fair, the school earned a fee and a gift to the school of some of the model hospital's furnishings when the fair closed. In providing postgraduate training in areas such as obstetrics after 1894, the school gave necessary credentials to graduates of smaller or less clinically

diverse schools, and earned fees for ITS. Similarly, beginning in 1905, affiliation brought pupils to ITS from smaller hospital schools. The students
helped carry the workload while they met newly imposed state registration
requirements. Conversely, the difficulty in managing the growing demands
at Presbyterian Hospital, plus 900 beds at the County Hospital, with 190
nurses led to the school's painful decision to give up the Presbyterian nursing service in 1903 and the loss of that income. Bitterly, Isabel McIsaac,
superintendent in 1903, reported to the school's board that the County
Hospital pay averaged $17.65/month/nurse at the same time that scrub-
women received $18.00 plus board, laundry, and lodgings.[12]

Fundraising continued to produce impressive results, however, that
allowed for expansion of existing school buildings and acquisition of new
properties. In addition, the interest on a legacy from John Crerar, previously used to endow private duty nursing for families that could not
afford to hire their own nurse, was allocated to cover general school
deficits from 1903 to 1905. In 1907, the Crerar Fund principal paid for
the next addition to the Nurses' Home.[13] By 1926 the school's real estate
and other assets reached a value of $500,000.

The University of Chicago

In December 1888, a few years after the founding of ITS, the Executive
Board of the new American Baptist Education Society voted to found a
college in Chicago which they hoped would ultimately become a university. Within six months, Baptist philanthropist John D. Rockefeller
agreed to be a major financial contributor to the enterprise, provided
that the president and two-thirds of the trustees were Baptists and that
both sexes would be "afforded equal opportunities."[14] Following the design
of the first University of Chicago which closed in 1886 (designated "The
Old University" in 1890), the second University of Chicago opened in
1892. Eager to equal its more prestigious competitors in the East, the
new university used Johns Hopkins University as a model. First President
William R. Harper pronounced research the university's primary work,
and "the work of giving instruction secondary." In 1915, the university's
second President, Harry Pratt Judson, stated that graduate work ought
to be the true intent of the university.[15]

Medical Training in Chicago

From its founding, the University of Chicago was intended to have a
school of medicine, separate from Rush Medical School founded in 1837.
At the spring 1897 convocation, President Harper expressed his belief
that the "greatest single piece of work which still remains to be done"

for education in Chicago and for the university was its own medical school. His vision required a well-endowed medical school that did not have to rely on student fees to survive and could, therefore, maintain a small student body, allowing the faculty to engage primarily in research. Such an institution would "occupy a place beside the two or three . . . that already exist . . . , whose aim it shall be to push forward the boundaries of medical science."[16] In his decennial report of 1901–1902 President Harper included plans to organize a nurses' training school as well.[17] By 1910, changes in medical education standards that preceded and followed the Flexner Report[18] ended medical apprenticeship training in the United States and medical education became university-based, lending support to Chicago's plan.

John D. Rockefeller Unites Several Interests

Rockefeller's personal role in university decisions was subtle but powerful. University records and memoirs reveal that Rockefeller's response to proposals had the effect of direct decision making. His financial support founded the university, the General Education Board, and the Rockefeller Foundation. All three of these institutions ultimately contributed money to the founding of the University of Chicago Medical School and Billings Hospital, which finally opened in October 1927. Dr. Franklin C. McLean, "chief designer and champion" of the project who listed a school of nursing in his "Ten Year Program," was named chairman, Department of Medicine.[19] Anna D. Wolf, a colleague of McLean's from the Rockefeller-funded Peking Union Medical College, was named superintendent of nurses and associate professor of nursing.[20]

Motivated by an interest in improving public health services, the Rockefeller Foundation funded the Commission for the Study of Nursing Education (1919–1923) that produced the Goldmark Report supporting university education for nurses.[21] Yale University's pioneering school of nursing, which operated as an autonomous unit at Yale and conferred the baccalaureate degree on its graduates, was also founded on a Rockefeller Foundation grant in 1923 and permanently endowed by the foundation in 1929. Realistically, however, the million dollars given to nursing must be viewed as meager compared to the many millions "poured into the medical school and other Yale institutes."[22]

During the years between Chicago's decision to found the medical program and the opening of the program, the Illinois Training School completed its negotiation with the university. Clearly in need of money and knowing the planned medical facility would need nurses, the university agreed to the ITS merger in 1926. In exchange for ITS assets worth $500,000, the University of Chicago would have its own school of nursing. The nurses would be granted bachelor degrees and placed under the university's broad institutional protection. University President Max Mason, who signed the memorandum of agreement for the university, was a Rockefeller associate who eventually joined the foundation staff. It is hard to imagine that the ITS merger was not known to and endorsed by Rockefeller or his representatives.

ITS Agrees to Merge

When the Illinois Training School Board made its agreement with the University of Chicago, 183 students, 179 graduate nurses, affiliated students from 70 smaller schools, and 162 attendants and orderlies provided all of the nursing care for patients in the Cook County Hospital. The hospital was, by then, the largest acute care hospital in the world with 2,500 beds serving 42,168 patients yearly.[23] Banks lending money to cover school expenses when the county government delayed its payments sometimes required ITS Board members to personally guarantee the borrowed money.[24] The always unpleasant political aggravation associated with dealing with the county commissioners grew ugly as the commissioners tried to deflect blame for hospital financial problems from themselves onto the school. Accusations of "padded payrolls and unlawful profits" made in the years surrounding World War I, a lawsuit from a disappointed nursing school competitor who wanted the Cook County contract, and public accusations of "having grown rich at the expense of the county" wore down the vigor of the board.[25]

The private structure of the Illinois Training School and the charitable intentions of its philanthropic sponsors seemed to fit neither the changing image of America in the 1920s nor the hurly-burly of city politics. Charity, once viewed as an appropriate "gift from richer to poorer members of the population," became in the twentieth century public service "made available to everyone under government auspices." The city hospital had become a "vehicle for [political] patronage and control"[26] incongruent with notions of nurses' cool hands stroking fevered brows. Across the nation, the deteriorating economy following World War I led to wholesale wage cuts and longer workdays in many industries, with resulting labor unrest. The inability of people to pay private duty nurses for home care of sick members worried families and reduced jobs for graduate nurses. Nonetheless, hospitals continued to admit large numbers of students to the training schools in order to have free pupil labor to deliver nursing care to hospitalized patients. When these students graduated, there were no jobs available to them in the shrinking markets of private duty and visiting nursing, resulting in a glut of unemployed graduate nurses. Prohibition provoked commonplace violation of the law, creating an uneasy social milieu for the remainder of the twenties. In such a context, the board sought to relinquish responsibility for its increasingly burdensome task of managing the Illinois Training School.

ITS's Plans Match Nursing's Collegiate Aspirations

In 1919, the ITS Board had sought university affiliation for the Illinois Training School, approaching first the University of Illinois.[27] The board's efforts coincided with recommendations for nursing's educational future being championed mainly by nursing faculty at Columbia's Teachers College, who held to the mainly Eastern and elite view that nursing should be professionalized. When the board chose Laura Logan to become dean of the Illinois Training School in 1924, Logan believed she was hired to facilitate the initiation of a collegiate program for nurses as she had previously attempted at the University of Cincinnati.[28] Logan, a Teachers College graduate, was part of the group of nursing leaders who were anxious to build on the Goldmark Report's 1923 recommendation to move nursing education into the university. Hoping the Goldmark Report would gain for nursing the status the Flexner Report had gained for medicine, the nursing group strongly supported the first collegiate programs at Yale, Western Reserve, and later at Vanderbilt University. Eager to escape hospital control through the separation of nursing education from nursing practice, Teachers College Nursing Division head Adelaide Nutting and her colleagues pressed universities and foundations to take advantage of the opportunity presented by Goldmark's recommendations.[29]

But other nurses opposed the move to collegiate education, fearing that "book learning" would replace carefully crafted clinical skill, and that graduates of lesser schools would be ". . . sacrificed to the hope of professionalization" and a search for "status" on the part of the nursing elite.[30] Hospital administrators and physicians countered the plans as not "practical" to the average general hospital, and even Goldmark believed the loss of nursing student workers to the hospital would necessitate training a new "hospital helper" as a replacement. Talk of creating substitute hospital workers in an already tenuous nursing economic market encouraged vulnerable graduate nurses to feel threatened and oppose the plan. In fact, had they fought to be the hired replacements, they could have solved their employment problems at the same time nursing solved its educational dilemmas. The nurses needed inspired leadership to show them this solution, but the leadership was preoccupied with battling hospitals, approaching foundations, and negotiating with universities. In the end, strong foundation support never materialized for university nursing education as it had for medical education.[31]

The Merger

Probably to enable students already in the school to complete their training under the conditions in which they entered, and to allow time for County Hospital to replace the nursing staff, the 1926 Memorandum of Agreement between the university and the training school identified December 1, 1929, as the date for the conveyance of property, which would initiate the merger. On October 29, 1929, "Black Tuesday," values on the New York Stock Exchange plummeted, the American economy collapsed, and the Great Depression followed. Nonetheless, ITS conveyed the school's assets to the university in March 1930.[32]

The early 1930s brought multiple crises to the university, its clinics and medical school. Financial desperation followed the reduction of income earned by the endowment after the crash. Outside consultants recommended "sharp decreases in the number of hospital employees and in salary and wage scales" and "sweeping reductions for the entire University." John D. Rockefeller withdrew from active participation, and his death followed in 1937. Dr. Franklin McLean, who relinquished the chair of medicine to assist new President Robert M. Hutchins (who had assumed duties late in 1929), was "removed from all clinical activity" by a successor. Flexner chastised the medical school for using paying patients for teaching, and the Chicago Medical Society accused the medical faculty of unfair competition for the same reason.[33] Besieged from all directions, the university did nothing about the nursing agreement until 1934. In the interim, the university pursued the matter through "discussions," summer quarter special graduate courses, and "survey" conferences.

Ultimately deciding that a nursing school was not feasible because the ITS endowment shrank in the crash and because the nation had an oversupply of graduate nurses, the university initiated a series of graduate courses for nurses who would become "teachers . . . supervisors and administrative officers" and "institutional executives." The university created a Committee on Nursing Education with representatives from all departments that contributed to nursing courses and assigned nursing to the Division of Biological Sciences.[34] In the future, the university transferred the Department of Nursing Education to the Division of Social Sciences, and ultimately discontinued the program in 1959.[35] Subsequently, the funds were used to support "salaries of nurse instructors responsible for various nursing education programs of the Hospitals and Clinics [and] Support of tuition for members of the Nursing staff who pursue formal nursing academic programs at institutions of higher learning on a part-time basis," a scheme which continues to the present day.[36]

The Memorandum of Agreement entitled the university to do what it did with the ITS money. The memorandum stated that the:

> . . . *University shall be free at all times to use the funds and properties herein contracted to be conveyed (except the scholarship fund for which a special use is hereinafter designated) in connection with and for the purpose of giving other or different courses of training for nurses than those herein described and to reorganize its School of Nursing and the courses of study to be given therein from time to time as in its discretion may be deemed wise and best in the furtherance of its educational work.*[37]

Similar discretionary power was given the university for the use of the scholarship money, as long as it was used "in the education and training of nurses."[38]

Though angrily discussed among interested nurses for years, no ITS graduate, faculty, or board member instituted legal action to seek full enforcement of the agreement. Each of the three nursing constituents went its own way, investing its time, energy, and loyalty in its own new venture.

Most of the old ITS faculty stayed on at Cook County Hospital and became faculty for the hospital diploma program that replaced ITS, with Logan remaining as dean. Logan's 1932 correspondence with the president of the University of Illinois at Urbana regarding a nursing training school for that university remains on file as eloquent testimony to Logan's unhappiness with the University of Chicago outcome.[39] The old ITS Board transferred allegiance to the new diploma school board or to the university. When the new University of Chicago Department of Nursing Education formed after 1934 with chair Nellie X. Hawkinson, it became a continuation program, offering baccalaureate education to RNs from the many powerful diploma programs that had developed at hospitals such as St. Luke's, Presbyterian, Michael Reese, and Cook County.

The nursing constituents who continued their support kept silent publicly, in persistent hope that the new university Department of Nursing Education would become a school some day. By the 1959 closure of the department, few participants remained to protest, and protest was not yet a nursing skill.

Timing Is Everything

The failure of the ITS Board to "strike while the iron was hot" in 1926 cost them the full realization of their plans. By 1930 changes in key university personnel, diminishing loyalties among ITS constituents, the absence of a unified national nursing education position, and a radically altered economic environment allowed opponents to prevent formation of a school. University opponents included educational "purists" who believed that undergraduate education should contain only broad liberal arts courses, not "vocational" courses such as nursing. With graduate schools forming at the university in other "women's fields" such as social work and library science during the same time period, and a major school of education already in existence, nursing may have found greater welcome at Chicago had its supporters sought graduate school status. Opposition to any sort of university education for nurses energized some members of the medical faculty and many nurses who believed that it constituted "Professional Snobbery."[40]

Ironically, ITS's reason for the delay in founding the school at the University of Chicago became moot since the Cook County School of Nursing formed instantly where the ITS had been. Where one day the school, faculty, students, catalogues, and all accoutrements carried ITS's name, the next day the very same courses, faculty, students, and catalogues bore the name Cook County School of Nursing. The work continued uninterrupted in the hospital and school. Nurses from Dean Logan to the lowliest student were absorbed into the new school. Though some resented it bitterly, many nurses became ardent supporters of the new diploma school, raising questions about nurses' loyalties. The nursing buildings were leased back from the university by the hospital for the new school to use, and the new board, which contained a number of former ITS Board members, belonged now as much to the hospital as to the school.

Not separate from Cook County Hospital, the Cook County School of Nursing endured successive political and economic encroachments. Payless months for some staff, unpaid milk bills at the hospital, unpaid rent for the nurses, orderly strikes, and all manner of criticism for patient care at Cook County Hospital marked the early 1930s.[41] Protesting conditions, Logan resigned in June 1932 along with nine other nurses who later returned. Logan suffered particular harassment from physicians who believed the nurses spent time in class "at a sacrifice of time that otherwise would be spent in bedside nursing." Called "Laura Hell-Cat Logan" by one physician, another doctor suggested physicians should ". . . make things sufficiently unpleasant so that a resignation" would be made, "although . . . a dismissal might be good for her."[42] Politicians, sharing physicians' views, planted news articles such as one accusing Logan of living the "high life in the Cook County School of Nursing with the indigent county footing the bills. . . ."[43]

Logan was not invited back to Cook County after her 1932 resignation as were the other nurses. She went on to superintend nursing diploma schools and hospital nursing divisions in New York, Boston, and St. Louis until her retirement in 1953. Logan's final efforts on behalf of the Illinois Training School bore some fruit as its successor school finally joined in 1949 with a university to become The University of Illinois-Cook County School of Nursing.

Formidable Divisions

Though the aspirations of certain national nursing leaders and constituents of the Illinois Training School to found a University of Chicago School of Nursing were not attained, ITS did buy for nurses an educational presence at the University of Chicago that they, most likely, would not otherwise have gained. Whether the outcome would have been different had ITS consummated its university agreement in 1926, when the participants and economics were right, can never be known. The merger agreement needed unified, assertive advocates to bring it to fruition. Lost in the valley between two women's movements, two world wars, altered national beliefs about benevolence, and roiling economic circumstances, the ITS Board, faculty, and graduates neither provided the necessary leadership nor protested the university's failure to comply.

Generations removed from its founders and their charitable ideals, tired of battling the county commissioners, stung by attacks on their honor, and eager for agreement, the ITS Board allowed clauses to be placed in the Memorandum of Agreement that enabled the university to evade its primary obligation to found a school. Not part of the era that believed it the responsibility of private, benevolent individuals to provide nursing to the needy, the board did not feel obliged to pursue the matter. Local nursing participants, because they were not board members, were not empowered to make their own contract or to control their own destiny. In addition, their primary loyalty to the hospital and patients led them to attach easily to the successor school, Cook County School of Nursing, abandoning their fight for defunct ITS aims. The national nursing community, engaged in a divisive debate over the proper place for educating nurses, did not unite behind the proposed program or formally protest its dissolution. With such formidable divisions and crippling political naiveté, even with its own money, the Illinois Training School could not attain full university acceptance for its nurses.

NOTES

1.   "Memorandum of Agreement" between the University of Chicago and the Illinois Training School for Nurses, June 10, 1926, p. 6. Original document, signed by Harold H. Swift, president of the University Board of Trustees and Emma Magnus Williams, president of the ITS Board, is held in a folder marked *Hospitals* Affiliation Agreements in the Office of Legal Counsel, The University of Chicago, 5801 S. Ellis Ave., Chicago, IL 60637.

2.   Harry F. Dowling, *City Hospitals: The Undercare of the Underprivileged* (Cambridge: Harvard University Press, 1982), p. 25.

3.   Thomas Wakefield Goodspeed, *A History of the University of Chicago—The*

First Quarter Century, (Chicago: The University of Chicago Press, 1916, 1972), pp. 12–13.

4.   First Annual Report of the Society of the Illinois Training School for Nurses attached to the Cook County Hospital, Secretary's Report, signed Mrs. Thomas Burrows. Midwest Nursing History Resource Centcr, 845 S. Damen St., Chicago, IL 60612.

5.   Margaret Marsden Lawrence (Mrs. Charles B.), paper read before the Fortnightly Club, n.d. (probably Summer 1880) as reported in Grace Fay Schryver, *A History of the Illinois Training School for Nurses, 1880–1929* (Chicago: The Board of Directors of the Illinois Training School for Nurses, 1930), p. 2.

6.   Schryver, p. 1. The original documents, deeded to the University of Chicago with all other school property (see Schryver, p. 176), are not found, see letters to author from Office of Legal Counsel dated October 8, 1987, and from The University of Chicago Library dated September 30, 1987.

7.   Mrs. Lawrence's paper, cf 5.

8.   Margaret M. Lawrence (Mrs. Charles B.) diaries, n.d. (probably 1882) as reported in Schryver, p. 12. See newspaper accounts of fraud and bribery among the commissioners for further evidence of the political interplay, e.g., *Sunday Tribune*, April 20, 1930; *Chicago Tribune,* June 18, 1887.

9.   Schryver, pp. 1–18.

10.   Schryver, pp. 17, 27.

11.   Schryver, pp. 18–19, 54, 62.

12.   Schryver, pp, 45, 49, 67–70, 74, 79–83.

13.   Schryver, pp. 64–6, 82, 85.

14.   Frederick Taylor Gates, "Introduction," in Goodspeed, p. 11.

15.   Goodspeed, pp. 146, 155.

16.   President Harper as quoted in Goodspeed, pp. 330–1.

17.   Goodspeed, p. 333.

18.   Abraham Flexner, *Medical Education in the United States and Canada* (New York: Carnegie Foundation, 1910).

19.   C. W. Vermeulen, M. D., *For the Greatest Good to the Largest Number, A History of the Medical Center, The University of Chicago, 1927–1977* (Chicago: The Vice-President for Public Affairs, The University of Chicago, 1977), pp. 31, 52.

20.   News About Nurses, *American Journal of Nursing*, 40(4) (April 1940): 449–50.

21.   *Nursing and Nursing Education in the United States*, Report of the Commission for the Study of Nursing Education, Josephine Goldmark, secretary. (New York: The MacMillan Co., 1923).

22.   Susan M. Reverby, *Ordered to Care: The Dilemma of American Nursing, 1850–1945* (New York: Cambridge University Press, 1987), p. 166.

23.   *46th Annual Report*, ITS, November 30, 1926, Redweld File-holder, Cook County School of Nursing Archives. In addition, 41,000 patients were examined and rejected, and 16,301 patients were seen in the dispensary that year.

24.   Letter from Mabel Magnus (Mrs. August) to Alice Wood (Mrs. Ira Couch Wood) dated February 1, 1921, File 1921 ITS, Cook County School of Nursing Archives. See also Chicago *Tribune* and *Herald* and *Examiner* newspapers, December

17, 1929, which reported that the county borrowed over one million dollars to run the nursing school, and the banks were refusing further loans.

25.   Speech by Mrs. August C. Magnus, October 1, 1929. Box 26, file 26–583, University of Illinois at Chicago, The University Library Special Collections, Department of Manuscripts, University Archives, Rare Books, 1733 Polk St., Chicago, IL. See also letter from Magnus to the University of Chicago Board, attached to memorandum and dated May 26, 1926. CC-SON Archives.

26.   Rosemary Stevens, *In Sickness and in Wealth* (New York: Basic Books, 1989), pp. 16, 22.

27.   Letter dated October 16, 1919, from Mrs. Ira Couch Wood sent to David Kinley, president of the University of Illinois at Urbana by Charles Thorne, director, Illinois Dept. of Public Welfare. His interested response was dated February 3, 1920, and another on February 10, 1920, suggested further study. File 43, Midwest Nursing History Resource Center.

28.   Laura Logan, letter of resignation to the Board of Trustees, Cook County School of Nursing, dated June 14, 1932, File 52, Midwest Nursing History Resource Center.

29.   Reverby, p. 164.

30.   Barbara Melosh, *"The Physician's Hand" Work Culture and Conflict in American Nursing* (Philadelphia: Temple University Press, 1982), pp. 42–3.

31.   Reverby, pp. 164–69.

32.   Documents signed by Elizabeth MacLeish and Helen Mordack, notarized by Howard B. Bryant, and attached to the Memorandum, cf 1.

33.   Vermeulen, pp. 34–9, 41–3,52–5.

34.   The Gift of the Illinois Training School for Nurses to the University of Chicago, *Illinois Training School Alumnae Report*, November 1933, pp. 2–3. Midwest Nursing History Resource Center. Reprint, *News Bulletin* of the University of Chicago.

35.   Frances C. Thielbar, chairman, Nursing Education, University of Chicago, letter to Mildred I. Tuttle, director, Division of Nursing, Kellogg Foundation, dated January 30, 1959. Center for the Study of the History of Nursing, The University of Pennsylvania School of Nursing, Philadelphia.

36.   Files entitled *Hospitals: Nursing Education, Loan, Endowment and Scholarship Funds* and *Nursing Education, Endowment Fund*, Office of Legal Counsel, University of Chicago. Confirmation of current use discussed in personal interview with Carolyn Smeltzer, EdD, FAAN, vice president for nursing, The University of Chicago Hospitals, October 18, 1989.

37.   Memorandum, cf 1, Section III, pp. 6–7. Originally, University Fund #6587, currently #65609.

38.   Memorandum, cf 1, Section IV, p. 8. Originally, University Fund #6588, currently #65610.

39.   File 49, Midwest Nursing History Resource Center, Letter dated February 5, 1932, from Pres. H. W. Chase of the University of Illinois at Urbana.

40.   Melosh, p. 68.

41.   File 52, Midwest Nursing History Resource Center, Letters from Dr. Nathan S. Davis III to Mr. McKibbin, dated November 23, 1932; from Dr. Wayne

Bissell to Dr. Nathan S. Davis III, dated September 10, 1932; and from Dr. Nathan S. Davis III to Dr. Ludwig Hektoen, dated March, 24, 1932.

43.   File 52, Midwest Nursing History Resource Center, News article dated January 22, 1932, in the *Daily News* and *Herald Express.*

Research for this chapter was supported by a National Research Service Award from the National Center of Nursing Research, National Institutes of Health, Professor Charles E. Rosenberg, Sponsor. The author gratefully acknowledges the assistance of many Chicago colleagues in the research for this chapter. Olga Church, Myra Levine, and Susan Dudas, faculty, University of Illinois College of Nursing; Mary Whelan, curator of the Midwest Nursing History Resource Center; Terry Norwood, Cook County School of Nursing Archives; and Samuel D. Golden, Esq., Office of Legal Counsel, University of Chicago.

8

Guarded by Standards and Directed by Strangers: Charleston, South Carolina's Response to a National Health Care Agenda, 1920–1930

Karen Buhler-Wilkerson

The year 1912 was a triumphal one for public health nurses who, declared their foremost leader, Lillian Wald, finally attained the position of their dreams. Wald's enthusiasm was for her own idea—the newly created Red Cross Rural Nursing Service, which promised to promote and actually establish "nursing for the people throughout the country." Her proposal called for the Red Cross to "standardize" public health nursing in towns and rural districts and to integrate the work of isolated nurses and nursing organizations under a "central body." In Wald's estimation it was a cause that "carried its own appeal."[1]

At its peak during the 1920s, nearly 3,000 Red Cross nursing services were launched across the country. For several years, combined overseas and home nursing programs made the Red Cross the largest single employer of nurses in the world. This success was short-lived, however, and within a few years local chapters were closing their nursing services at an alarming rate. By 1930, 2,323 of these services had been discontinued. At the outset, Wald presumed they would make some mistakes in the organization of this "great movement," but she never anticipated such a dramatic collapse. The enthusiastic beginning and precipitous decline of the Red Cross nursing service is one of the more interesting stories of our ongoing American aversion to nationally organized health care.[2]

Note: This chapter was originally published in *Nursing History Review* I (1993): 139–54. Copyright (c) 1993 by The American Association for the History of Nursing. Reprinted with permission.

This historical account is a case study with its focus in Charleston, South Carolina, where the Ladies Benevolent Society (LBS) had been caring for the sick poor in their homes since 1813—as they saw best. While this may be a "peculiarly" southern story, it illustrates how, in the absence of locally perceived need, national agendas for health care find little sustenance or support at home.[3]

"THE GREATEST MOTHER": THE AMERICAN RED CROSS

Wald first proposed her "vast" scheme for country nursing to the Red Cross in 1908. Despite their initial lack of interest, Wald eventually secured the support of New York businessman and frequent sponsor Jacob Schiff. Even with Schiff's support, however, the Red Cross began to share Wald's zeal only when Schiff and Mrs. Whitelow Reid offered to provide the money necessary to begin the nursing service.[4]

A special committee was immediately appointed. It recommended approval of the project, suggesting a trial year conducted under the supervision of the Red Cross Committee on Rural Nursing. The committee members were well known to Wald and her nursing colleagues; most were strong supporters of nurses of "professional caliber." At their first meeting, held in November 1912, the nurse members were given the task of making recommendations for the nursing service. Taking advantage of this opportunity, they immediately convinced the other members that, due to the nature of the rural nurse's work, she would have to possess the highest qualifications. Their suggestions included not only the requirement that all applicants complete a four-month course of training under the supervision of a recognized visiting nurse association, but also the development of scholarships and loan funds necessary to underwrite this requirement. The committee's rapid acceptance of the nurse members' recommendations suggested that, at least for the moment, the Rural Nursing Service would develop under the careful control and protection of the nursing leadership.[5]

Despite the hopes of many, the recently renamed Town and Country Nursing Service remained a modest undertaking. Beyond the rather fundamental problem of finding qualified nurses, few local groups had the funds needed to establish a nursing service. By 1917, eighty-five affiliations with a total of ninety-seven nurses had been established in twenty-one states. The earliest programs were in the eastern states, followed by those in the South and the West. Their work mirrored that of the public health nurse in most urban settings; nurses did bedside care of the sick, preventive services for children and mothers, and tuberculosis cases, plus a few "sanitary inspections." But unlike big cities where health department nurses did most of the preventive work and visiting nurse association nurses did the bedside care, in these smaller communities the Red Cross nurse cared for everyone—sick or well.[6]

World War I interrupted this experiment, but these developmental years provided the opportunity for the Red Cross to establish the parameters of its peacetime mission. By April 1919 the Red Cross had resumed its ambitious plans for a "new era of health" by sending thirty-one Red Cross nurses out on the Chatauqua Circuit as a "publicity stunt."[7] Expanding on Wald's original idea, the nursing service was now conceived as "the basis and backbone of the Red Cross endeavor." The Red Cross developed policies and procedures for adoption by local chapters and planned to provide properly qualified, guided, and supervised nurses. Each chapter was expected to promote popular interest and pay the nurse's salary. Thus, the Red Cross plan called for national direction but local financing.[8]

Controlling the local chapters' activities rapidly proved more difficult than stimulating their interest. Most had a residue of funds from their war efforts and a score of workers anxious to replace war duties with another big cause. The "great boom," as Mary Gardner, temporary director and frequent critic of the service dubbed it, was overwhelming; overnight hundreds of chapters with money in hand established Red Cross Public Health Nursing Services. Insiders, who took to calling the Red Cross the "greatest mother," would later admit that these were "alarming" years when events proceeded almost out of control.[9]

Hoping to establish some uniformity, at least in its nursing staff, the Red Cross remained committed to only hiring nurses with postgraduate training in public health nursing. But the demand for nurses speedily outran the supply. Beyond this obvious problem, sending young and inexperienced city-bred and city-trained nurses to the country to harmoniously adapt their services to local conditions was an arrangement fraught with difficulties. According to Red Cross historian Portia Kernodle, a "kind of friendly feud" developed between some chapters and the distant national Red Cross over standards and policies. The "autocratic rulings of the Red Cross so necessary in war" were increasingly unacceptable to the local chapters that wanted to run their nursing service in a manner suited to local conditions. They preferred to hire a nurse "they knew and liked" regardless of her training. By 1922, despite the efforts of the Red Cross to maintain high educational standards, only 48 percent of the nurses employed by local chapters had any postgraduate training.[10]

The Red Cross also failed to keep its commitment to provide the personal visits, national correspondence, and definite standards that conveyed to isolated nurses a sense of support and encouragement. With shrinking budgets, the number of divisional offices and field personnel were reduced and visits to local chapters dramatically curtailed. Managing only an annual visit, nursing field representatives provided little guidance, support, or supervision. Predictably, in their absence other new programs began to compete with nursing for increasingly limited chapter funds.[11]

The American Medical Association and the National Organization for Public Health Nursing, as well as local health departments and tuberculosis associations, questioned and even disapproved of the Red Cross's new enterprise. Critics claimed that chapters initiated nursing services with insufficient funds or staff, inadequate community support, and without cooperative agreements with existing agencies, health officers, or local physicians. Public Health Nursing leader Mary Gardner viewed the Red Cross plan for expansion from the top as of dubious virtue. Demand for nurses, Gardner suggested, should come from the community. Only then could programs develop slowly, fostering essential community support and understanding as they grew.[12]

As if external faultfinding was not enough, opposition and criticism of the nursing service began to come from within the Red Cross. Somewhat surprisingly, Mabel Boardman, a longtime supporter of the program, publicly accused the Red Cross of "exceeding its rights and endangering its proper obligations." She regarded the Red Cross as an organization for meeting emergencies and thought it was stretching the meaning of the Red Cross charter too far to think of disease as a disaster that the Red Cross must attempt to prevent. While Boardman's remarks caused a minor sensation in the Red Cross, as with the opinion of other assailants they were discussed and duly dismissed.[13]

By the latter part of 1921, the number of Red Cross nursing services in operation peaked at 1,243, and local chapters' devotion began to waver as war surplus funds were used up. During the three years between January 1921 and December 1923, Red Cross nursing services closed at an average rate of 410 a year. By January 1924, only 804 services and 967 nurses remained. Although the withdrawal rate of Red Cross chapters lessened, the end was not yet in sight. According to Kernodle, an "original understanding or misunderstanding" partially caused the failure of some chapters to find the means to continue their nursing services when war funds were gone. Chapters were expected only to "demonstrate" the value of their service for a year or two and then some other agency (e.g., health department) would take it over. In most communities (64 percent) this transfer of responsibility never materialized and the services were allowed to lapse.[14]

THE SOUTHERN DILEMMA

The gap between Red Cross standards and pressure to keep up with demand for nurses was most pronounced in the southern division. There, in the words of Red Cross Division Director Jane Van De Vrede, southern people were generally unwilling to accept the policies of any "national body." The rather slow development of this work in the South resulted, she claimed, from the combination of the regions "marked conservatism in accepting all innovation" and Red Cross adherence to its ideals and policies: insistence on highly trained nurses and centrally derived decisions. This combination made it nearly impossible to supply nurses from local resources because southern training school graduates did not meet the eligibility requirements for Red Cross enrollment or admission to postgraduate public health nursing programs. Even those who qualified for training and scholarships were, according to Van De Vrede, reluctant to leave the South to attend these programs.[15]

Beyond the disparity between supply and demand, Van De Vrede also claimed that "the great number of negroes forming a dependent population which must be carried outright in any welfare undertaking" was another deterrent to the development of this work in the South. Apparently, the implication was that if white southerners established a nursing service they would immediately be confronted with caring for the significant health care needs of the black population. They therefore simply chose to avoid these rather complex issues in segregated communities. Whatever the cause, by 1920, with 50 percent of the southern chapters anxious to begin nursing services, only 5 percent (twenty-four) had been supplied a nurse.[16]

"IN CHARLESTON, WE TRUST THE PEOPLE WE KNOW"

The Charleston Red Cross story strikingly elucidates the local dilemmas created by this well-intentioned national agenda, even when methods and outcomes precisely match those anticipated by the Red Cross planners. Three months after the 1918 Armistice, the Charleston Red Cross Chapter launched its new nursing service with adequate funds ($26,000) and requisite "machinery and spirit" (9,427 members). Enamored with the Red Cross idea of "making a great contribution to the welfare" of their community, they immediately called a meeting of all (nineteen) organizations in the city interested in health matters to seek their endorsement. The participants unanimously voted to "back up" the program as outlined by the Red Cross and promised their cooperation.[17]

A memo from Red Cross national headquarters describing these developments mentioned that "the Benevolent Society, which has supported colored visiting nursing since 1902 will also coordinate their service with the chapter, but without merging identity." The memo concluded with the hope that Charleston's nursing agencies would soon "see the wisdom of standards set by the Red Cross and act accordingly." Clearly, the memo writer at national headquarters had no idea of this organization's standing in Charleston society. Founded in 1813 by the wives, sisters, and daughters of the city's most prominent families, the Ladies Benevolent Society (LBS) was not an organization to be ignored. Evidently, the Red Cross, unaware of "local conditions," chose to categorize the work of the LBS as "colored" visiting nursing, because both of their nurses were black. In fact the LBS cared for both black and white patients and had, after several years of experimentation, found black nurses to be the most acceptable caregivers within the homes of Charleston's sick poor, black or white. After contracting to care for sick Metropolitan Life Insurance policyholders in 1911, the LBS grew tremendously with nearly nine hundred patients being cared for in 1920.[18]

The LBS Board's initial response to the Red Cross plan was "to wait and see." While they perceived the Red Cross to be a potentially competitive organization, publicly they expressed great interest in any endeavor to make theirs a healthy city.[19]

The Red Cross plan was to divide Charleston into four districts, providing a nurse for each and a supervisor to oversee the whole program. As in so many chapters across the country, plans were completed six months before qualified staff became available and as a result the office was not fully operational until February 1920. Despite this slow start, at national headquarters they were "all very proud of this chapter's activities, and the fine way the Charleston Committee on Nursing Activities [had] gone about organizing a very difficult piece of work."[20]

By April the chair of the Nursing Activities Committee became concerned that, despite their good start, sufficient work had not been done to warrant the large amount being spent by the chapter on this program. She was also distressed by the "great deal of unrest among the nurses" caused, she discovered, by a supervisor "not fitted for her position." A month later, the supervisor had handed in her resignation and Marie Lebby had agreed to replace her.[21]

Despite the mismatched supervisor and a total turnover of the staff, the nursing service somehow continued at a reasonably productive level that first year. The chapter looked forward to the future, confident that Marie Lebby would know how to get their program under control because, remarkably, she was a southerner, a lady, and a nurse.

A LADY IS A LADY, EVEN IF SHE'S A NURSE!

Marie Lebby came from Charleston. After graduating from Rollins College and making her debut, she felt little enthusiasm for her expected role as a southern lady. Wanting to "do something useful," she decided to go to medical school, but her family would not "hear of it" and practically

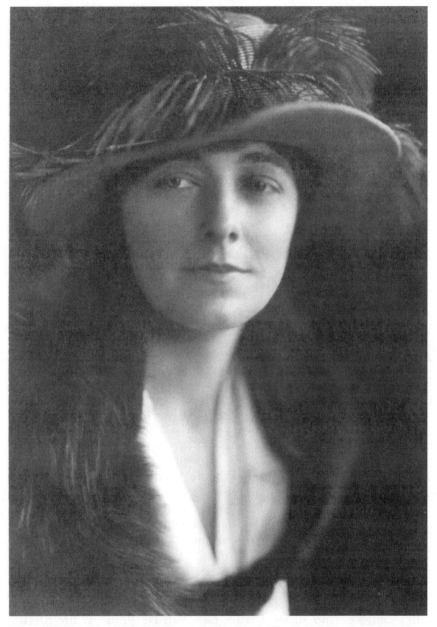

Marie Mikell Lebby (Mrs. Thomas C. Boushall), Public Health Nursing Supervisor, Charleston, South Carolina Chapter of the American Red Cross. (Courtesy of Mrs. Granville Valentine)

disowned her. Eventually they agreed to let her go to nursing school at St. Luke's Hospital in Richmond where she would be under the watchful eye of family friend and "gentleman" Dr. Stuart McGuire. Much to her relief, Lebby found that, unlike Charleston, "in Virginia women from some of the best families were nurses."[22]

After graduation, Marie Lebby joined Base Hospital 45, serving with Stuart McGuire in France. Returning to New York, she completed the postgraduate public health nursing course at Columbia University. Anxious to return to the South, Lebby was delighted when her teacher, the well-known nurse leader Adelaid Nutting, "commanded" her to return to Charleston to straighten out their problems. Nutting wanted Lebby to take over the Charleston Red Cross Service and show them what a real nurse—meaning a lady with the right education—could do. Lebby returned home in June of 1920, working intermittently and part-time as an acting-supervisor for the Red Cross that summer.[23]

While the LBS had greeted the Red Cross plans for a nursing service with ambivalence, they welcomed Marie Lebby's arrival. Much to their relief, they found that Lebby recognized "the unique position of the Ladies Benevolent Society." She was anxious to cooperate with them and confident that the domains of the two nursing services need not overlap. Reassured that she "understood," they appointed her to their board. While Charlestonians may not have approved of "Miss Marie" becoming a nurse, local lore has it that, at least in this case, "a lady is a lady, even if she's a nurse."[24]

The Red Cross was equally pleased with Lebby "who gained for the service many friends among the doctors who, up to that time, were not quite sure what we were trying to give the city." While delighted with Lebby's public relation skills, the Red Cross must have found her intermittent availability discouraging. By September 1920, the Red Cross Board decided they had "demonstrated" public health nursing for Charleston long enough and planned to propose at the January City Council Meeting that the city health department "undertake the responsibility of Public Health Nursing in the city." Despite the health department's interest and a supportive "mass meeting," the city failed to appropriate the necessary funds.[25]

By spring of 1921, Charleston's Red Cross was in crisis. Their treasury was down to $10,519, their chairman had resigned, Lebby was planning to marry a Richmond banker, they had only one nurse left on staff, and they could get no support from Jane Van De Vrede at the Atlanta Divisional Office. That April, determined to terminate their demonstration, Marie Lebby asked the LBS Board to consider taking over the Red Cross Nursing Service. She added that, if they did not, she "would form another organization" for that purpose. In a special meeting called by the LBS Board later that month, Georgia Jatho, chair of the Red Cross Nursing Activities Committee, presented their proposal as a great opportunity for the LBS, but one that required acceptance of the methods and standards established by the Red Cross nationally. Concretely, this meant that the LBS each year would have to raise $8,000 to $10,000 for an office, staff, literature, and nursing supervisor consistent with Red Cross standards. Accepting the Red Cross's methods also meant the work "would be entirely in the hands of a nursing supervisor" and the LBS Board would simply receive monthly reports from her. Jatho was confident that if the LBS did not undertake this work, it would be assumed by another organization and this would be "a great misfortune as it meant the death of the LBS." Lebby contended that Charleston was not rich enough to support two nursing organizations, and therefore, "either one must die or both must hobble on."[26]

The LBS Board took this "golden opportunity" and threat seriously. They consulted with several businessmen, had numerous "animated discussions," and presented the matter to the membership. In the end, they declined the Red Cross challenge "to write for our city a new page in history," accepting instead "the possibility of destruction or a very restricted future."[27]

As they proved in other decisions, the LBS Board was unwilling to trade methods acceptable within Charleston's peculiar traditions for the methods and standards of outsiders. Initially, almost half the LBS Board demonstrated some interest in the Red Cross plan; it was LBS Superintendent Catherine Ravenel's warnings that "all would change" that coalesced opposition. Most distressing was the need to "give up every detail" into the hands of a nursing supervisor. According to Ravenel, all reports would go to the supervisor, who would form all committees, and the board's only responsibility would be to "supply the money." Observing what was happening elsewhere in South Carolina, it must also have been clear to Ravenel that "qualified" supervisors usually came from northern postgraduate public health nursing programs. Accordingly, she cautioned careful consideration, warning that not only would they be giving up the "well organized work which we have striven so hard to establish," but they would also be turning over the LBS's future to the judgment and vision of a "stranger." Sharing Ravenel's sentiments that "a stranger coming here to supervise would find conditions and people very different from elsewhere," the membership unanimously voted to simply place the Red Cross proposal in the minutes as an "informational item." With hardly enough money in the treasury to get through the year, the LBS chose, in the words of Marie Lebby, "to close their eyes to the possibilities and drift on."[28]

Unsuccessful in their negotiations with the LBS, the Charleston Red Cross came to realize that the failure of local organizations to take up this work seemed related to "some objection to the Red Cross supervision." In response, the board sought a "purely local organization" to carry on the service free of Red Cross standards and policies. By January 1922, the task of "safeguarding the health of the community" had been taken up by the newly created Charleston Public Health Nursing Association. The local Red Cross chapter voted to show their support by providing $1,500, selling the new organization the "property" used by the Nursing Activities Committee at half price, and turning over all current nursing records. Watching with "keen interest" and much relief the continuance of their nursing service elsewhere, the Red Cross focused its attention on discovering whether it was viable in any peacetime capacity.[29]

In December 1924 the work and staff of the Charleston Public Health Nursing Association was, in turn, taken over by the recently reorganized Charleston County Health Department. That same year the Metropolitan Life Insurance Company (MLI) opened an independent nursing service in Charleston, having just terminated its contract with the LBS because of complaints from policyholders who "did not like the colored nurses." The record does not explain why the LBS allowed the termination of this beneficial relationship rather than hire a white nurse to care for these grieved patients. Whatever the explanation, discontinuing their contract meant the ladies of Charleston had chosen a very different future for their organization.[30]

By 1925 Ravenel characterized the work of the LBS as "much restricted." Their calls now came from old patients, those the Health Department nurses could not reach, and "those who shrink from asking for city help." Yet, despite this inevitable outcome, simply supplementing the work of the other nursing organizations was more acceptable than having the LBS's mission taken over by outsiders. In the aggregate, the outcome for Charlestonians was a rather confusing collection of small nursing organizations—each driven by its own fragmented perception of community need. Operating mostly in isolation, their interactions remained casual at best. For those seeking nursing care, centralizing all public health nursing services within the LBS might have provided a more rational approach to their needs. For the LBS, however, fragmented and diminished services proved more acceptable than compliance with the dictates of outsiders such as the Red Cross or the MLI.[31] The ladies of Charleston held to the principle that appropriate methods of caring and spheres of usefulness were intimate matters defined at home within locally acceptable boundaries—not by a national agenda guarded by homogenized standards and directed by strangers.

Charleston's story echoed across the country as cities and local voluntary health organizations experimented with the Red Cross's national agenda for health. It confirmed the failure of the Red Cross's scheme for a national nursing service on many fronts. This vast plan to give the

Red Cross a peacetime mission and extend the work of the public health nurse across the country to small-town America was valued only by a few reformers like Wald. Standards that sent strangers to small towns where they only "trust the people we know" quickly caused difficulties. Nurses, once again dispatched to do the impossible, were courageous and enthusiastic, but inescapably found themselves unemployed.[32] Most significant, however, was the local chapter members' unwillingness to finance health services that ranked low in perceived importance to their local citizenry.

Acknowledgments

This study was supported by the National Center for Nursing Research, National Institutes of Health. I wish to thank the staff of the South Carolina Historical Society, the Carolina Low Country Chapter of the American Red Cross, the archives of the Metropolitan Life Insurance Company, the National Archives Civil Research Branch, the Waring Historical Library of the Medical University of South Carolina, and Marie Lebby Boushall and her daughter, Mrs. Granville Valentine, for their invaluable assistance.

NOTES

1.   The collection of the American Red Cross, National Headquarters is at the National Archives, Washington, D.C. Lavinia Dock et al., *History of American Red Cross Nursing* (New York: Macmillan, 1949), 1213–15, 1220–21, and Portia B. Kernodle, *The Red Cross Nurse in Action, 1882–1948* (New York: Harper and Brothers, 1949), 71–72.

2.   Dock, 1214, 1220–22, and Kernodle, 256–86. For these statistics, see "Public Health Nursing, Changes in Service, July 1, 1919 to June 30, 1930," folder no. 140.18, Public Health Nursing, American Red Cross, National Archives (hereafter cited as PHN, ARC, NA).

3.   For an excellent discussion of the "peculiar South," see Drew Gilpin Faust, "The Peculiar South Revisited: White Society, Culture, and Politics in the Antebellum Period, 1800–1860," in *Interpreting Southern History: Historiographical Essays in Honor of Sanford W. Higginbotham,* ed. John Boles and Evelyn T. Noyes (Baton Rouge: Louisiana State University Press, 1987), 78–119.

4.   Dock, 1212–15, and Kernodle, 72.

5.   For an extensive review of the evolution of Red Cross standards and programs, see Dock, 1211–92, and Kernodle, 71–89. For a more extensive overview of public health nurses efforts toward the creation of standards, see M. Louise Fitzpatrick, *The National Organization for Public Health Nursing, 1912–1952: Development of a Practice Field* (New York: National League for Nursing, 1975).

6.   Dock, 1291–92. In 1916, 47 percent of Red Cross visits were for bedside care of the sick, while "instructive" visits to children, infant welfare, prenatal and tuberculosis cases, sanitary inspections, and "other" made up the remaining calls. Rural nurses were also caring for a significantly smaller number of patients than

their urban counterparts and tended to make more visits to each patient. For a comparison, see Karen Buhler-Wilkerson, *False Dawn: The Rise and Decline of Public Health Nursing, 1900–1930* (New York: Garland Publishing, 1989), 153–55. The Red Cross nursing service changed its name several times, reflecting its evolving mission and/or organizational changes. During World War I it became the Bureau of Public Health Nursing and in the 1920s it was renamed the Public Health Nursing Service.

7.   Chatauqua was called the "canvass college of America." It was a very popular traveling program of "enlightenment and entertainment" presented two to three times a day for several days or even weeks under a large tent. Programs ranged from travelogues to plays. Kernodle, 238–41.

8.   Buhler-Wilkerson, *False Dawn*, 221–28; Dock, 1293–1351; and Kernodle, 256–86. For Red Cross instruction to chapters, see "The Organization and Administration of a Public Health Nursing Service," 1 March 1919, Form A 701, folder no. 15, PHN, ARC, NA.

9.   Ibid. "Public Health Nursing, Changes in Service, July 1, 1919 to June 30, 1930," folder no. 140.18, PHN, ARC, NA. Elizabeth Fox, who succeeded Gardner as director, mentioned the "mother" role in her monthly report, 3 June 1929, folder no. 140.18, PHN, ARC, NA. Gardner "temporarily" rescued the Red Cross by becoming director on 1 April 1918, when the previous director resigned over the Red Cross's failure to "push forward" with the service. Fannie Clements to Frank Persons, 26 March 1918, folder no. 140.12, PHN, ARC, NA. See also, Mary Gardner, "Under the Red Cross," *The Public Health Nurse* 20 (November 1928): 597–99 (hereafter cited as *PHN*), and Elizabeth Fox, "The Development of the Red Cross Bureau of Public Health *Nursing*," *PHN* 12 (February 1920): 175–81.

10.   Kernodle, 278–81. "The Organization and Administration of a Public Health Nursing Service," folder no. 151, and "Report of Public Health Nursing Service, July 1, 1920 to June 30, 1921," folder no. 140.18, PHN, ARC, NA. "Report of the Western Office," May 1919, National Organization for Public Health Nursing, roll no. 27, National League for Nursing Records Collection, New York.

11.   This commitment is described in Dock, 1267–68; Kernodle, 267–68, 272, 281–82. Concurrently, the nature of the nursing programs was increasingly limited to bedside care as their preventive programs were taken over by official agencies whose growth was supported by the Rockefeller Foundation, the Children's Bureau, and the Sheppard Towner Act. This trend was financially supported by the Metropolitan Life Insurance Company, which contracted with surviving Red Cross chapters for a considerable portion of the bedside care they provided for policy-holders living in rural areas and small towns.

12.   Kernodle, 275–78, and Buhler-Wilkerson, *False Dawn*, 221–28. For an example of the variety of letters written by the Red Cross in its effort to assure other organizations that it did not "contemplate the invasion of territory where other organizations are engaged in work of this character," see Rupert Blue (Surgeon General) to Mrs. Ira Perkins, Chief, Child Conservation Section, Council of National Defense, Washington, 3 April 1919, Public Health Service, General File, 1897–1923: 3815, box 372, National Archives. Much of the visiting nurse leadership's "chronically sore and morbidly disposed" feeling toward the Red

Cross developed over what they called the Red Cross's "ruthless ambition" at the expense of public health nursing during World War I. See for example, Ella Crandell to Mary Beard, 2 February 1919, roll 31, Wald Collection, New York Public Library, New York.

13. Buhler-Wilkerson, *False Dawn*, 225, and Kernodle, 241, 276–78, 285.

14. Kernodle, 263, 281–83. Between 1920 and 1930 there were 2,959 nursing services created by the Red Cross; 2,393 of these were discontinued, 383 (13 percent) turned over to public agencies, 41 (1 percent) turned over to private agencies, and 1,899 (64 percent) closed due to "lack of funds, interest, etc." As of 30 June 1930 only 636 (22 percent) were still in operation. "Public Health Nursing, Changes in Service, July 1, 1919–June 30, 1930," folder no. 140.18 PHN, ARC, NA.

15. Van De Vrede was born in Wisconsin and moved to Georgia in 1908. "Qualified" nurses were graduates of a two-year nursing course in a general hospital with a minimum of fifty beds (must include men), members of an organization affiliated with the American Nurses Association, registered to practice, and graduates of a recognized postgraduate course. In 1919 there were thirteen educational institutions giving this course that ranged from four to nine months. The only course available in the South was in Richmond, which gave a three-month course. The Red Cross provided scholarships that were paid back through a year of service. Exceptions were made, and eventually supervised experience was recognized as adequate preparation; Dock, 1235–56. Since membership in an organization "affiliating" with the American Nurses Association was required and most black nurses in the South were excluded from these organizations, there were few, if any, "qualified" southern black nurses. They could join the National Organization for Public Health Nursing; Darlene Clark Hine, *Black Women in White: Racial Conflict and Cooperation in the Nursing Profession, 1890–1950* (Bloomington: Indiana University Press, 1989), 91–95. See Jane Van De Vrede, director, Bureau of Public Health Nursing, "Southern Division Report of the Bureau of Public Health Nursing; July 1919 to January 1, 1920," folder no. 149.18, PHN, ARC, NA.

16. Ibid.

17. Dock, 1295–99. Records of the Charleston, S.C., Red Cross Public Health Nursing Service are at the Carolina Low Country Chapter office in North Charleston. Red Cross Executive Committee 13 March 1919, Red Cross, Charleston Chapter (hereafter cited as RC, CC). See memo written by Virginia M. Gibbs and sent by Elizabeth Fox to all Division Directors, Public Health Nursing Service, 1 March 1920, folder no. 140.18, PHN, ARC, NA.

18. Ibid. The Ladies Benevolent Society Collection records (hereafter cited as the LBS Papers) are at the South Carolina Historical Society, Charleston, S.C. The LBS claims to be the country's oldest women's organization, since the Female Benevolent Society of Wiscasset, Maine, which was founded in 1805 no longer exists. Margaret Simons Middleton, "The Ladies Benevolent Society of Charleston, S.C.," *The Yearbook of the City of Charleston* (YCC) (Charleston, 1941), 216–39. For a more detailed discussion of the LBS's history see, Karen Buhler-Wilkerson, "Caring in Its Proper Place: Race and Benevolence in Charleston, S.C., 1813–1930," *Nursing Research* 41 (January/February 1992): 14–20.

19.   Minutes of the Board, 14 February 1919, LBS Papers.

20.   Ibid., and Gibbs Memo, 1 March 1920, LBS Papers.

21.   At the end of the first eleven months, the staff of three to five nurses had made 9,182 visits at a cost of $7,641. They cared for an average of 342 patients a month, making approximately 8 to 10 visits a day. Annual Report Red Cross Nursing Activity Committee for 1921 and April and May 1921, Monthly Report of the Red Cross Board, RC, CC. See also American Red Cross Department of Nursing, Bureau of Public Health Nursing monthly reports for 1920, PHN, ARC, NA.

22.   Interview with Marie Mikell Lebby (Mrs. Thomas C. Boushall), February 1991 in Richmond, Va. At the time she was one hundred years old. She is still living and pleased to have her story told.

23.   Ibid. Lebby's father would not let her accept a Red Cross Scholarship for her studies or spend her salary on things such as expensive clothes, because he was concerned people would think he could not support her. She apparently went off with her family for several weeks that summer to the mountains where she helped with a well baby clinic.

24.   The quote is a comment made by Betty Hamilton, a family friend and neighbor, who has known the Lebby family for years; interview with Karen Buhler-Wilkerson, January 1991, Charleston, S.C. Minutes of the Board, January 1921, 14 February 1919, LBS Papers.

25.   Lebby's public relations activities were discussed at the 6 January 1921 meeting. Lebby was finally expected to join the Red Cross on a full-time basis November 1920, but found it impossible to assume these duties. She did agree to stay on part-time until they could secure a permanent supervisor, which they would do "as soon as we know where we stand financially." Report of the Nurses Activities Committee, 4 November 1920. The proposal came from the Nurse Committee to the Executive Committee, 29 November 1920. These plans were discussed with Jane Van De Vrede, the head of the Division Office, who reminded the board that they must insist on the city following the standards required by the Red Cross at the 2 December 1920 Board Meeting. The mass meeting is discussed in the 28 January 1921 meeting. See Board Minutes, RC, CC.

26.   Between 1913 and 1931, twenty-eight Red Cross Chapters were operating public health nursing programs in South Carolina. By 1936, only two remained; 48 percent had discontinued operations within the first four years of operation. Almost half had been organized in 1920. See Rosa Hayward Clark, "History and Development of Public Health Nursing in S.C." (South Carolina State Board of Health, February 1942), 14–17, 34. The idea for the LBS to take over the Red Cross service originated with Lebby. See Minutes of the Nursing Activities Committee, 4 April 1921, RC, CC. The Red Cross proposal for takeover was first presented to the LBS Board by Marie Lebby. A week later, Georgia Jatho, chair of the Nursing Committee of the Red Cross, met with the LBS Board to further discuss their plan. See Minutes of the Board, 8 April 1921 and 15 April 1921, LBS Papers.

27.   See Minutes of the Society, 21 April 1921, 6 May 1921, and 1 June 1921, LBS Papers.

28.   Ibid.

29. The Red Cross decision to abandon their standards was reported in the 26 May 1921 minutes, RC, CC. The vote to support the new organization is reported in the 5 January 1922 minutes of the Annual Meeting. The discussion of the future role of the chapter is reported in the 1924 Annual Report, Charleston Chapter Red Cross. See Clarke, 34. The fortune of the Charleston Chapter of the Red Cross continued to decline. By 1923 their membership had dropped to 1,472 and there was only $3,486 in the treasury, Annual Report, 1924, RC, CC.

30. Leon Banov, *As I Recall: The Story of the Charleston County Health Department* (Columbia, S.C.: R. L. Bryan Co., 1970). When the Charleston County Health Department took over the Charleston Public Health Nursing Association's work, they employed four nurses, a supervisor, and several other workers who had previously been employees of this association. This was reported in the Annual Meeting Records, February 1924, RC, CC. See also Clarke, 24–27. See the Reports for the Department of Health, YCC, 1920, 1922, and 1924. A little over a year later, hearing of MLI's objection to the LBS's "colored nurses," the same association wrote that they would refrain from offering their services to MLI until they found it impossible for LBS to comply with MLI's demand that "white nurses be employed." Minutes of the Board, 9 February 1923, LBS Papers. It is unclear if MLI contracted with the Charleston Public Health Nursing Association to care for their policyholders, but in May of 1924 the company opened an independent nursing service. The Metropolitan Life Insurance Company's nursing service was caring for around 200 cases and making 1,854 visits annually while the LBS visited about 230 cases, making 1,394 visits annually. Louise Tattershall, *Public Health Nursing in the United States: January 15, 1931* (New York: National Organization for Public Health Nursing, 1931).

31. Annual Report Book, 1906–1930, see Reports for 1923–1930 for Patient Data, see especially drafts of the Annual Report for 1924, p. 83; "The Ladies Benevolent Society Elects Its Officers for Ensuing Year," Report of the Annual Meeting for 1925; "The Ladies Benevolent Society Meets," Annual Report for 1923, p. 82, LBS Papers. Ravenel, who had presided over the annual meetings for forty-four years, was unable to attend the 1930 meeting. Ravenel died on 6 March 1933 and had conducted business from her bedroom through the Junior Superintendent for some time before her death. Middleton, 239.

32. In Charleston this saying is such a tradition that one of the local TV stations uses "In Charleston, We Trust the People We Know" as their advertisement. For a Canadian version of the complex local situations nurses are sent to save, see Meryn Stuart, "'Half a Loaf Is Better Than No Bread': Public Health Nurses and Physicians in Ontario, 1920–1925," *Nursing Research* 41 (January/February 1992): 21–27.

9

"Strange Young Women on Errands": Obstetric Nursing Between Two Worlds[1]

Judith Walzer Leavitt

Today when most American women deliver their babies in the hospital, they can predict and even help to shape the patterns of care they receive from their nurses and physicians. But many of the first generation of women to give birth in the hospital—from the 1930s into the 1950s—did not find that the hospital met their needs and expectations. Some complained bitterly that they did not feel welcome in this new institutional setting, blaming both nurses and physicians for their feelings of alienation. One woman wrote that she felt "alone among strangers" in the hospital; another remembered that "No one kind reassuring word was spoken by nurse or doctor."[2] Birthing women sometimes heaped their harshest judgments on their nurses. Ann Rivington's story of her 1933 confinement in a city hospital pointedly focused the brunt of her ire upon her nurses:

> I went there with no false expectations of luxury or coddling, with no fond hopes of ease or comfort even. But a certain adequate minimum of care I did consider my right . . . [I was] left lying in the emergency room. . . . The nurses were cynical and cruel to everyone on the ward. . . . We were all obsessed with a mad desire to get away.[3]

Six years later, in an article recounting her hospital delivery, Lenore Pelham Friedrich wrote that "the early morning waking, the constant running in and out of strange young women on errands such as count-

---

Note: This chapter was originally published in *Nursing History Review* 6 (1998): 3–24. A publication of the American Association for the History of Nursing.

ing blankets, are painful memories to nearly every sensitive maternity patient."[4] Many women perceived that their nurses showed a distinct lack of sympathy for the discomforts and pain of labor and delivery. Why did these birthing women view their hospital-based obstetric nurses so negatively? Why did they not see their nurses as helpmates during this stressful time? This paper explores parturient women's negative impressions of the hospital nurses who staffed the maternity wards from the 1930s through the 1950s to analyze how and why one group of women reported a seeming lack of empathy emanating from another group of women in the hospital setting.

Before the 20th century, almost all American women had their babies at home.[5] A few poor urban women (probably not more than 5% of the total) went to charity hospitals or medical school dispensaries in the late 18th and 19th centuries, but this was rarely because of choice. Women considered their own homes, where they could be surrounded by familiar women friends and relatives, to be the most desirable birth setting, and both midwives and doctors entered this domestic woman-centered environment to attend labor and delivery. The system worked well because it met social expectations and in most cases it resulted in live deliveries. Furthermore, it allowed women who had some financial options to combine traditional practices with medicine's ever-evolving innovations. Women could avail themselves of physicians' medical expertise while keeping their comforting bedroom location and their women helpers. Increasingly by the turn of the 20th century, trained private-duty nurses, new medical technology, and obstetrical expertise were available in women's homes. Birthing women could, in short, get what seemed to be the best of both worlds of women's tradition and men's medicine. Anita McCormick Blaine, for example, whose economic and social position in Chicago allowed her to choose optimal care when she first became pregnant in 1890, determined to have her baby in her childhood home surrounded by friends and relatives. "Every chair and table speaks to me of dear familiar times," Anita wrote to her mother, "I never can be able to tell you what peace comes to me from being in this home of all my girlhood now . . . I am so grateful that my sweet baby can come to me here." While a woman friend and a trained nurse supported her, and her husband waited outside the room, a physician administered chloroform and delivered her child. Blaine wanted and got the traditional home birth experience accompanied by the most that medicine and nursing at the time had to offer.[6]

In the 20th century, middle- and upper-class women like Anita Blaine and the growing number of physicians who specialized in obstetrics increasingly found fault with these home-based childbirth practices. The application of the new knowledge about bacteriology and germ transmission particularly made home deliveries difficult to manage. From both birthing women and their physicians came pressure to change procedures and to modernize birth by moving it to the hospital.[7]

In part women's desires to go to the hospital in the first third of the 20th century reflected merely one more instance of a movement that had begun in the 18th century, when male physicians first began attending normal births in this country. Since that time, women who could afford them sought out the newest technological and medical advances in obstetrics. Middle-class women invited male physicians into their home birthing rooms to use forceps, ether, and chloroform and to perform surgical operations because they believed this would help them become living mothers of living children. Motivated in large part by fears of death and long-lasting debility that seemed the all too common results of childbirth, women embraced innovations in childbirth because many believed that "science" could deliver on its promise for an improved birth experience. The expectation that death or postpartum debility could just as likely result from childbirth as could life and health led women on a long search for better and safer births. In the 18th and 19th centuries the quest for improved birthing conditions led women to seek medical help in their homes. In the 20th century, it led American women into hospitals.

Modern streamlined hospital birth, under the observation and control of specialist nurses and doctors, seemed like the answer to women's prayers for physical comfort and safety. Some hospitals were so enticing that author Betty MacDonald, giving birth in the 1920s, recalled, "The prospect of two weeks in that heavenly place tempted me to stay pregnant all the rest of my life."[8] The hospital offered what many considered to be the safest application of the newest technological and scientific methods of birth. Furthermore, the environment, the food, the total care from the nurses all made the hospital stay seem like a vacation from domestic chores. Because of the dual attraction of new medicine and comfort, of safety and convenience, upper- and middle-class women increasingly sought an institutional location for their confinements. By 1940, 55% of America's births took place within hospitals; by 1950, hospital births had increased to 88% of the total; and by 1960, outside of some isolated rural areas, it was almost unheard of for American women to deliver their babies at home.

Seeking the newest and best way to have babies and convinced that hospitals had superseded traditional ways of giving birth, women wanted to believe that progress had finally come for them. The popular literature on childbirth in the 1920s and 1930s reveals their hopes that this almost universal experience of womankind could be made less dreadful through science. Articles in women's journals were filled with heartrending personal examples of women whose lives would have been saved if they had been in the hospital for their confinements. For example, *Good Housekeeping* told the story of Ann Hamilton, a young woman of "pioneer stock" who "loved America, its traditions, its ideals, and its promises for the future in which her children would have their part." Hamilton had a protracted labor at home in 1920 attended by a general practitioner who "did his best, but . . . had nothing with which to work" and by a neighbor who "was not a trained nurse and did not know what to do." Her 60-hour labor ordeal resulted in her death, and in the death of her baby.[9] Through such emotion-laden examples, the possibilities of scientific obstetrics captivated birthing women, who, like the rest of the population, were determined to join the march of medical progress.

The hospital, lauded as the newest and best place for delivery, looked doubly attractive to women who could not create a supportive home atmosphere. As one woman put it: "Sure! It would be nice to have babies born at home! But who is going to bathe the baby . . . bring the mother's tray . . . change her sheets? Who?" In the 1920s and 1930s it became increasingly difficult to assemble and maintain home birth attendants. Home birth did not hold the same comforts and sustenance that Anita McCormick Blaine had found so reassuring in 1890. The "hospital is equipped with every modern device for the safe delivery of babies," wrote one mother, "nursing and medical attention is available at any hour of the day or night. How much simpler—and more restful—to be in a hospital where babies are an accepted business." Another woman found, "My stay in that hospital was like a lovely vacation." "I can't tell you the relief I feel as I walk out my door headed for the hospital to have a baby," wrote another. "I have nothing to worry about . . . and have only to concentrate on giving birth. All this peace of mind, plus expert medical attention, makes me wonder why anybody would consider it a "privilege" to have her baby at home."[10]

So growing numbers of women went to the hospital to give birth. Mothers-to-be learned they could plan when they would have a baby, and doctors could predict the course of labor because they controlled it with drugs and instruments. "The old way [of having a baby] was no fun," wrote one father about the 1916 birth of his first daughter. Twenty-two years later, in 1938, his second wife gave birth to another daughter, who "was born the new way—the easy, painless, streamlined way." His wife reflected in the *Reader's Digest*, "It's a good hour's ride by auto from our house in the country to the hospital in New York and for weeks I had nightmares of a mad dash in the dark over a sleety road, and all the stories I'd ever read of babies being born in taxicabs filled me with terror. So it was with vast relief I heard the doctor say: 'Come in to the hospital next Tuesday night and you'll have your baby Wednesday.' Just like that. It was like ordering something from a store." She and her husband took in a matinee and dinner before she checked into the hospital. The next morning pituitrin induced her labor, Nembutal and scopolamine deadened her perceptions and memory of it, and the doctor delivered her baby. "Why, I wouldn't mind having another baby next week," she said, "if that's all there is to it."[11] Increasing numbers of middle-class women turned to the hospital and the specialist for their births, believing, as one of them put it, "the vexation of hospital routine shrinks to infinitesimal importance beside the safety of the delivery room."[12] Second only to surgical suites in beckoning patients, maternity wards and maternity hospitals promised women the ultimate in modern and safe birth experiences.[13]

In most hospital deliveries, women left their families and friends at the door of the labor room and faced their birthings virtually alone, as one account of birth in the 1930s indicated:

> *Arriving [at the hospital], she is immediately given the benefit of one of the modern analgesics or pain-killers. Soon she is in a dreamy, half-conscious state at the height of a pain, sound asleep between spasms. . . . She knows nothing about being taken to a spotlessly clean delivery room, placed on a sterile table, draped with sterile sheets; neither does she see her attendants, the doctor and nurses, garbed for her protection in sterile white gowns and gloves; nor the shiny boiled instruments and antiseptic solutions. She does not hear the cry of her baby when first he feels the chill of this cold world, or see the care with which the doctor repairs such lacerations as may have occurred. She is, as most of us want to be when severe pain has us in its grasp—asleep. Finally she awakes in smiles, a mother with no recollection of having become one.*[14]

Not all hospitals followed these specific procedures, of course, but each did have its own practices and routines. Many birthing women opted for this kind of medicalized delivery. As Erva Slayton said, "I really selected the hospital from choice."[15]

But many other women, and these numbers increased from the 1930s through the 1950s, realized that physical removal of childbirth from their homes into medical institutions and the common use of analgesics and instruments often did not result in experiences they would have chosen. Margaret Budenz, in labor with her third child in 1943, was upset when her doctor told her that "books were not allowed in the labor room." A woman from Elkhart, Indiana, wrote, "So many women, especially first mothers, who are frightened to start out with, receive such brutal inconsiderate treatment that the whole thing is a horrible nightmare. They give you drugs, whether you want them or not, strap you down like an animal." A woman from Columbus, Ohio, concurred that a new mother was "foiled in every attempt to follow her own wishes."[16]

Many normal deliveries are turned into nightmares for the mothers by "routine" obstetrical practices. I have had two such experiences. My [next] baby will be born at home, despite the sterile advantages of a hospital confinement, for I feel the accompanying emotional disadvantages are just not worth it.[17]

In the hospital the familiar supports disappeared, and in their place came only the impersonal bustle of starched skirts, the thermometer poked in the mouth, and the whispers of unfamiliar people speaking among themselves. One woman remembered her 1935 confinement as a "nightmare of impersonality" during which she felt "helpless" and "like a pawn in a strange game." Others remembered being "all alone," "abandoned" and "lonely . . . knowing no one." One woman found her hospital experience so traumatic that, she wrote, "Months later I would scream out loud and wake up remembering that lonely labor room and just feeling no one cared what happened to me . . . I was treated as if I was an inanimate object."[18]

Obstetrical nurses often received the brunt of the blame for these alienating experiences. Hospital nursing had expanded alongside the exploding numbers of hospitals in the early 20th century, and, during the 1930s and 1940s, graduate nurses began replacing student apprentices as staff (or floor) nurses. In 1929, 4,000 graduate nurses worked in staff positions, but by 1941—only 12 years later—their number had grown to over 100,000, more than the number of private duty nurses and students combined.[19] Hospital nursing differed significantly from home-based private duty nursing, whether obstetrical or medical. In homes nurses worked for a single physician and took care of individual patients. Isolated from their fellow nurses and on call around the clock, they worked alone. In hospitals nurses worked with many physicians and were responsible for multiple patients simultaneously. They worked, in 1941, 48-hour weeks, often, however, in split shifts. They had the company of other nurses. The generation that switched from home to hospital nursing sometimes equated being back in the hospital with their student days and resented their sudden lack of autonomy. On the other hand, many came to understand and appreciate the benefits of the companionship of their peers.[20]

The biggest adjustment hospital-based graduate nurses faced was the loss of a one-to-one relationship with their patients. There were positive parts to this transition, however. Nursing historian Barbara Melosh has noted, "Institutional nursing released nurses from the vestiges of personal service that clung to private duty. As one former private-duty nurse commented, 'I don't have to entertain the patient and help trim last year's hat!'" Melosh demonstrated how nurses turned this to their workplace advantage:

Responsible for more than one patient, the nurse could limit the demands of any one person. She could excuse herself from one room to answer real or imaginary summons from another quarter, or seek a brief refuge from the entire floor by retreating to the nurses' station or the nurses' lounge. . . . By disciplining patients to their proper roles, nurses avoided many of the disadvantages of private duty and could negotiate some respite from the quickening pace of hospital work.[21]

The reverse of such possible benefits was that in moving further from patients' beds, nurses felt a loss of what had drawn them to nursing in the first place, the personal interactions and caring for people. They still, as historian Susan Reverby pointed out, "changed dressings, performed complex procedures, or prepared patients for the operating room." Nevertheless, they spent more and more time "coordinating patient activities, handing out medications, writing nursing notes, performing clerical duties, and organizing the work of an increasingly complex staff. The nurse became tied to the nurses' station, whereas patients became disembodied voices on an intercom system or a cup of pills on a medication chart."[22]

The biggest change for maternity nursing was that most hospitals did not allow nurses to follow patients from early labor throughout their hospital stay. Instead they compartmentalized maternity care into labor, delivery, and postpartum duties, and different nurses cared for babies in the separate nursery.[23] Hospitals strictly defined and structured maternity care, especially to try to prevent the occurrence of puerperal infections.[24] Supervisors mapped out careful procedures and required nurses to follow strict protocol. One nurse called it a "rigid, mechanized system of caring for mother and baby. . . . Assembly-line thinking helped to create the problem of impersonalized, assembly-line care." She concluded that the nurse was caught between her "two masters—physician and institution" and had to comply with the regulations or risk losing her job.[25]

Hospitals required nurses to focus on procedures such as shaving and giving enemas, while at the same time they had to try to remain obedient to doctors.[26] Mildred Green, a 1931 nursing graduate, recalled that as a staff nurse, because of all the prescribed routines, she did not have very much time to spend with mothers. She remembered that nurses

saw the necessity of seeing that [the patient] got her medication if it was ordered. That she got fluids. That her blood pressure was checked. That the fetal heart tones were checked. That every half-hour or so someone went in and checked frequency and strength and duration of contractions and that they were properly recorded. You kept track of her bladder to see whether it was full or not. . . . You watched for signs of progression of labor and watch for the blood to show . . . the nurses were in disgrace if you didn't get the mother to the [delivery] room on time.[27]

The ideal of obstetric nursing emphasized that nurses must carefully follow routines and act as physicians' associates. As C. M. Hall wrote, "In obstetric nursing, as in all fields of nursing, the student nurse is taught to be an intelligent associate to the physician . . . to prepare for his every need, to anticipate his wants, to carry out his orders accurately and intelligently."[28]

Barbara Melosh and Susan Reverby have described how hospital nursing in these years came under the rule of the efficiency experts, most especially Frank and Lillian Gilbreth and Frederick Winslow Taylor. While a positive evaluation of the move for efficiency might emphasize nurses' "link between service and science" (as Melosh called it)[29] or see it as "new techniques of scientific management" (in Reverby's words),[30] the new focus on time and motion efficiency also significantly depersonalized maternity care. Nurses' ward work was reduced to its smallest components, and at the same time, women's labor, delivery, and postpartum weeks were routinized in a strict and formal schedule. Nurses awakened hospitalized postpartum women for early temperature taking, and nurses monitored and forced women to follow strict rules about eating, defecating, and exercising. Women stayed in bed exactly 10 days following delivery, they dangled their legs on the 11th day, they sat in a chair on the 12th day, they walked on the 13th, and went home on the 14th. Nurses adhered to routine, bed-panning pre- and postpartum women alike every four hours, whether they needed it or not. They fed babies, too, on a rigid four-hour schedule. They kept assiduous records of each and every activity. The resulting task-oriented style of nurses' work contributed to the impersonal, assembly line kind of care that parturient women described as annoying and hateful. As routines governed nurses' ward work, individual care, and certainly individual patient need, receded.[31]

Bacteriological understanding of the causes of puerperal infection led to a lot of attention to scrupulous cleanliness in hospital maternity routine, and it fell to nurses to maintain good aseptic techniques. But the high priority on cleanliness often blurred the line between nursing and housekeeping. Despite Florence Nightingale's insistence that "nurses should not scour, it is a waste of power," maternity nurses in early 20th-century American hospitals were often involved in cleaning, scrubbing and waxing floors, folding laundry, cleaning and sterilizing equipment. As one nursing historian put it, "Care of laboring women had to compete for nursing time with care of the supplies and cleaning the rooms. During very busy times with many laboring women, the cleaning tasks mounted proportionally and nurses had to scurry to keep rooms and instruments ready for the next anticipated births."[32]

Eleanor Waddel, a 1946 nursing graduate who spent her career in Wisconsin, recalled that in addition to watching over many patients,

We didn't have cleaning women, you know. . . . I also took care of the . . . water sterilizer. . . . I knew how to pack those . . . we made our own sponges. We made our own Kotex . . . if there was any cleaning that needed to be done, we did it . . . we were carrying commode buckets a great deal. . . . We washed all of our bloody linens. Everything. You could have ten deliveries [and] all the bloody linen was washed and we did it. We washed it. Who mopped the floors? When I worked nights, every morning before I went off duty I mopped the whole delivery room suite and took the mop to the roof . . . these are the things you do. You know, this is part of your job. I mean, if you have the time the walls get washed."[33]

One nurse recalled her cleaning duties as a student nurse in obstetrics as more onerous than similar duties on other services and offered this as the reason she did not want to go near obstetrics wards as a graduate. Obstetric nursing students "made dressings, cleaned, packaged, and sterilized supplies, sharpened needles, and patched holes in rubber gloves. [We] mended and folded laundry, scrubbed, scoured and polished floors, walls, and fixtures." She stated, "I just detested obstetrics as a student! To me, obstetrics was autoclaves, formula room, cleaning the delivery room and zonked out women."[34] Another nurse recalled of her obstetric service, "We didn't do one-to-one nursing, we made rounds on people to see if they needed hypos and did vital signs. That was done every four hours . . . we just had an incredible amount of other duties we had to accomplish to keep the place running, linen, making packs, gloves, it was just incredible. You tried to balance all those insurmountable tasks along with watching patients."[35] Between the routines and the cleaning duties and the numbers of simultaneously laboring patients, what time did hospital obstetric nurses have for individualized patient care?

From the birthing woman's point of view, these impersonal routines defined nurses' behavior, and in the process nurses seemed to lose their compassion, humanity, or even common sense. Elsa Rosenberg, herself a nurse, delivered a baby in a different hospital from the one in which she trained and practiced. She said that when the nurses realized she was Jewish, they "gave a back-log of complaints against their previous Jewish patients." Although bothered by such categorizing and stigmatizing of patients, Rosenberg was even more disturbed by the care she received at the hands of these nurses. She related that during her labor the nurses came by regularly, with pen in hand, "stood at the door and called in, no one looked at my pad to check the bleeding, they would poke their heads in and ask if the pains had started yet and then dash madly off before you could ask them anything." Finally a student nurse came inside the room to time her contractions. "She did not examine me, she tucked the sheets in very tight around me, since she said the doctor would be coming in to see me and the bed was to be tidy, she wouldn't let me draw up my legs, or move because the bed was to remain tidy." Rosenberg thought herself nearing full dilatation, but she could not convince the floor nurse or the student that her labor had moved along so quickly.

> *[The student nurse] went and sat on the window sill. It was January 25th and the window area was cold, so she turned up the heat. My bed was right next to the radiator and I just couldn't take the heat, but SHE was cold. I kept screaming that the baby was coming, and she said to me, "Mrs. Rosenberg, this is your first baby, the first baby takes from 12 to 18 hours of pain and you have only been in pain a matter of minutes, so you had better make up your mind that you are going to tolerate a little bit of pain."*

When the supervisor next appeared in the doorway, the student nurse repeated to her that Mrs. Rosenberg thought she was ready to deliver but that she needed to labor 12 to 18 hours before delivery, obviously reciting facts she had learned from the book or classroom. Needless to say, Rosenberg was fully dilated, her perineum bulging, the baby's head crowning, and she was experiencing an urgent urge to push when the nurse finally checked her. They rushed her to the delivery room, while the student nurse held her legs together, and instructed her not to push. But Rosenberg wrote, "Well, I didn't want my legs held together to stop the baby, and possibly cause damage by stopping the oxygen and if the baby was going to come, it was going to come when it was ready and not to suit their timetable, so I gave the [student nurse] a punch that sent her sprawling, and then I spread my legs and pushed!"[36]

Parturients wrote many such stories about nurses who held back babies until physicians could be summoned. "I was strapped on the delivery table," wrote a woman from Marietta, Georgia. "My doctor had not arrived and the nurses held my legs together. I was helpless and at their mercy. They held my baby back until the doctor came into the room." A Wisconsin woman related that "When the nurse finally examined me she called for another nurse to call the doctor immediately while she strapped my legs together and gave me ether to hold the baby until the doctor arrived." A California woman wrote, "The doctor dropped by at 6:45, cast me a scornful glance and went out to make house calls. One hour later my legs were released from the stirrups and held together by a nurse, who sat on my knees, up on the delivery table, mind you, because the baby was coming too fast. A few minutes after 8 o'clock, the doctor arrived and allowed my baby to be born."[37]

It was hard for birthing women to understand the pressures their nurses were under absolutely to obey physicians' orders. The nurses knew all too well that failure to wait for specific physician instructions, even if that meant holding the women's legs together, could jeopardize their careers. While there are many stories of nurses risking physicians' wrath and delivering babies themselves without being so instructed, many other nurses felt unable to act outside of specific orders, knowing such action could lead to their dismissal. Nurses' priorities were established by others.[38]

Various complaints about obstetrics nurses' insensitive behavior toward their patients reached the public. Ann Rivington delivered one of her children in a city hospital in New York in the 1930s, and wrote her story in the popular magazine *American Mercury*. She understood that the care she received in a public hospital would be less than a woman might expect in a private hospital or ward. But, she insisted, "We were the mothers of citizens," and should have access to a required minimum of care. "Why, for example, was I left lying in the emergency room more than half an hour before I was examined?" she asked. "If everybody had been busy, I could have accepted the situation without a thought. But all the while two internes and three nurses sat in the room eating ice-cream and gossiping, while I lay in pain and uncertainty."[39] Rivington admitted that some of the nurses she witnessed during her stay in the hospital tried to be kind despite their heavy work loads, but she described them more often as acting with "callous indifference" and "cruelty." She wrote about a nurse "sitting in the corridor reading a popular magazine, . . . deaf to [women's] cries for help." She told the poignant stories of her fellow postpartum ward mates.

> *There was, for example, the case of the young Irish girl and the bed-pan. . . . At a quarter to two in the afternoon, she first asked for a bed-pan. Visiting hours began at three. It was not until half past two that the pan was brought to her, and when three o'clock came, the nurse had not yet taken it away. Instead, a screen was placed around the girl's bed, and she was told that as punishment for the trouble she had caused she might wait till five o'clock, when all the guests were gone.*

Rivington thought that nurses treated immigrant and African American women most cruelly. She related a tale of a Black woman on her ward:

> *I noticed that the nurse who was supposed to cleanse her body would scarcely touch her. She was forced to handle her own bed-pan, though it was against the rules for her to do so. One day she complained. "You're a smart nigger, aren't you?" said the nurse. "You're dirty anyhow. All the filth comes from your part of town." The girl answered pluckily, "I ain't bein' smart. You treat us like dogs around here, but we're human, that's all." "I'll call Dr. X—," the nurse threatened. "All right. Go ahead and call him." . . . The doctor was not called. But from that moment the girl was singled out for*

special unkindness and neglect. "They don't wash me at all no more," she confided to me, "but you know what I do? I sneak out of bed and wash myself, late at night. I can't stand to be dirty."[40]

Rivington told the story with great admiration for the woman whose behavior only brought on more "withering sarcasm that only a very courageous soul could withstand."

The revelations in two compilations of maternity ward stories printed in the *Ladies' Home Journal* in May and December, 1958, added fuel to this fire of protest against obstetric nurses. One woman wrote about her experiences in a Chicago suburban hospital: "I wonder if the people who ran that place were actually human. My lips parched and cracked, but the nurses refused to even moisten them with a damp cloth. I was left alone all night in a labor room. I felt exactly like a trapped animal. . . . Never have I needed someone, anyone, as desperately as I did that night." Another woman wrote, "I remember screaming, "help me, help me!" to a nurse who was sitting at a nearby desk. She ignored me." And the woman who wrote, "I have listened to nurses laughing at other new mothers who were crying out in pain, I have heard other mothers being slapped and threatened with dead babies and misfits. I heard these things while I waited for the births of my second and third babies. What happens to the women who are threatened this way and then do deliver a misfit or a stillborn? Do they spend the rest of their lives blaming themselves? Do the words of these sadistic nurses . . . forever ring in their ears?"

Some registered nurses added their voices to the chorus in the popular women's magazine. One related, "I have seen nurses . . . become impatient (or worse) with a patient and express their feelings, often within her hearing. 'She got herself in this fix and now is a poor time to change her mind'" Another nurse admitted, "I have seen careless and callous treatment of obstetrical patients, along with indifference and discourtesy. . . . I have seen nurses be careless in screening patients from public view during procedures requiring their bodies to be exposed, to the outrage of the patients' feelings of modesty. I have heard such unthinking remarks as 'You had your fun, now you can suffer' made by a nurse to a mother in great distress."[41]

Antisemitism, racism, cruelty, and callous disregard for individual needs: This does not sound like nursing! Nor does it in any way resemble the nursing texts or literature from the period. Nurses were nowhere being taught to act like these stories indicate they did. How should historians interpret these repeated reports of indifferent, cruel, and even seemingly sadistic nurses?

Barbara Melosh offered this explanation: "No doubt harried nurses on understaffed wards did sometimes become curt and impatient, and when they were forced to cut corners, they did not always have time to dispense 'TLC' (tender loving care). But the tone of many comments about the new breed of nurses also suggests another interpretation." Melosh believes "the nurse had grown too scientific and gained too much control of her patient to satisfy sentimental expectations of nursing as womanly duty."[42]

I agree that the significant routinization of nursing activity during these years accounts for some of these negative reactions. No longer was maternity nursing a one-on-one interaction, in which a birthing woman could expect singular attention from her attendant. No longer were women in their own homes where they might expect to be the center of attention, surrounded by people who knew and loved them. No longer were nurses able to give their full attention to any individual woman in labor. The hospital and the medical routines, in the name of science, had superseded this personal, home-based kind of care. And we can understand why birthing women, especially at the height of their labor pains or in the throes of their postpartum adjustment, might miss this individual attention and interpret anything short of it as inadequate to their needs. But this interpretation that patients were reacting to nurses who were only acting scientific or controlling falls short, I think, when applied specifically to maternity wards for two reasons: one, it does not recognize that women had come to hospitals specifically seeking so-called scientific care because they viewed it as superior to what was available to them at home, and two, patients on other wards in the hospital did not complain quite like maternity patients did, which seems to mean that there was something specific in the obstetric interaction itself that explains these negative perceptions. Furthermore, the complaints, when we look at them closely, were not about cold scientific care, they were about lack of care and insensitive treatment; they were the cries of women who felt ignored and in danger.[43]

The early generations of birthing women who went to the hospital were women who would have tolerated a lot to be assured of safe deliveries, of coming out of the encounter as the "living mother of a living child." If they had been convinced that the routinized and lonely care they received in the hospital was safer than what they had been used to at home, they might have resigned themselves to it. They were a pro-science group; they wanted science to work for them to make birth more comfortable and safer. Hospitals had promised safer childbirth, but in the years before antibiotics, their maternal mortality statistics were actually no better than those recorded for home deliveries.[44]

What did science contribute to the obstetric encounter? First, bacteriology taught physicians and nurses the importance of what they called at the time "scrupulous cleanliness." Postpartum infections killed more new mothers than any other single cause, and asepsis had proved its value. Nurses, as the primary attendants on birthing women in the hospital, had to take major responsibility in this area, which was an onerous burden, especially given the numbers of patients over whom they watched and the way deliveries seemed to stack up over the course of a day. But perhaps even more onerous for those nurses who had entered the field to care for people was the imperative of record keeping so that anyone could trace back and find the problem if something went wrong. The kind of detail that was asked for precluded nurses from their caring tasks and instead relegated them to an intense concentration on putting down the right numbers in the right places on patients' charts. To birthing women—who complained that nurses stood in the doorway and didn't make eye contact as they asked their rushed questions—it seemed as if successful births were only to be measured through physical and quantitative measures. It seemed as if the new hospital procedures, in these respects, left women alone while their attendants scurried about "on errands." Science seemed to create a wedge between birthing women and their female attendants.

It was science the birthing women sought when they came to the hospital to give birth. It was science that helped to define nursing duties. But science did not actually define all of nurses' interactions with birthing women in the hospitals from the 1930s through the 1950s. First, the science of obstetrics, if we can call it that, was still quite underdeveloped in this period, and obstetricians like Joseph B. DeLee still battled to get basic methods established.[45] Women who went to the hospital, and the nurses who worked there, both certainly understood that it was not "scientific" to sit on a woman's legs to delay the birth of her baby. Second, science was not the only set of principles governing the hospital maternity ward setting. Social issues remained of overriding importance in this period.

Much of the hostility and negativity in obstetric nurses' interactions with birthing women can best be explained by the very different expectations and needs the two groups of women brought to their encounters. Birthing women brought with them to their hospitalized births (consciously and unconsciously) a cultural memory about their own or their friends' and relatives' home-based birth experiences that allowed them to realize what some of the problems were in the hospital setting. They knew, for example, that the course of labor could not always be predicted. They knew from their own experiences that women should not be left alone during the long and difficult hours of labor. They came to the hospital expecting nurses to substitute for the family and friends in home deliveries in addition to adding the benefits of medical advances. At home people had been around them constantly, checking labor progress not just in degrees of dilatation but in emotional responses. These traditional birth attendants provided psychological support, emotional support, and practical physical support. Around the birthing bed, they held the parturient, they coached her, they told stories about their own deliveries, they answered worried questions. They provided what historians have called a "social" cushion of help for the woman as she wended or struggled her way through labor and delivery. This support system was rooted in society's gender system, where women helped other women through such trying gender-shared experiences. Traditional births created a set of gendered expectations that birthing women carried with them into the hospital. Despite all their longings for the benefits of science, they did not—could not—leave behind these other expectations of how women should behave toward one another, especially at such a critical time as labor and delivery. This is not "sentimental expectations of nursing as womanly duty" as Barbara Melosh put it, but deep, age-old commitments women had to one another that formed the very core of their community interactions and identity. These were the powerful gendered expectations that birthing women brought with them to the hospital, where they got transferred to nurses in this new 20th-century context. But in the hospital context these gender bonds cracked and broke under the strain of hospital routine.

The women who were writing to *Ladies' Home Journal* and to each other about the callous and cruel nurses they encountered in the hospitals wrote from this point of view and with these memories and these needs. To them, the nurses should have fulfilled both the tasks of the new science and the tasks of the old social childbirth. But instead, birthing women found that nurses, usually the only women present during labor and delivery in the hospital, seemed to ignore the social aspects of birthing women's expectations; sometimes it seemed even as if they gave short shrift to the scientific ones! The routines, the formalities—keeping the bed neat for the doctor, producing charts, and making sure the doctor delivered the baby even when that meant holding it back—seemed to take over considered judgment about what constituted good obstetrical care and they certainly overruled individualized, genderized, "social" care. The nurses' responses to women's cries for traditional support seemed like rejection and seemed to underscore the bad feelings of an increasingly alien hospital environment.

The nurses whom these birthing women encountered in the hospital had a very different perspective. The married, largely unemployed, upper-middle or middle-class birthing women who wrote most of the accounts that we have available to us met mostly unmarried, often younger, working- or middle-class women who were trying to earn their living in a difficult and competitive arena.[46] The two groups did not share many of life's experiences. Nurses worked for their living in a very hierarchical,

male-dominated medical system. The nurses struggled under two masters—the physicians, who placed strict expectations on them based on
medical knowledge and their own ideas of the personal service they
needed, and the hospitals, which imposed highly regulated notions of
efficient behavior routines. The gender system the nurses knew best was
the one that defined women's roles as subservient to men, the nurses'
role as determined by male medicine and hospital administrations. The
gender hierarchy in medicine and nursing was so stark that it actually
defined how the two professions regarded each other. Nurses lived with
the male/female, doctor/nurse distinction. How could they be expected
to traverse the labor room minefield to meet yet another set of gendered
expectations? Yet meet the traditional ideas that birthing women brought
into their labor rooms they did.

Obstetric nurses were, thus, struggling against and contending with
two gender systems. Their particular situation as women caring for women
during a time of the quintessentially female act of bringing forth the next
generation separated them from their nursing colleagues on other wards,
who dealt with male patients or with women hospitalized for reasons
other than bearing children. At the same time as they were judged by
their patients on criteria established outside medicine, outside the hospital, even outside nursing—in the domestic world of the home, ruled
by traditional women's values and activities—obstetric nurses lived very
much in a world that was ruled by medicine, by the hospital, and by tight
nursing codes. If they resisted hospital and medical requirements, they
risked losing their jobs; if they did not, they risked the opprobrium of
their women patients. The obstetric nurses of this period truly were caught
between the two worlds and the two gender systems.

The strident and angry tone of the birthing women's criticisms of
obstetric nurses as well as the nurses' own reported sarcasm and cruelty
can, I think, be accounted for by these reasons. The two groups of women
came at different moments in their lives from very different experiences
into the same world, the hospital, where, even in the same room, they
occupied very different spaces. Their femaleness did not provide enough
of a commonality for them to see the world through the others' eyes or
for their communication to be easy. Their differences, sometimes in
marital status, socioeconomic class, work experience, and needs, and
often even motherhood itself, were too great for them to be expected
easily to span the gap and understand one another. Their differences
in terms of defined status in the delivery room were most significant:
the nurses were employed and at work, in thrall to their job definitions,
while the birthing women labored to deliver their babies in a space not
their own. And science, which might have helped to bridge the distance
between them, since it represented values and ideals both groups sub-

scribed to, was not yet well enough developed in the field of obstetrics to provide the needed glue.

Birthing women and obstetric nurses from the 1930s through the 1950s lashed out against each other when they felt their goals misunderstood and their needs ignored. Both groups felt their own vulnerability in a male-dominated world of hospital medicine. Nurses displayed a lack of sympathy to women in pain when the parturients disrupted their already overcrowded and precarious schedules. Their apparent callous disregard stemmed from frustration about their lack of power and control over their own working conditions. Caught up in the tensions decreed by hospital rules and routines, an out-of-order bedpan request seemed to threaten to topple the whole foundation. Nurses had to give priority to their own concerns about their positions within the male-dominated, gendered work environment that bound them. To the extent that birthing women were critical of the nurses, they acted from their own positions of vulnerability, having moved outside their own homes where they had been in control of their birth experiences into this new world of institutions in which they were no more than objects on an assembly line. They sought their own traditional gendered connections when they moved from their homes into the hospital. The timing of the meeting—the early years of hospital-going birthing women and the early years of graduate nurses on hospital staffs—occurred when both groups were still groping for their own voice and place in the new context of the hospital. The dual vulnerabilities turned some of their encounters into confrontations.

The title of this chapter, "Strange Young Women on Errands," evokes the mountain of tradition and expectations that stood between birthing women and their hospital nurse attendants in this period. To birthing women the use of the word *strange* referred to traditional birth practices that suggested that unfamiliar people did not belong in the birthing room. A woman would by choice invite only women she knew and trusted to be with her at such a vulnerable time. *Young women* also referred back to tradition when unmarried women had been denied access to birthing rooms because of their presumed innocence and lack of experience. Only their own marriage and pregnancy would entitle them entrance into this women's sorority based on intimate female experience. *Errands* also was a word not congenial to the birth setting: women attendants were supposed to focus solely on the service to the parturient. They should not be running irrelevant errands like counting blankets. Even while hoping for science's benefits, birthing women in this transition generation groped for the security of what they knew best, women's traditional connections to one another.

Yet the nurses the women met in the hospital maternity wards had very different interpretations of those same words. To them *strange* defined their relationship with all their patients in the hospital environment, who they would not know personally. *Young women* merely stated who they were, some of them in hospital nursing only for a short time in their lives, usually before they married and had children. *Errands* was a word that could be used to describe many of the nurses' job routines as established for them by the physicians and hospitals for whom they worked. One group of women saw these words as problematic, the other saw them as commonplace.

The natural childbirth movement, which grew out of these alienating experiences, ultimately brought these two groups of women together. Sara Williams, Margarete Sandelowski, Margot Edwards, Mary Waldorf, and others have examined that period of childbirth history and have demonstrated how birthing women and their nurses after about 1960 came to see how strongly linked were their interests and destinies.[47] The story of hospital obstetric nursing as patient advocacy opened a very different chapter in nursing history than the one I have been describing here. Modern-day obstetrics is still very much influenced by gendered expectations, experiences, and interactions, but now birthing women and the nursing attendants see their common gender as a building block instead of a barrier. Today's nursing practices have grown out of the adversarial relationships that existed between nurses and birthing women for a time between 1930 and 1960. It took the period of conflict, perhaps, to produce today's more collaborative approaches. Out of pain do we bring forth children. From conflict we learn the benefits of cooperation.

Acknowledgments

I would like to thank Sarah Pfatteicher for her timely research assistance, Karen Walloch for her useful reading and comments, and the anonymous reviewers for their helpful suggestions. I especially want to thank Sara Williams. Her University of Wisconsin nursing MS thesis, "Caught in the Middle: Maternity Nurses and the Natural Childbirth Movement" (1987), and interviews with Madison-area nurses, the transcripts of which are in the State Historical Society of Wisconsin, were extremely valuable in the preparation of this chapter.

NOTES

1.　This is a revised version of a paper presented at the Twelfth Annual Conference on Nursing History, Little Rock, Arkansas, September 29, 1995. I am grateful to Pegge Bell, Joan Lynaugh, and Karen Buhler-Wilkerson for making the talk possible. I very much appreciate the helpful responses of the conference attendees and especially the suggestions for revision offered by Joan Lynaugh, Karen Buhler-Wilkerson, and Laura Ettinger.

2.　The problematic of this chapter developed out of my book, *Brought to*

Bed: Childbearing in America 1750–1950 (New York: Oxford University Press, 1986), specifically from a brief discussion on pp. 190–194. In this paper, to help the reader, I will provide the original references for the quotations used in both places. The first quotation is from a Montana woman quoted in Gladys Denny Shultz, "Journal Mothers Report on Cruelty in Maternity Wards," *Ladies' Home Journal* 75 (May 1958): 44–45. The second is from personal communications to the author from women answering a *New York Times Book Review* author's query of July 1983 (Clohessy, September 9, 1983).

3.   Ann Rivington, "Motherhood—Third Class," *American Mercury* 31 (February 1934): 160–165.

4.   Lenore Pelham Friedrich, "I Had a Baby," *Atlantic Monthly* 163 (April 1939): 461–465. See also "I Had a Baby Too: A Symposium," in *ibid.* (June 1939): 764–772.

5.   This account of the move to the hospital is derived from my book *Brought to Bed.*

6.   I examine Blaine's childbirth experience in *Brought to Bed*, 58–59, 89–90, 172–173, 201–202. The quotation is from Anita McCormick Blaine to Nettie Fowler McCormick, Aug. 24, 1890, Series 2B, Box 46, Nancy Fowler McCormick papers, Wisconsin State Historical Society.

7.   The issues surrounding the move to the hospital are explored in *Brought to Bed*, passim, and in my "The Medicalization of Childbirth in the Twentieth Century," *Transactions and Studies of the College of Physicians of Philadelphia* 11 (1989): 299–319.

8.   Betty MacDonald, *The Egg and I* (Philadelphia: Lippincott, 1945), 163.

9.   Rose Wilder Lane, "Mother No. 22,999," *Good Housekeeping* 88 (May 1926): 270.

10.   Women quoted in M.F. Ashley Montagu, "Babies Should Be Born at Home!" *Ladies' Home Journal* 72 (Aug. 1955): 52–53, and in Shultz, "Journal Mothers Report on Cruelty," 44.

11.   J.P. McEvoy, "Our Streamlined Baby," *Reader's Digest* 32 (May, 1938): 15–18.

12.   "I Had a Baby Too: A Symposium," *Atlantic Monthly* 163 (June, 1939): 768.

13.   Philip A. Kalisch and Beatrice J. Kalisch, *The Advance of American Nursing* (Boston: Little, Brown and Company, 1978), 343.

14.   Roy P. Finney, *The Story of Motherhood* (New York: Liverright, 1937), 6–7. See also Alan Frank Guttmacher, *Into This Universe: The Story of Human Birth* (New York: Blue Ribbon Books, 1937), 192–267.

15.   Erva Slayton to Mrs. Slayton (mother), Jan. 1, 1919. Slayton Family Collection, Michigan Historical Collection, Bentley Historical Library, University of Michigan.

16.   Margaret R. Budenz, *Streets* (Huntingdon, Ind.: Our Sunday Visitor, 1979), 266; quoted in Shultz, "Journal Mothers Report on Cruelty," 44–45.

17.   Shultz, "Journal Mothers Report on Cruelty," 45.

18.   Quotations are from personal communications to the author from women answering the *New York Times Book Review* author's query of July 1983. Quotes here from Katherine S. Egan, Aug. 25, 1983; Marilyn Clohessy, Sept. 9, 1983; Elsa Rosenberg, July 30, 1983; and others from letters by women who wish to remain anonymous.

19. Susan M. Reverby, *Ordered to Care: The Dilemma of American Nursing 1850–1945* (Cambridge: Cambridge University Press, 1987), 188.

20. See Reverby, *Ordered to Care*; Barbara Melosh, *"The Physician's Hand": Work Culture and Conflict in American Nursing* (Philadelphia: Temple University Press, 1982); Kalisches, *Advance of American Nursing*.

21. Melosh, *"The Physician's Hand,"* 191.

22. Reverby, *Ordered to Care*, 195.

23. Joan Lynaugh suggests that "obstetric units actually were the first hospital units to segment care and move patients along an assembly line from labor and delivery to maternity floors, while sending the product (baby) to the nursery." Not until the 1960s did other services organize patient care in this way. Joan Lynaugh to author, June 5, 1996.

24. See *Brought to Bed*, 182–189, for a discussion of some of the debates about hospital maternity safety records in this period.

25. Mary E. Hilliard, "Evolution of a Maternity Nurse," *Nursing Forum* 4 (1965): 6–29.

26. Joyce E. Roberts, "Maternal Positions for Childbirth: A Historical Review of Nursing Care Practices," *JOGN Nursing* 8 (1979): 24–32.

27. Mildred Green oral history, 1986, conducted by Sara Jane Williams (Sara Monkres), transcript in "The Maternity Nurses Oral History Project," 1986, State Historical Society of Wisconsin Archives, Mss 783, Box 1: MAD 4/39/C1.

28. C. M. Hall, "Training the Obstetrical Nurse," *AJN* 27 (1927): 373–379. See also Margarete Sandelowski, *Pain, Pleasure, and American Childbirth: From the Twilight Sleep to the Read Method, 1914–1960* (Westport, Conn.: Greenwood Press, 1984), 62.

29. The phrase is Susan Reverby's title to chapter 8 of her book: "Nursing efficiency as the link between service and science," in *Ordered to Care*.

30. The phrase is Barbara Melosh's, *The Physician's Hand*, p. 173.

31. See Reverby and Melosh, and Sara Jane Williams, "Caught in the Middle: Maternity Nurses and the Natural Childbirth Movement," MS (Nursing) thesis, University of Wisconsin, 1987.

32. Williams, MS thesis, 50.

33. Sara Williams interview with Eleanor Waddell, 1986, transcript in the SHSW archives.

34. Quoted in Williams, MS thesis, 68–69.

35. Quoted in Williams, MS thesis, 74–75. Apparently maternity wards were slower to relieve nurses of these tasks than other parts of the hospital. See, for example, Nan H. Ewing, "Obstetrical Nursing in a General Hospital," *AJN* 24 (1924): 44–46.

36. Elsa Rosenberg to author, in response to *New York Times Book Review* author's query, July 1983.

37. All quoted in *Ladies' Home Journal*, 1958.

38. On nurses' authority, see Reverby, *Ordered to Care*, and Melosh, *The Physician's Hand*.

39. Ann Rivington, "Motherhood—Third Class," *American Mercury* 31 (1934): 160–165.

40. Rivington, "Motherhood—Third Class," 163.

41.   Gladys Denny Schultz, "Cruelty in the Maternity Ward," and "Journal Mothers Report Cruelty in the Maternity Ward," *Ladies' Home Journal* May 1958, 45, 152–155; December 1958, 58–59, 135–138.

42.   Melosh, *"The Physician's Hand,"* 193.

43.   There is the added question about how scientific nurses' practices were in this period, a question too large to address here. See Susan M. Reverby, "A Legitimate Relationship: Nursing, Hospitals, and Science in the Twentieth Century," in *The American General Hospital: Communities and Social Contexts*, eds. Diana Elizabeth Long and Janet Golden (Ithaca: Cornell University Press, 1989), 135–156; and Sylvia Rinker, "*To Spread the 'Gospel of Good Obstetrics': The Nursing of Obstetric Patients, 1890–1940*," paper delivered at the Twelfth Annual Conference on Nursing History, Little Rock, Arkansas, September 29–October 1, 1995.

44.   See the graphs and statistics on this point in *Brought to Bed*.

45.   For a discussion of DeLee's attempts to make obstetrics more scientific, see Judith Walzer Leavitt, "Joseph B. DeLee and the Practice of Preventive Obstetrics," *American Journal of Public Health* 78 (1988): 1353–1359.

46.   Melosh, *"The Physician's Hand"*; and Reverby, *Ordered to Care*.

47.   See Williams, MS thesis; Margot Edwards and Mary Waldorf, *Reclaiming Birth: History and Heroines of American Childbirth Reform* (Trumansburg, New York: Crossing Press, 1984); and Sandelowski, *Pain, Pleasure, and American Childbirth*.

10

The Physician's Eyes: American Nursing and the Diagnostic Revolution in Medicine

Margarete Sandelowski

(THE) NURSE SHOULD BE THE DOCTOR'S EYES IN HIS ABSENCE[1]

The emergence of trained nursing in the United States in the 1870s and its capture[2] in hospitals by the 1930s did not merely coincide with the diagnostic revolution that fundamentally transformed American medicine in this period; they were tightly linked. During this time, hospitals were increasingly sold to potential patients as sites for the sympathetic and scientific care embodied in the new trained nurse and the new diagnostic technology housed there. Although barely (if at all) mentioned in histories of medical technology and hospitals, nurses were more than footnotes in the story of how technologically mediated diagnosis became a distinguishing feature of medical practice and hospital care. Nurses played a crucial role in this transformation, sharing with physicians the use of such new devices as the thermometer and often performing much of the physical, mental, and "sentimental"[3] labor engendered by x-ray and laboratory tests. Nurses made hospitals more hospitable, not only to patients but also to the new devices and device-mediated techniques that became the sine qua non of medical practice. In this chapter I focus on nursing and the new diagnostic technology in the formative years—from 1873 to the early 1930s—of both modern American nursing and tech-

Note: This chapter was originally published in *Nursing History Review* 8 (2000): 3–38. A publication of the American Association for the History of Nursing.

nologically mediated medical diagnosis. I use the term technology to refer not only to devices but also to the social interactions, divisions of labor, and human purposes around these devices.

THE DIAGNOSTIC REVOLUTION IN MEDICINE

Historians of medicine and medical technology have emphasized the enormous impact on medicine of the introduction of such sense-extending devices as the stethoscope, ophthalmoscope, laryngoscope, and fluoroscope and of such device-mediated techniques to measure, monitor, analyze, and record body functions as clinical thermometry, electrocardiography, and chemical assays of urine, blood, and other body fluids. They also have described the initial reluctance many physicians expressed toward using them.[4] The new diagnostic technology enhanced physicians' abilities to investigate and diagnose disease and their prestige as the preeminent practitioners of science. Indeed, physicians derived much of their cultural authority from their association with a technology that was seen to embody science.[5]

However, physicians feared not only "losing touch"[6] with patients (in the dual senses of losing contact with them and losing the skill of "digital observation"[7]) but also losing their authority and exclusive claim to the knowledge and skill that using this technology required and the knowledge about disease it offered. Physicians were concerned that reliance on technology would undermine their efforts to practice and to present medicine as an intellectual and independent, as opposed to manual and collaborative, pursuit. In the early 19th century, physicians associated technology with the manual labor, instrumentation, and barbarities of surgeons from whom they were eager to disassociate themselves. By the end of that century, however, physicians were recognizing that the new diagnostic devices, like surgical instruments, allowed physicians not only to improve medical practice and advance medical science but also to be seen as actively and concretely doing something to earn the social standing, authority, and remuneration they sought.

Eager to "purge subjectivity"[8] from, and to incorporate science into, the practice of medicine, physicians increasingly relied on what they perceived as objective instrument- or machine-generated information. They became less comfortable with patient descriptions and their own unaided senses as the sole or even primary basis for diagnosis. However, in the process of augmenting their diagnostic power and cultural authority the new technology had the effect of separating physicians from their patients. Physicians were socially separated from patients by acquiring increasingly specialized and arcane knowledge not readily accessible to anyone but themselves. What the doctor heard and saw through the magic and science of the stethoscope and microscope could not easily be heard, seen, or understood by others. Physicians' new knowledge, which set them apart from and elevated them above patients and other professional competitors seeking access to the patient's bedside, constituted an advantageous separation.

Yet, generalist physicians were also physically separated from patients as medical diagnosis was increasingly accomplished at a distance from the patient and through the efforts of specialists, including other physicians, nurses, and technicians. For example, although the stethoscope brought physicians closer to patients' bodies than they had been, it also maintained a space between the patient's body and the physician's ear. René Laennec, the inventor of "mediate auscultation"[9] via the stethoscope in the early 19th century, was reportedly motivated by the desire not only to hear the sounds of body organs but also to avoid the close physical contact with patients that placing an ear to the body entailed but which social mores made suspect. The microscope, in turn, permitted diagnosis to occur without any patient present at all. And, laboratory and x-ray diagnosis increasingly required what the general physician in practice typically or often did not have, namely, the time and expertise of specialists to conduct these tests and to interpret their results.

Historians have described and even glorified physicians' relations to the new diagnostic technology, but its relations to nursing remain virtually unexplored. Did the technology play as central a role in redefining nursing as it did in redefining medicine? That is, was the diagnostic revolution as revolutionary for nursing? While diagnosis, in some form, had always been central to medical practice and the physician-patient relationship, was it as critical to nursing practice and the nurse-patient relationship even in the new era of diagnosis? What did nurses gain and lose with the advent of new diagnostic techniques? What were nursing's concerns around these techniques? What did nurses contribute to the diagnostic revolution in medicine and what, in turn, were the immediate and long-term effects of this revolution on nursing?

I begin to address these questions here. I focus on what nurses and physicians perceived as one of the most essential functions of the nurse, namely, to serve as the physician's eyes. Physicians appropriated nurses' eyes as proxies for their own even as they were appropriating nurses' hands to carry out patient care. Nurses were trained and expected to collect, record, and interpret information vital to the diagnosis—and, therefore, to the treatment and prognosis—of disease under the putatively watchful eyes of physicians, without making any claims to participating in diagnosis. The trained nurse's eyes were, if not the first, then the most critical instruments in physicians' new diagnostic armamentarium.

TRAINED NURSING AND THE TRAINED SENSES

In the formative years of American-trained nursing, nursing observation was largely an embodied relation with patients in which nurses relied on their trained senses of sight, touch, and smell. Indeed, the "trained nurse" (typically conceived and, therefore, referred to here as female) was distinguished from other female caregivers, in part, by the "trained senses" she directed toward the "close observation" that promised to elevate nursing above "mechanical, routine, nonintelligent practice and place it upon a scientific, professional basis."[10] In contrast to the behaviorist cast the idea had in the 1920s and 1930s, the psychodynamic and interpersonal casts it acquired after World War II (WWII), and the phenomenological and narrative casts it has today, knowing the patient[11] used to mean knowing the patient largely in the flesh. Nursing was primarily an intimate corporeal relation involving the physical bodies of patients and the physical senses and ministrations of nurses. Listening to patients, in the sense of eliciting and interpreting their stories to know them by heart—as well as by sight, smell, and touch—had yet to become a prevailing and integral part of the rhetoric or fabric of the nurse-patient relationship.[12] Indeed, Florence Nightingale viewed too much talking on the part of both patients and nurses as physically taxing and, therefore, as indicative of poor nursing practice.

Florence Nightingale and the Observation of the Sick

Nightingale had established observation as the habit and faculty that enhanced the utility of and legitimized the need for trained nurses. Nightingale believed that a woman who could not cultivate this habit ought to abandon the pursuit of nursing, even though she might be kind. In 1860 in the classic primer *Notes on Nursing*, she instructed:

> *The most important practical lesson that can be given to nurses is to teach them what to observe—how to observe—what symptoms indicate improvement—what the reverse—which are of importance—which are of none— which are the evidence of neglect—and of what kind of neglect.*[13]

For Nightingale, acquiring the habit and faculty of observation was no simple feat. Speaking "the whole truth and nothing but the truth"— whether in court or at the bedside—required "many faculties combined of observation and memory."[14] There was no more "final proof"[15] in the fact that a person had told the same story many times than there was in the fact that one story had been corroborated by many people. Nightingale had no patience with nurses who, albeit unknowingly, imparted false information about patients to physicians. False information often resulted from asking the wrong (that is, "leading" instead of "pointed")[16] questions.

Nightingale carved out an essential role for nursing in the diagnosis and treatment of conditions leading to poor health and sickness, even as physicians were increasingly claiming diagnosis and treatment exclusively for themselves. Moreover, in an era when most physicians were just beginning to understand the specific etiologies of disease and the importance of clearly differentiating one disease or disorder from another, and to adopt the view that specific treatments should be matched to specific diagnoses,[17] Nightingale's ideal nurse was an expert in a kind of differential diagnosis not heretofore practiced by either nurses or physicians. This nurse was able to discriminate among symptoms deriving from disease itself, from the therapies chosen to treat these diseases, from deficiencies in the patient's life circumstances that might have initially contributed to the disease, and most important, from failures of the nurse "to put the patient in the best condition for nature to act upon him."[18] The trained nurse could differentiate, for example, among defects in cooking, choice of diet, choice of hours for taking food, and in the appetite as causes of "want of nutrition"[19] in the patient. The trained nurse also understood that each of these defects, in turn, required different remedies. The remedy for the first defect was to cook better, for the second was to make other choices in diet, for the third was to offer patients food when they wanted it, and for the fourth was to show patients what they liked.[20]

Nightingale admired nurses who had developed a precision of eye virtually equal to the measuring glass, although she maintained that nurses' eyes could not fully substitute for the accuracy of this device. An observant nurse could tell at a glance how many ounces of food her patient had consumed, even if the amount was very small. Nurses also had to learn the "physiognomy,"[21] or look, of various diseases and how they appeared in combination with the looks of individual patients. Nightingale promoted nursing observation as the artful and idiographic corrective to the scientific "averages" that threatened to seduce nurses away from "minute observation"[22] and physicians away from the particularities and peculiarities of individual cases.

In summary, Nightingale's nurse cultivated the habit and faculty of observation to achieve the good nursing care upon which good medical care depended. In the days before the development of specific pharmacologic agents or public health measures targeted directly at the causes of disease and before the refinement of aseptic surgical techniques, medical care often entailed little else but nursing care. The trained nurse had knowledge only nurses could possess by virtue of their constant presence at the bedside, and it was this very privileged knowledge that physicians needed for accurate assessment and management of patient conditions. Nightingale's observant nurse not only enhanced the comfort and promoted the health of her patients, but she often also saved their lives and saved the day for physicians who might otherwise be misled by the limited information available to them from their abbreviated contacts with patients.

American Trained Nursing and the Powers of Observation

Nightingale's instructions concerning observation and its importance in nursing and medical practice were incorporated and developed in the earliest lectures to and instructional texts for American students of nursing.[23] American instructors also pointed to observation as a critical feature distinguishing trained nursing from uneducated womanly ministrations to the sick. They emphasized the value of trained nursing and the shortcomings of medicine by repeatedly reminding students that it was nurses who provided accurate descriptions of patient conditions "to those who have had no opportunity for persistent observation."[24] The physician was completely dependent on the nurse for what only she could know and for what he had to know. As Clara S. Weeks, the author of one of the most influential early textbooks of nursing, concluded:

> *The nurse, who is with her patient constantly, has, if she knows how to make use of it, a much better opportunity of becoming acquainted with his real condition than the physician, who only spends half an hour with him occasionally.*[25]

Indeed, according to Weeks, the "very excitement"[26] of (or agitation caused by) the physician's visit often so altered patients' conditions that they might look better or worse to the visiting physician than they really were. In addition, patients often told nurses things they did not tell their doctors. Nursing observation was especially crucial in the cases of infants, delirious patients, and others who could not or ought not—in order to conserve their energy—speak for themselves. The trained nurse was the physician's eyes, but she did not so much extend a largely sighted physician as a virtually blind one. Indeed, he saw very little without her.

Authors, such as Weeks, who sought to establish nursing as a valued profession for women, recurringly reminded students of nursing of the responsibility and power that lay in the nurse's eyes and in the constancy of her vigilance at the bedside. The physician depended on the nurse's "powers of observation"[27] and in that dependence lay her professional power. Accordingly, nurses were taught to take careful notice of their patients and the conditions surrounding them. Didactic texts emphasized the physical condition of the patient, physical manifestations indicating aberrant mental states, and the physical environment of the sick room. Nightingale's admonition to nurses to learn the laws of health and to observe the total life circumstances of their patients could be more closely adhered to in home and public health nursing, where nurses had the opportunity to see the larger family and other social circumstances of their patients that contributed to ill health. In the hospital, however, nurses were confined largely to observations of the physical and proximate causes of disease and discomfort, that is, to what could be immediately seen, felt, smelled, or heard from outside the body and to such factors in the physical environment as ventilation, lighting, and noise.

Nurses' "relation to symptomatology"[28] was a major topic of instruction from the earliest days of trained nursing. Nurses were taught to differentiate between subjective and objective symptoms, between symptoms and signs, between real and feigned symptoms, between leading and misleading symptoms, and between symptoms and signs significant for nursing care and those significant for medical care. They were to note and record the degree, character, duration, frequency, time of occurrence, apparent cause, modification, and significance of an array of symptoms and signs, such as pain, palpitation, dyspnea, cough, expectoration, and vomiting. Nurses were to appraise the condition of every visible portion of the body, using parameters appropriate for that part. For example, they were to observe the color, volume, degree of moisture, coating, markings, motion, and manner of protrusion of the tongue. They were to note the rate, volume, strength, rhythm, and tension of the pulse.[29] Before technological intrusions into the living body were routine in clinical practice, learning the subtleties of symptomatology and of patient expression, posture, mood, and temperament was especially critical. What could be discerned from the outside comprised virtually all the information available to the general nursing or medical practitioner.

Practicing close observation entailed not only cultivating the sensory faculties but also understanding and managing its effect on patients. Being under the constant scrutiny of professional strangers, whether in the home or hospital, was new to patients unused to either trained nursing in the home or to hospital care. While being looked after was likely comforting to most patients, being looked at could be disturbing and even result in error. Nurses were admonished not to let patients know they were being observed because this could generate misleading symptoms.[30] Nurses learned to observe patients while they were ministering to their needs; that is, they learned to take opportunities, such as the bath, to note conditions of the body. They also learned to observe one patient while caring for another. Nurse trainee Mary Clymer noted the difficulty she had "trying to have my eyes in 13 while my hands make a bed in 11."[31]

In short, the close observation expected of the trained nurse required knowledge of symptoms and signs and their various relations to disease, treatment, and environmental conditions, the cultivation of all the nurse's senses with an emphasis on the practiced and disciplined eye, savvy in patient relations, and the ability to communicate and increasingly record observations in a manner likely to be of most use to both patient and physician. If the key to good nursing was observation, the key to accurate medical diagnosis and patient recovery was the close observation of the trained nurse. The trained nurse was to be all-seeing: to take all of the "visual opportunities"[32] available to her and to maintain "visual control"[33] of her patients and the sick room. Except for the candle, gas, stopwatch (to count the pulse), and, later, electric light, nursing observation in the late 19th century was largely an in-the-flesh practice unmediated by technological devices.[34]

THE INSTRUMENTAL EYE

While nurses were learning the importance of observing the sick, medical practice in the latter decades of the 19th, and early decades of the 20th, century increasingly involved new technological means of observing living patients, of looking into and through them in addition to looking at and over them. From the middle of the 19th century, physical diagnosis with and without sense-extending devices such as the stethoscope increasingly prevailed. After 1900 the primacy and value of physical diagnosis were increasingly challenged by the x-ray and the analytic, graphic, and quantitative techniques of laboratory diagnosis, electrocardiography, and sphygmomanometry.[35] In order to harness the benefits of this new technology, physicians had to share its use with nurses (and, eventually, also with a host of new technicians whose jobs were created in response to it). These new "instruments of precision"[36] and symbols of medical science not only complicated the nurse's work but also blurred the boundary line between nursing and medical practice.

Clinical Thermometry

Clinical thermometry became part of American medical practice in the latter part of the 19th century. Although the mercury thermometer had been invented early in the 18th century, its initial design made it impractical as a clinical tool. Thermometers were originally rather large devices, about a foot long and bent at a right angle, which had to be carried in a holster under the arm, much as "one might carry a gun."[37] Moreover, because thermometers did not maintain temperature readings at their maximum level once they were removed from the body, physicians had to read them while they were still placed against the body. The invention of portable and self-registering devices that maintained the temperature at its maximum reading after removal from the body, the 1871 translation of Carl Wunderlich's scientific treatise on medical thermometry,[38] and the 1873 translation of Edouard Seguin's manual on medical and family thermometry,[39] contributed to the virtually complete replacement in American clinical practice, by the end of the 19th century, of the hand with the thermometer to discern patient temperature. The glass or metal thermometer replaced the "hand-thermometer,"[40] or the hand, as the thermometer.

In contrast to other diagnostic devices, such as the stethoscope, laryngoscope, and microscope, which nurses assisted physicians in using and/or only occasionally used themselves, the direct use of the thermometer was soon delegated to nurses. Indeed, nurses became the most likely and frequent users of this device, charged with taking temperatures in the physician's absence and with maintaining the thermometers themselves. The thermometer was rather quickly incorporated into routine nursing practice and, almost as quickly, came to be associated with, and even to represent, nursing. The earliest American textbooks of nursing and lecture notes indicate that nurses were expected to use the thermometer in their daily practice, that is, at the very least, to take and record the temperature.[41] Advertisements for preprinted blank temperature charts appear in the back of texts written for nurses, indicating that nurses were responsible for maintaining legible records of patients' temperatures.[42] The thermometer was a prominent feature of what nurses, physicians, and advertisers considered to be part of the nurse's "uniform," "armamentarium," "chatelaine," and "nurse's case."[43] Companies manufacturing thermometers marketed them directly to nurses and as suitable gifts for nurses (see Figure 1).[44] Early popular verbal and pictorial depictions of nursing, as well as advertisements for nursing itself, often presented the nurse with a "thermometer in her hand"[45] The thermometer was soon even incorporated into the image nurses had of themselves and their functions. In her widely read 1893 textbook on nursing, Isabel Hampton encouraged the nurse to think of herself as the "ward thermometer and barometer (alert for) any change in the ward atmosphere."[46] Nurses not only used thermometers; they were thermometers.

Thermometry was depicted also as a womanly "handicraft,"[47] and the thermometer itself was depicted as a means "second to none"[48] in the practice of the womanly arts of mothering and nursing. Seguin, who popularized "family thermometry," viewed the handling and intelligent reading of the thermometer and the accurate recording of the temperature as necessary to learning the "ABCs of motherhood."[49] The thermometer was necessary also to "that part of nursing which mainly consists in spy-

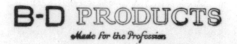
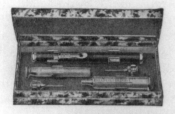
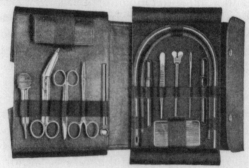
Figure 10.1 Becton, Dickinson ad marketing thermometers as suitable gifts for nurses.

ing the subtle and bold invasion of disease, and of measuring . . . its deadly strides into the vitals of the innocent."[50] Women were the sentries who would be first to detect and "measure the strength of the enemy on the stem of [their] thermometers."[51]

The earliest instructions that nurses received about the thermometer show varying detail and increasing complexity, with information ranging from the procedural—that is, how to take, read, and record the temperature in adults and children—to the scientific—that is, the theoretical basis for clinical thermometry and the meaning of various temperatures and temperature profiles in the progression of disease. In Bellevue Hospital's 1878 *Manual of Nursing*, only one paragraph on the thermometer appears at the end of the book as an addendum, and it contains information on how to take an oral temperature, a reference to axillary and rectal temperatures, and what the normal axillary temperature is.[52] The Connecticut Training School's *Handbook of Nursing*, published in 1879, contains somewhat more information and a reference to Seguin's work.[53]

Fourteen years later, in 1893, in the first edition of *Nursing*,[54] Hampton devoted a chapter to temperature, linking variations in temperature to variations in pulse and respiration, and differentiating normal from abnormal temperatures, and addressing diurnal variations in temperature and factors (such as the placement of thermometers and the temperature and nature of foods) that could raise or lower temperature. Hampton classified temperatures, ranging from the "temperature of collapse" at 95°–97°F to "hyperpyrexia"[55] at over 105°F, and she differentiated among continuous, intermittent, and remittent fevers. She included "specimen charts"[56] showing temperature, pulse, and respiration in typhoid fever, pneumonia, and malaria. Hampton taught nurses how to convert Fahrenheit to Centigrade and Centigrade to Fahrenheit temperatures, how to test a thermometer for accuracy, how to take mouth, axillary, and rectal temperatures, and how to clean and store thermometers. Reprising concerns raised by physicians about the dangers of substituting instruments for the trained senses of the clinician, Hampton advised nurses not to rely solely on the thermometer. Even though ascertaining temperature by touch alone could be highly misleading (as skin temperature was not a reliable indicator of body temperature), touching the patient was still an essential component of nursing observation that allowed the detection of conditions that might go unnoticed without it.

Didactic instructions for nurses concerning thermometry became more detailed over the years, providing more information on the scientific basis for clinical thermometry and its relation to the diagnosis and course of disease and detection of patient responses to treatment. Since many so-called medical treatments entailed nothing but nursing care (as in "fever" nursing[57]), the thermometer was as much an instrument of nursing—assisting the nurse to evaluate the effectiveness of her ministrations—as it was an instrument of medicine. As Bertha Harmer noted in the first edition in 1922 of probably the most widely read series of textbooks of nursing,[58] it was not enough for the nurse merely to be able to take the temperature. She had to know what caused various temperatures to occur and the nursing measures that would lower and raise temperature to normal levels. The nurse did not merely take the temperature; she used the thermometer to diagnose, monitor, and rediagnose patient conditions.

As thermometry became routine in clinical practice and virtually the sole province—in the hospital—of the nurse, instructional texts for nursing included increasingly more information on "making temperature taking safe."[59] The "safety work"[60] of clinical thermometry included the maintenance and disinfection of thermometers, ensuring the accuracy of thermometer readings, and preventing harm to patients. Both instructional texts teaching nurses about thermometers and advertising texts promoting the sales of competing brands of thermometers indicate that breakage was a constant concern.[61] Nurses considered themselves fortunate if they were not required to pay for the thermometers they broke.[62] Since the same thermometer typically had to be shared among patients, nurses were also increasingly concerned with the best methods to clean thermometers. Clinical thermometry was one of the earliest focal points of scientific investigation by nurses as they evaluated the effectiveness of various procedures for disinfection of thermometers. Most notable in this area of research was the 1929 Martha E. Erdmann and Margaret Welsh report of the studies in thermometer technique they had conducted between 1927 and 1928.[63]

The safety work of clinical thermometry also included preventing situations likely to cause injury to patients from broken thermometers or from false temperature readings. Nurses were cautioned about hysterical or malingering patients who deliberately sought to elevate temperature readings by placing the thermometer against something hot while the nurse was not looking. There were also other uncooperative patients who did not or could not keep the thermometer in place for the length of time required to register its maximum reading. Nurses were warned never to leave patients unattended with thermometers in place unless they were certain that it was safe to leave a patient unsupervised or that the patient was physically able, or could be trusted, to be left alone.[64] Although clinical thermometry did not create the view that patients were themselves often unreliable partners in restoring them back to health, it reinforced and extended the view of thermometry as a practice that depended on the cooperation of the patient.

Clinical thermometry served also to influence the aesthetics of nursing (and of hospital nursing, in particular), affecting the order and structure of work on the ward and the appearance of nursing care. As physicians became more interested in the scientific investigation of disease and in establishing patterns of temperature in various diseases, they ordered temperatures to be taken more frequently. Whereas temperatures might have initially been taken once or twice a day, increasingly, temperatures had to be taken four or more times in a 24-hour period. Under ideal conditions, thermometers required 3–5 minutes to register temperature in the mouth but up to 15 minutes to register temperature in the axilla, often a preferred mode of taking the temperature. Moreover, the normal diurnal variations in temperature made it necessary to take temperatures at times when body temperature tended to be at its lowest and highest levels. Physicians also expected all temperatures to be taken and recorded before their scheduled morning and/or evening rounds. Accordingly, the practice soon arose of assigning one nurse—the "temperature nurse"[65]—to take and record all the temperatures on a ward. This early manifestation of functional nursing—that is, giving one task to one nurse for her to complete on all patients—stood in sharp contrast to the home or private duty model of nursing where one nurse provided all the care that one patient required. The "temperature nurse" was a new factor that detracted from the exclusivity of the traditional nurse-patient relationship.

Thermometers also figured prominently in the development of specialized equipment trays that became a characteristic feature of nursing care. These trays were a means for the nurse to be efficient and organized in gathering and arranging the materials needed to conduct procedures at the bedside and to give a finished appearance to her work. In instructional and advice literature concerning the thermometer and other trays, nurses were told to consider not only functionality and safety in their work but also symmetry and neatness in presenting equipment to patients and physicians. Indeed, symmetry and neatness were critical features of the rotating system nurses used to distinguish between clean and dirty thermometers and, thereby, to prevent inadvertently using a dirty thermometer.[66]

In summary, from the beginning of American trained nursing the thermometer became both fact and symbol of nursing practice. The thermometer was an instrument that helped the nurse to diagnose and monitor patient conditions and to detect defects in nursing and medical care. As an instrument increasingly linked in professional, popular, and advertising literature with nurses, the thermometer represented both the precision of science and the ministrations of the trained nursing. Moreover, the thermometer forged a link between nursing and technology, whereby nurses came to understand themselves not only as users of scientific instruments but also as functioning like them.

(Stetho) Scopic Examinations

In the case of the thermometer the practice of taking and recording the temperature eventually fell to the woman or nurse in the home and to the nurse in the hospital. In contrast, scopic examinations, or physical examinations conducted with such eye- and ear-extending instruments as ophthalmoscopes, laryngoscopes, and stethoscopes, remained largely in the physician's domain through the 1930s. If nurses participated in scopic examinations at all, it was primarily to hold patients in position for the examination, to ensure their cooperation, and to see to it that the proper equipment was at the physician's hand.[67]

Nurses' use of the stethoscope in this period was confined largely to listening to the fetal heart, although the practice of regular fetal auscultation, conducted with increasing frequency as labor progressed to delivery, had yet to become standard obstetric practice.[68] Nurses sometimes also used stethoscopes to take blood pressure, but taking the blood pressure did not become part of routine nursing practice until the 1930s. Nurses were instructed about blood pressure, but didactic literature and procedure manuals directed toward them indicate that taking the blood pressure was not something they were expected to do at all or on a regular basis.[69] Although there were physicians in the first decade of the 20th century who still viewed blood pressure measurement as a dangerous substitute for digital observation (or palpation) of the pulse,[70] blood pressure was typically conceived as a component of the physical examination of patients that only physicians conducted.

Moreover, in contrast to clinical thermometry, the labor involved in scopic examinations was not so easily divided and delegated. One user could not simply take and record scopically derived information for another user to interpret as these instruments did not permanently register any number or graphic analogue to the temperature. Unlike the temperature scale, which anyone with reasonable visual acuity could see on a thermometer, the use of scopic devices depended on having the specialized scientific knowledge and perceptual skill to see or hear device-mediated objects and sounds, an interpretive skill apart from the skill of interpreting what these objects and sounds meant for the diagnosis of disease.

Because these instruments entailed interpretive skills that were taught exclusively to physicians, they remained outside of the sphere of the nurse. In addition, the belief seemed to prevail that scopic examinations were not appropriate for nurses to learn, as they were at the heart of the diagnostic encounter between physician and patient. One physician reported in 1888 being rebuked for teaching a nurse stethoscopic examination of the chest to detect heart complications in a case of rheumatism. Nurses, he was warned, would get into trouble for having "too much knowledge for a nurse."[71] The stethoscope, especially, seemed to symbolize medicine and the art and new science of physical diagnosis, much as the thermometer became a symbol of nursing.[72]

X-ray and Laboratory Diagnosis

In the first 3 decades of the 20th century, patients were increasingly subjected to x-ray and laboratory examinations to diagnose and monitor their ailments or to detect disease that had not as yet produced any discernible ailments. In this period, patients entered hospitals not only to receive medical treatment and nursing care for illness or injury but also to find out whether and why they were sick. Moreover, x-ray and laboratory tests were increasingly used to assign and confirm diagnoses already made and as ritual screening components of hospitalization. By the 1930s, being admitted to a hospital entailed having an x-ray taken, having blood drawn, and providing a urine sample.[73] X-ray and laboratory technology embodied the new scientific hospital, and x-ray and laboratory units and equipment were prominently featured in annual reports and other materials promoting hospitals.[74]

As a consequence of their increasing reliance on x-ray and laboratory testing, physicians in general practice became increasingly dependent on specialist physicians, nurses, and others to use this technology. Roentgenographic and laboratory tests exemplified, perhaps more than any other technological innovations, the extent to which diagnosis became an interdependent and collaborative process involving physicians, nurses, technicians, and patients, rather than a discrete moment in exclusively physician time. Unlike clinical thermometry and scopic examinations, these tests entailed many activities that could be demarcated from each other and then delegated. Exactly what components of this new diagnostic work nurses performed depended on such factors as the extent of x-ray and laboratory testing conducted in the hospitals in which they worked and the availability of house physicians, specialist physicians, and technicians to do the work. For example, smaller hospitals typically offered less extensive in-house testing, but they also had fewer or no house physicians or other ancillary personnel to do this work. Shortages of personnel were especially acute after World War I (WWI).

Accordingly, nurses' work in x-ray and laboratory diagnosis variously included the before, during, and after care of equipment and of patients at the bedside or in the units in which the tests were conducted, the transportation of patients to these units, the collection, labeling, storing, and delivery of specimens, the creation and maintenance of written records of these examinations, and/or the conduct of the examinations themselves. Urinometers to measure the specific gravity of urine, litmus paper to determine its pH, and other devices to measure albumin and sugar were part of the nurse's outfit and responsibilities from the earliest days of trained nursing.[75] Nurses also performed a promotional function for hospitals by taking visitors (during annual events such as Hospital Day) on tours through laboratory and x-ray units and showing off the new scientific equipment housed there.[76]

In addition to carrying out the various tasks associated with x-ray and laboratory testing on the unit, nurses were employed in x-ray and laboratory departments themselves as roentgen associates, administering barium for fluoroscopic examinations of the gastrointestinal tract and maintaining records. Nurses were also employed as x-ray technicians and microscopists in hospitals and physicians' offices, obtaining and developing x-ray pictures and conducting chemical assays of blood, urine, sputum, and other specimens. As students, nurses were rotated through x-ray and laboratory departments and had available to them elective training in x-ray or laboratory work in their last year of school and in postgraduate courses.[77]

There were both nurses and physicians who promoted x-ray and laboratory work as nursing specialties. Nurses advocating nurse specialization saw this work as an opportunity to gain knowledge and skills that would make them more marketable to physicians and hospitals. In an era when most nursing positions in hospitals were still filled by student nurses and when graduate nurses were increasingly competing with each other for decreasing positions in the home and in public health, the "needy"[78] x-ray and laboratory fields offered employment to the equally needy graduate nurse. The routinization of x-ray and laboratory diagnosis also legitimized the need for more science education in nursing curricula to make nurses more able assistants. The work that this new kind of diagnosis generated made knowledge of anatomy, physiology, physics, chemistry, and bacteriology even more essential. Moreover, by virtue of the association of x-ray and laboratory technology with the much revered science, nurses who were knowledgeable in these fields could further differentiate themselves not only from untrained nurses but also from the trained nurses who knew nothing of these fields. Both nurse and physician advocates of nursing specialization in these fields promoted roentgen and laboratory work as especially fitting for nurses showing a "scientific turn of mind."[79]

For nurse and physician proponents of nurse specialization in x-ray and laboratory work these fields offered an interesting departure from, and often better working conditions than, bedside nursing.[80] They argued that the hours of work were generally more regular and convenient, that the pay was sometimes better, and that the nurse won a reprieve from the daily complexities and physical exertions of caring for sick people that tended to shorten her working life. Yet, although a departure from traditional bedside nursing, the work permitted the nurse to draw from her nursing background to alleviate the discomfort and fear that patients, especially children, experienced as they encountered these strange new tests.

Indeed, as nurse advocates proposed, this work demanded not only the technical skills associated with applying the technology but also the skills of the trained nurse in managing patients' emotions and in protecting the privacy these tests often threatened. Patients reportedly had many misconceptions and fears about these tests and were embarrassed by having to remove their clothes for x-ray and other procedures. Nurses' observations during these examinations were also critical to the accurate interpretation of test results and, therefore, to accurate medical diagnosis. X-ray and laboratory work was deemed especially suited to the nurse who wanted to keep in touch with nursing, but who was less "adapted" by virtue of "physique or personality" to do continuous bedside nursing.[81] Nurses were, therefore, considered "natural(s)"[82] to assume the new work these tests generated as they were already serving in hospitals, had a great deal of knowledge about patients and diseases, and were already trained to be assistants to physicians.

Physician proponents of nurses in x-ray and laboratory fields, in particular, viewed nurses as especially suitable to assume the work of busy, absent, and unavailable physicians. Physicians could not have large caseloads of patients and the revenues they generated and also perform all the work the new diagnosis demanded. Accordingly, some of them turned to nurses as an available, cheap, and compliant alternative to house physicians. Lamenting the post-WWI shortage of interns in small hospitals, one North Carolina physician, Edmundson Boice, advocated the delegation of such "laborious" and "routine"[83] tasks as urinalysis, blood counts, and medical histories to nurses. Like other physicians, he had delegated these tasks to a "good nurse"[84] and was very satisfied with the results. According to Boice, a good nurse could assume more and more tasks until she was "almost as much assistance as a well-trained house physician."[85] Arguably, by not having to compete for house physicians, hospitals risked lowering standards and losing the new ideas these physicians brought with them. Also, these house physicians could be paid less because this work would not be their life. A house physician worked for the experience, not the $25 per month he earned. In contrast, a nurse worked for what she earned, and she had to make laboratory work her life.

However, according to Boice, delegating these tasks to nurses was ultimately the cheaper alternative since, once they were trained, there was no longer the cost of training a new house physician every year.

Although x-ray and laboratory work was promoted in the immediate post-WWI period and the 1920s as good for both nurses and physicians, nurses appear not to have entered these fields as specialists in numbers sufficient to meet the demand.[86] By the 1930s, advocates of nurse specialization promoted these fields to nurses for whom they were still "unknown land."[87] One physician reportedly lamented what he perceived as the timidity of most nurses who lacked the "ability and thirst for progression" that becoming a "roentgenologist's assistant"[88] could satisfy. Nurses apparently still feared the dangers to health and fertility that x-ray work entailed. (Roentgenologists were reportedly initially reluctant to permit nurses near x-ray machines because of this danger.)[89] Moreover, this work was not always as interesting as advertised, typically involving routine and monotonous procedures. Also, this work was often simply added on to the nurse's ward work without any additional pay.[90] For all of its difficulties, most nurses likely preferred the intimacy of bedside care to the "science" of laboratory or x-ray work and did not see this work as essentially nursing work. Indeed, there is some indication that nurses saw x-ray and laboratory diagnosis as interfering with nursing work and the order of the ward.[91]

THE "OVER-WORKED EYE"[92]

Especially after 1900, nurses acquired much of the labor of the new diagnosis. Instructional texts for nurses increasingly devoted more attention to the nurse's assistive role in medical diagnosis. By the 1930s, "assisting [the] physician in examining patients . . . and [in] making diagnostic tests" was one of twelve "aspects of nursing skill"[93] identified in a comprehensive activity analysis of nursing. In successive editions of the classic Harmer (and, later, Harmer and Virginia Henderson) textbooks on the principles and practice of nursing, what was topically referred to in 1922 as "nursing procedures"[94] used in the treatment of disease was, by 1939, described under the heading of "assisting with diagnostic procedures."[95] The Ewald Test Meal, for example, was a nursing procedure used to treat alimentary tract diseases in 1922, but in 1939 it was a diagnostic procedure that nurses assisted the physician in performing.

Physicians increasingly depended on nurses to detect and act on problems early as the nurse was likely to be the first one to discern an aberration in temperature or to find albumin in a patient's urine and, therefore, to spare the patient dangerous delays in treatment. Yet, although (or, perhaps, because) diagnosis was becoming a process to which nurses, patients, and others increasingly contributed, physicians sought to reserve the act of diagnosis exclusively for themselves. A recurring theme in instructional texts for nurses was that they were never to cross the line between nursing observation and medical diagnosis.[96] As one physician warned:

> *Outside of correct reports, the nurse has nothing to do with diagnosis or prognosis. And, beyond executing orders and recording bedside notes, (she) has no part in the treatment.*[97]

Nurses were repeatedly admonished in didactic texts that diagnosis was not their business, even as they were increasingly being offered and sought more scientific knowledge about disease and clinical experience in various components of diagnosis and as physicians were increasingly expecting nurses to perform de facto acts of diagnosis. Nurses were supposed to be able to distinguish between normal and abnormal conditions and to look for reasons for any abnormal findings. However, nurses were never to use the words normal or abnormal in reporting or recording patient conditions, and they were to refrain from offering their opinions on etiology or diagnosis.[98] Ethel Johns and Blanche Pfefferkorn summarized the paradoxical position of the nurse in relation to diagnosis by observing that:

> *While the nurse is debarred from making a diagnosis, she is tacitly permitted to arrange into a pattern any significant symptoms upon which such diagnosis may be based.*[99]

Dividing and Denying the Labor of Diagnosis

The new diagnostic technology reinforced the processual, as opposed to episodic, nature of diagnosis. This technology also both reinforced and blurred the line between the diagnosis that was supposed to be the physician's exclusive domain and the observation that was the nurse's shared domain.

A case in point involves the practice of clinical thermometry. When thermometers were first introduced into clinical practice, there seems to have been some concern among physicians about whether nurses or family members could be entrusted with their use. Physicians soon discovered, however, that the kind of information they needed for the diagnosis, treatment, and scientific study of disease required a graphic record of temperatures taken regularly and at critical moments in the progression of a disease, which, in turn, required someone at the bedside at the right times to obtain this information. Wunderlich, whose treatise was extremely influential in persuading physicians of the need for the thermometer in medical practice, contended that a major impediment to

the practical utility of the thermometer was that it was too time-consuming for the physician to take all the temperatures he required.[100]
Seguin had also noted that there was no part of the physician's work that
required so much help as thermometry.[101] If only 1–2 temperature readings were needed, a physician could obtain these himself when he visited his patients. Indeed, if he could not, Seguin advised that the physician
not take the case.[102] However, if 6–7 daily temperature readings were
needed, the physician needed help; it was not necessary that he take the
temperatures himself but only that he knew who took the temperatures
and how they were taken. The physician's knowledge of pathological
thermometry was sufficient to enable him to control or estimate the temperature readings obtained.

Moreover, anyone with good sight could be taught quickly to take accurate temperatures. Indeed, Wunderlich noted that persons unencum-
bered with the specialized knowledge of physicians were likely to make
even fewer errors than the physician in obtaining an accurate temperature because they had no preconceived opinions to prejudice them.[103] In
a similar vein, Seguin observed that

> *As astronomic observations are often better recorded by honest, attentive
> assistants than by astronomers, so a medical student, a nurse, (or) a rela-
> tive can be made a useful assistant to the medical thermometrician.*[104]

Yet, while Wunderlich noted the value and even necessity of assistants
in performing the work of medical thermometry, he also believed that
the "mere reading of temperature degrees helps diagnosis no more than
dispensing does therapeusis."[105] Physicians minimized the skilled safety
work involved in obtaining temperatures from children and delirious
and fearful patients. Moreover, clinical thermometry was itself a technique that permitted the labor of diagnosis to be separated into unequal
parts, with nurses increasingly assuming what were perceived as the
largely mechanical tasks of taking and recording temperatures and of
maintaining thermometers and physicians assuming what was perceived
as the higher-order interpretive task of evaluating what the temperatures meant. By placing the tasks of diagnosis in a hierarchy and reserv-
ing the label of diagnosis only for physician acts of interpretation,
physicians could deny that nonphysicians played any part in thermo-
metric diagnosis, even as nurses were interpreting and expected to interpret temperature readings.

X-ray and laboratory technology also entailed an actual and rhetorical division and denial of labor. Nurses were seen as naturals to do much
of the work of diagnosis without usurping the physician's preeminent
role in diagnosis. Physicians in general practice were especially worried
about the encroachment of x-ray and laboratory physician specialists (for

example, pathologists and roentgenologists), who were competing for access to and revenues from patients by claiming the diagnostic act for themselves. Concerned over the abuse of medical specialization and overuse of the new diagnostic technologies, rank-and-file physicians were concerned that laboratories and x-ray units be seen as tools for the general physician—who knew the patient—to make diagnoses, not as diagnostic entities themselves.[106] Nurse specialization in these fields seemed neither to threaten physician access to patients nor, more importantly, their exclusive claim to diagnosis. The effect of this division and denial of the labor of diagnosis was to downplay the technical, interpersonal, and machine-body tending expertise of nurses and their frequently greater skill in these components of the application of the new technology to the patient.

Easy Enough for a Nurse to Do

The delegation to nurses of tasks considered easy enough for a nurse to do belied the actual complexity of these tasks. An especially good illustration of the complexity of tasks left to nurses was the Ewald Test Meal. This test was commonly used to diagnose gastrointestinal ailments and included a carefully sequenced and timed orchestration of events, which could involve up to four patients undergoing the test at the same time. According to Elizabeth Connolly, the superintendent of nursing at the North Carolina Sanatorium, 14 student nurses had successfully conducted 365 tests between 1921 and 1923. In her description of the procedure,[107] the test first involved patient preparation, which included instruction about the test and fasting. On the day of the test, with the patient resting in a recliner the nurse passed a rubber tube with a "bucket" (or tip designed to catch the gastric contents) into the stomach. This process often induced gagging in the patient, which the nurse reduced by spraying the throat with a 2% solution of cocaine. Once the tube was in the stomach, the nurse aspirated its contents with a syringe, taking care that the plunger not fit its barrel too snugly. Too tight a fit could cause the lining of the stomach to be damaged as it was sucked into the tip of the tube. The nurse then gave the patient the Ewald meal of bread and water, with or without the tube still in place. Removing it at this point meant that the nurse would have to reinsert it later rapidly enough to conform to the timing of events the test required. With a clock in full view the patient was given four minutes to finish the meal. If the nurse was supervising four patients at 2:45, this meant that patient 1 was required to finish the meal between 2:45 and 2:49; patient 2 was to finish between 2:49 and 2:53; patient 3 was to finish between 2:53 and 2:57; and patient 4 was to finish between 2:57 and 3:01. Exactly 11 minutes after the patient had finished the meal, the nurse aspirated the stomach contents. Patient 1 would have her or his stomach aspirated at 3:00, patient 2 would be aspirated at 3:04, patient 3 would be aspirated at 3:08, and patient 4 would be aspirated at 3:12. The nurse then placed the aspirated specimens into test tubes. She had to assure herself that the specimen was not bile-tinged, as that indicated that the bucket had passed out of the stomach into the duodenum, thereby invalidating the test. The nurse then removed the tube from the patient, taking care not to leave the bucket inside the stomach or esophagus and to avoid the laryngeal or pharyngeal spasms that often occurred during this process. Such spasms could greatly impede the tube's passage out of the patient. Tugging at the tube would both frighten the patient and further impede removal of the tube.

THE "OVER-TRAINED NURSE"

Assisting physicians with the new diagnosis required nurses to have new knowledge and skills in the application of devices and in enlisting patient cooperation for tests that could be uncomfortable, time-consuming, and/or frightening. However, even before technologically mediated diagnosis characterized medical practice, physicians were ambivalent about what nurses needed to know and, more important, should be taught to conduct the kind of close observation and reporting they required to prescribe treatment. On the one hand, many physicians saw nurses as Baconian data collectors, whose only frame of reference was to obtain the "raw data" the physician required. On the other hand, nurses were not just to report whatever they saw without interpretive comment but also to discern the likely reason for a symptom, to know what a symptom meant, and to take the required action.[108] Nurses were in the bizarre position of having to be mindful of symptoms without speaking their mind about them. Nurses were to "know . . . as much as the physician about the meaning of symptoms," yet they were to have no "tendency to become medical women, or to set up their own opinions in practice."[109]

Physicians' ambivalence about nurses' powers of observation and the education required to cultivate them is evident in the vigorous debate about the "overtrained nurse."[110] At times juxtaposed with the "undertrained"[111] physician the idea of the overtrained nurse emerged almost simultaneously with the actual appearance of trained nurses. A general concern of physicians who engaged in this debate was how much knowledge nurses should have for the good of patients and, perhaps, more important, for the good of physicians. Arguing that both a little and a lot of knowledge were dangerous to both patients and themselves, physicians were especially concerned that nurses not assume that either diagnosis or treatment was in their sphere.[112]

Especially troublesome to physicians most anxious about nursing education were examination questions for nurses that required answers only a physician should know and often did not.[113] As one physician argued, what patients required was not a nurse who could write a thesis about urinalysis or how to test for hydrochloric acid in stomach contents but, rather, one who could fluff their pillows, feed them, and report on their condition to the doctor. Indeed, advances in medical science and technology were causing both physicians and nurses to lose sight of the true and nonscientific function of the nurse.[114] As one physician summarized it:

> *We do not want a scientific person; we do not want a person with theories of her own, or with a smattering of other people's theories . . . Of what use is it for [the nurse] . . . to hear lectures on the eye and the ophthalmoscope, subjects which occupy the earnest and constant study of highly educated men, and can be pursued to advantage by those only who give their whole time and attention to them?[115]*

CONCLUSION: THE NURSE'S EYES

Nurses played a central role in the technological transformation of medical practice and hospital care by putting the new diagnostic technology into use. Carl Mitcham differentiated between two views of technology as activity, that is, between activities that bring artifacts into existence and activities that put them to use.[116] Although nurses played no known part in the invention of the diagnostic devices addressd here, they did play a critical role in their application. Nurses performed key components of the work of medical diagnosis, variously obtaining device-mediated information from patients and recording, interpreting, and acting on this information. Nurses directly applied new devices and techniques to patients and they provided the before and after care of patients, and devices. The new "medical gaze" of the physician, accomplished with the aid of diagnostic technology, was, in part, "articulated through and mediated by" the nurse's eyes and hands.[117]

Yet, although nurses were essential to medical diagnosis, medical diagnosis was arguably not central to nursing. Instrumental diagnosis did not redefine nursing as it did medicine, where diagnosis replaced treatment in this period as the central point of the physician-patient encounter.[118] Nurses' encounters with patients around observation were still largely in-the-flesh; with the possible exception of the thermometer, there is little evidence that nurses used the information derived from these devices to alter nursing practice.[119] The new diagnostic technology seems to have altered the form more than the content of nursing work.

However, the new diagnostic technology complicated the work of the nurse and ideas about what nursing practice appropriately entailed.

Nurses had more work to do in this realm, but whether this work drew nurses away from their traditional ministrations is still a matter for debate.[120] Perhaps less debatable—as it pertains to the development of modern American nursing—is that by blurring the dividing line between nursing observation and medical diagnosis, diagnostic technology was instrumental in both reinforcing and subverting the rhetorical and actual dividing line between nursing and doctoring. Clinical thermometry and x-ray and laboratory diagnosis, by their very material designs and the physical operations they entailed, reinforced the lines between medicine and nursing by permitting tasks to be divided into physical, mechanical, and interpretive components, which, in turn, could be delegated to non-physicians or (at, the very least, rhetorically) reserved for physicians. Scopic techniques, by virtue of their not being so divisible (and, there-fore, delegatable), also reinforced these lines.

These diagnostic techniques also subverted those lines by requiring the execution of tasks physicians often had insufficient time or skill to perform. While the delegation to nurses of tasks physicians considered easy enough for a nurse to do degraded the skill these tasks required, it also appears to have given nurses the opportunity to obtain more scien-tific knowledge and technical skill and to enter the new terrain of tech-nological diagnosis. The diagnostic revolution required nurses to become skilled in tasks neither rhetorically nor legally delegated to them, as physi-cians expected nurses to stand in for them as doctors—that is, as diag-nosticians—in their absence. By virtue of their absence and the constant presence of the nurse at the bedside, physicians had no choice but to depend on nurses, and nurses, in turn, had no choice—if patients were to be safe—but to perform de facto acts of diagnosis. Diagnostic tech-nology did not create but rather illuminated the importance of this spa-tiotemporal asymmetry between medicine and nursing that favored nursing power.[121]

By making diagnosis central to medicine in this period the new tech-nology also disempowered nursing. Before the diagnostic revolution in American medicine the focus of the physician-patient encounter was less on discerning the reason for an ailment than in alleviating its miseries. In the days prior to safe surgery and effective pharmacologic agents, med-ical treatment largely entailed good nursing care. With the new focus on diagnosis, even in the continuing absence of effective treatments for the diseases diagnosed, physicians gained power and control as the physi-cian's diagnosis (obtaining it, confirming it, and/or being treated for it) was what brought patients into hospitals. In the new era of diagnosis, nursing seemed less autonomous and more dependent on medical diag-nosis for its existence.

Accordingly, although nurses shared the use of many of the new diagnostic devices with physicians, they had different relations to them with different effects. Like the term technology itself, the nursing relation to the new diagnostic technology was "equivocal."[122] Nurses did not lose the close bonds they had with patients, which had arguably always been more intimate than physician-patient relations. They also did not gain the cultural authority that the new diagnostic technology conferred on physicians. Although they acquired new knowledge and skill, what nurses gained most of all was new (and, arguably, more) work to do. Diagnostic technology was also critical in elasticizing the sphere of the nurse; that is, this technology did not so much expand the sphere of influence of the nurse as permit her scope of responsibility to expand or contract according to whether physicians or others were available to perform the various tasks required by the technology. Whether a nurse did virtually all of the work associated with a diagnostic procedure or very little of it depended on the availability of other personnel and economic constraints. Yet, although the nurse's scope of responsibility was not fixed, there were certain duties that were relatively constant; nurses generally always cleaned up, and they always gained the cooperation of patients.

In an important sense the "doctor-nurse game" Leonard Stein described in 1967[123] began, in part, with the diagnostic revolution in medicine. However, it was then, as it remains even to this day, a game of words. Indeed, nurses would do well to understand language as practice and words as creators (as opposed to carriers) of meaning and reality. The denial of nonphysician diagnosis was largely a rhetorical move that became well entrenched in social custom, the law, and the popular imagination. The emergence of the nursing diagnosis movement in the 1960s was, in part, an effort to let physicians claim medical diagnosis while renaming and claiming the diagnostic work nurses actually performed.[124] The contemporary resurgence of the nurse practitioner has resurrected the debate about whether and what kind of diagnoses are in the nurse's proper sphere.

However, nurses promoting the nurse diagnostician with the argument that nursing and medical diagnoses are clearly defined and different entities would do well to consider the implications for nursing of the "conceptual acrobatics"[125] required to maintain this difference. Nurses promoting the nurse practitioner as the cheaper alternative to perform simple diagnostic acts would do well to remember that, in the history of nursing, skill has often appeared, not as an "objectively identifiable quality" but rather as an "ideological category" over which nurses have repeatedly been "denied the rights of contestation."[126]

NOTES

1.   Robert A. Kilduffe, "The Nurse and Her Relation to Symptomatology, I: The Pulse," *Trained Nurse and Hospital Review* 65, no. 6 (1920): 498.

2.   Rosemary Stevens, *In Sickness and in Wealth: American Hospitals in the Twentieth Century* (New York: Basic Books, 1989). According to Stevens (p. 12), nurses were "captured by the hospital and institutionally subsumed."

3.   Anselm Strauss et al., "Sentimental Work in the Technologized Hospital," *Sociology of Health & Illness* 4, no. 3 (1982): 254–77.

4.   The classic work in this field is Stanley Joel Reiser, *Medicine and the Reign of Technology* (Cambridge, U.K.: Cambridge University Press, 1978). See also by Reiser, "Technology and the Eclipse of Individualism in Medicine," *The Pharos* 45, no. 1 (1982): 10–15; "The Science of Diagnosis: Diagnostic Technology," in *Companion Encyclopedia of the History of Medicine*, ed. W. F. Bynum and Roy Porter (London: Routledge, 1993), 2:826–51; and, "Technology and the Use of the Senses in Twentieth-Century Medicine," in *Medicine and the Five Senses*, eds. W. F. Bynum and Roy Porter (Cambridge, U.K.: Cambridge University Press, 1993), 262–73. Other key scholarship in this field includes the works of Joel D. Howell and Audrey B. Davis. See Howell's "Early Use of X-ray Machines and Electro-cardiographs at the Pennsylvania Hospital, 1897 through 1927," *Journal of the American Medical Association* 255, no. 17 (1986): 2320–23; *Technology and American Medical Practice. 1880–1930: Anthology of Sources* (New York: Garland Press, 1988); "Machines and Medicine: Technology Transforms the American Hospital," in *The American General Hospital: Communities and Social Contexts*, ed. Diana Elizabeth Long and Janet Golden (Ithaca, N.Y.: Cornell University Press, 1989), 109–34; and, *Technology in the Hospital: Transforming Patient Care in the Early Twentieth Century* (Baltimore: Johns Hopkins University Press, 1995). See Davis, *Medicine and its Technology: An Introduction to the History of Medical Instrumentation* (Westport, Conn.: Greenwood Press, 1981); and "American Medicine in the Gilded Age: The First Technological Era," *Annals of Science* 47 (1990): 111–25.

5.   For the growing importance of "science" in this period, the association of new diagnostic instrumentation with science, and physicians' effective use of the rhetoric of science, see Merriley Borell, "Training the Senses, Training the Mind," in *Medicine and the Five Senses*, ed. W. F. Bynum and Roy Porter (Cambridge, U.K.: Cambridge University Press, 1993), 244–61; Charles E. Rosenberg, *No Other Gods: On Science and American Social Thought*, rev. ed. (Baltimore: Johns Hopkins University Press, 1997); S. E. D. Shortt, "Physicians, Science, and Status: Issues in the Professionalization of Anglo-American Medicine in the Nineteenth Century," *Medical History* 27 (1983): 51–68; and, Ronald G. Walters, ed., *Scientific Authority and Twentieth-Century America* (Baltimore: Johns Hopkins University Press, 1997).

6.   Hughes Evans, "Losing Touch: The Controversy Over the Introduction of Blood Pressure Instruments into Medicine," *Technology and Culture* 34, no. 4 (1993): 784–807.

7.   Evans, "Losing Touch," 799.

8.   Reiser, "Technology and the Eclipse of Individualism," 12.

9.   Reiser, "Science of Diagnosis," 829.

10. Bertha Harmer, *Textbook of the Principles and Practice of Nursing* (New York: Macmillan, 1922), 45.

11. See, for example, Patricia Benner, ed., *Interpretive Phenomenology: Embodiment, Caring, and Ethics in Health and Illness* (Thousand Oaks, Calif.: Sage, 1994); Donald A. Laird, *Applied Psychology for Nurses* (Philadelphia: J. B. Lippincott, 1923); Hildegard E. Peplau, *Interpersonal Relations in Nursing* (New York: G.P. Putnam's Son, 1952); and, Christine A. Tanner et al., "The Phenomenology of Knowing the Patient," *Image: Journal of Nursing Scholarship* 25, no. 4 (1993): 273–80.

12. David Armstrong, "The Fabrication of Nurse-Patient Relationships, *Social Science & Medicine* 17, no. 8 (1983): 457–60.

13. Florence Nightingale, *Notes on Nursing: What It Is and What It Is Not* (New York: Dover, 1969/1860), 105.

14. Nightingale, *Notes*, 106.

15. Nightingale, *Notes*, 106.

16. Nightingale, *Notes*, 109.

17. Charles E. Rosenberg, *The Care of Strangers: The Rise of America's Hospital System* (Baltimore: Johns Hopkins University Press, 1987); and John H. Warner, *The Therapeutic Perspective: Medical Practice. Knowledge, and Identity in America. 1820–1885* (Cambridge, Mass.: Harvard University Press, 1986).

18. Nightingale, *Notes*, 133.

19. Nightingale, *Notes*, 110.

20. Nightingale, *Notes*, 111.

21. Nightingale, *Notes*, 116.

22. Nightingale, *Notes*, 124.

23. See, for example, Bellevue Hospital, *A Manual of Nursing* (New York: G. P. Putnam & Sons, 1878), 23–35; Harmer, *Textbook*, 45–49; Isabel Hampton Robb, *Nursing: Its Principles and Practice for Hospital and Private Use*, 3rd ed. (Cleveland, Ohio: E. C. Koeckert, 1906), 253–69.

24. Philadelphia General Hospital, *Nursing Procedures*, 1924, Center for the Study of the History of Nursing, University of Pennsylvania, School of Nursing, p. 120 (hereafter cited as CSHN).

25. Clara S. Weeks, *A Textbook of Nursing* (New York: D. Appleton, 1890), 80.

26. Weeks, *Textbook*, 80

27. Robb, *Nursing*, 41.

28. See, for example, the following series written by a physician: Robert A. Kilduffe, "The Nurse and Her Relation to Symptomatology, I: The Pulse," *Trained Nurse and Hospital Review*, 65, no. 6 (1920): 498–501 (hereafter cited to as TNHR); "The Nurse and Her Relation to Symptomatology, II: The Temperature," TNHR 66, no. 1 (1921): 13–16; and "The Nurse and Her Relation to Symptomatology, III: The Respiration," TNHR 66, no. 2 (1921): 109–12.

29. See, for example, the series by Myer Solis-Cohen, "How to Observe Symptoms," TNHR 35 (July 1905): 8–11, (August 1905): 83–85, and (September 1905): 140–42; and, Eugene A. Smith, "The Observation of Symptoms," *Trained Nurse* 1, no. 1 (1888): 52–55.

30. See, for example, Weeks, *Textbook*, 80.

31. Log, 26 August 1888, Mary U. Clymer Papers, CSHN.

32.   Agnes B. Meade, "Training the Senses in Clinical Observation," TNHR 97, no. 6 (1936): 540–44. Quote on p. 540.

33.   John D. Thompson and Grace Goldin, *The Hospital: A Social and Architectural History* (New Haven, Conn.: Yale University Press, 1975), 232. "Supervision/observability" (p. 231) competed with "privacy" (p. 207) in the history of hospital design. That is, as more patients were housed in private rooms, nurses found it harder to maintain visual control of patients and the environment surrounding them. With the increasing replacement of the ward with the private room a nurse could no longer stand at one point in a ward and see everything she needed to see.

34.   In Linda Richards, *Reminiscenses of Linda Richards: America's First Trained Nurse* (Boston, Mass.: Whitcomb & Barrows, 1911), 18–19, Richards suggested an important early environmental impediment to nursing observation. Concerning night duty at Bellevue Hospital, she recalled:

> No sooner had the day nurses left the wards than the gas was turned so low that the faces of the patients could not be distinguished. One could only see the dim outlines of figures wrapped in gray blankets lying upon the beds. If any work was to be done, a candle must be lighted, and only two candles a week were allowed each ward. If more were used, the nurse had to provide them . . . The captain of the watch . . . at 5 A.M. . . . turned off all the gas, leaving us in total darkness. Richards had this practice reversed by promising that nurses would use no more gas than they required to fulfill their duties.

35.   See, for example, Borell, "Training the Senses"; Malcolm Nicolson, "The Art of Diagnosis: Medicine and the Five Senses," in *Companion Encyclopedia of the History of Medicine*, eds. W. F. Bynum and Roy Porter (London: Routledge, 1993), 2:801–25; and, Reiser, "Science of Diagnosis."

36.   S. Weir Mitchell, *The Early History of Instrumental Precision in Medicine*, (New Haven, Conn.: Tuttle, Morehouse, and Taylor, 1892).

37.   Martha E. Erdmann and Margaret Welsh, "Studies in Thermometer Technique," *Nursing Education Bulletin* 2, no. 1 (1929): 8–33. Quote on p. 11. See also, on the history of clinical thermometry, Logan Clendening, "The History of Certain Medical Instruments," *Annals of Internal Medicine* 4, no. 2 (1930): 176–89; J. Gershon-Cohen, "A Short History of Medical Thermometry," *Annals of the New York Academy of Sciences* 121 (1964): 4–11; Hugh A. McGuigan, "Medical Thermometry," *Annals of Medical History* 9, no. 2 (1937): 148–54; and Reiser, *Medicine and the Reign of Technology*, 91–121.

38.   Carl A. Wunderlich, *On the Temperature in Diseases: A Manual of Medical Thermometry*, trans. W. Bathurst Woodman (London: New Sydenham Society, 1871).

39.   Edouard Seguin, *Family Thermometry: A Manual of Thermometry for Mothers, Nurses, Hospitalers, Etc., and All Those Who Have Charge of the Sick and the Young* (New York: Putnam, 1873); and *Medical Thermometry and Human Temperature*, 2nd ed. (New York: William Wood, 1876). Excerpts of Sequin, *Family Thermometry* are reprinted in *Temperature, Part 1: Arts and Concepts*, ed. Theodore H. Benzinger (Stroudsburg, Pa.: Dowden, Hutchinson & Ross, 1977), 316–335.

40.   Seguin, *Medical Thermometry*, 253.

41. See, for example, Amanda Beck, *A Reference Handbook for Nurses* (Philadelphia: W. B. Saunders, 1905), 50; Harmer, *Textbook*, 134–151; and Lecture 21 November 1887, Mary U. Clymer Papers, CSHN.

42. See the ads at the back of Bellevue Hospital, *Manual of Nursing*, and Emily M. A. Stoney, *Bacteriology and Surgical Technique for Nurses* (Philadelphia: W. B. Saunders, 1900).

43. See, for example, Frank S. Betz Company, *Surgical Instruments and Supplies*, 1918, Medical Trade Ephemera Collection, College of Physicians of Philadelphia, p. 37; Anna M. Fullerton, *Surgical Nursing* (Philadelphia: P. Blakiston's Son, 1899), 255; E. Hibbard, "A Nurse's Requirements," *Trained Nurse* 2, no. 5 (1889): 188–89; Emily A. M. Stoney, *Practical Points in Nursing for Nurses in Private Practice*, 2nd ed. (Philadelphia: W. B. Saunders, 1897), 25; and, H. W. Weed Company, *Illustrations of Surgical Instruments*, 1902, Medical Trade Catalog Collection, Division of Medical Sciences, National Museum of American History, Washington, D.C., p. 2115.

44. See the Becton, Dickinson ad located before the table of contents, *American Journal of Nursing* 27 (April 1927).

45. See, for example, Alice Ward Bailey, "Hospital Life," *Scribner's Magazine* 3 (1888): 698–715; Emily Bax, "Are Nurses Overpaid?" *Hygeia* 9 (1931, August): 727–31, quote on p. 727; Katherine DeWitt, "Hospital Sketches," *American Journal of Nursing* 6, no. 7 (1906): 455–59.

46. Isabel A. Hampton, *Nursing: Its Principles and Practice* (Philadelphia: W. B. Saunders, 1893), 93.

47. Seguin, *Family Thermometry*, 4.

48. Seguin, *Family Thermometry*, 5.

49. Seguin, *Family Thermometry*, 19.

50. Seguin, *Family Thermometry*, 19–20.

51. Seguin, *Family Thermometry*, 20.

52. Bellevue Hospital, *Manual of Nursing*, 143.

53. Connecticut Training School for Nurses, *A Handbook of Nursing for Family and General Use* (Philadelphia: J. B. Lippincott, 1879), 107–9.

54. Hampton, *Nursing*, 167–85.

55. Hampton, *Nursing*, 170.

56. Hampton, *Nursing*, 184.

57. J. C. Wilson, *Fever Nursing* (Philadelphia: J. B. Lippincott, 1899).

58. Harmer, *Textbook*, 138.

59. Helen W. Faddis et al., "Making Temperature Taking Safe," *Pacific Coast Journal of Nursing* 24, no. 2 (1928): 73–74.

60. A contemporary concept with historical relevance described by Shizuko Fagerhaugh et al., "Chronic Illness, Medical Technology, and Clinical Safety in the Hospital," *Research in the Sociology of Health Care* 4 (1986): 237–70.

61. See, for example, the Becton, Dickinson ad, TNHR 66, no. 1 (1921): 73; the Faichney Instrument ad, *Hospital Management* 21, no. 2 (1926): 88; and Minnie Goodnow, *The Technic of Nursing* (Philadelphia: W. B. Saunders, 1928), 148.

62. Daisy Barnwell Jones, *My First Eighty Years* (Baltimore: Gateway Press, 1986), 250. A student at Johns Hopkins in the late 1920s and early 1930s, she described having fallen and, as a result, broken 32 thermometers for which she

did not have to pay. This book is available at the North Carolina Collection (hereafter referred to as NCC), University of North Carolina at Chapel Hill, N.C.

63.   Erdmann and Walsh, "Studies in Thermometer Technique," 8–33. See also Ruth Ashburn, "A Bacteriological Study of Clinical Thermometer Technic," *American Journal of Nursing* 30, no. 3 (1930): 336–42 (hereafter cited as AJN); A. Frances Fischer and Catherine Simonds, "A Modern Hospital Takes its Temperatures," AJN 29, no. 1 (1929): 89–90;

64.   See, for example, Goodnow, *Technic*, 148; Harmer, *Textbook*, 150; and Weeks, *Textbook*, 67.

65.   Hampton, *Nursing*, 50.

66.   See, for example, Faddis et al., "Making Temperature Taking Safe," 74; Harriet M. Gillette, "A Practical Thermometer Tray," AJN 26, no. 11 (1926): 840; and "A Method of Taking Temperatures," AJN 27, no. 10 (1927): 810.

67.   See, for example, Minnie Goodnow, *First-Year Nursing: A Textbook for Pupils During Their First Year of Hospital Work*, 2nd ed. (Philadelphia: W. B. Saunders, 1919), 138.

68.   See, for example, Joseph B. Cooke, *A Nurse's Handbook of Obstetrics*, 10th ed. (Philadelphia: J. B. Lippincott, 1924); Joseph B. DeLee, *Obstetrics for Nurses*, 9th eds. (1913; reprint, Philadelphia: W. B. Saunders, 1930); and Carolyn Conant Van Blarcom, *Obstetrical Nursing*, 3rd eds. (1922; reprint, New York: Macmillan, 1922 and 1933).

69.   See, for example, Robert A. Kilduffe, "The Blood Pressure: A Consideration of Its Technique and Significance," TNHR 68 (March, 1922): 228–30; Louise Gliem, "High Blood Pressure: Its Care and Treatment," AJN 24, no. 12 (1924): 1184–89; Veronica F. Murray ("Technic of Taking Blood Pressure," AJN 34, no. 11 (1934): 1057–64; Charles C. Sutter, "Blood Pressure," AJN 15, no. 1 (1915): 7–13; William S. Middleton, "Blood Pressure Determination: A Nursing Procedure," AJN 30, no. 10 (1930): 1219–25; and Irving Wilson Voorhies, "What Is Blood Pressure?" TNHR 61 (1918, July) 6–8. The Philadelphia General Hospital School of Nursing did not include the taking of blood pressure in its procedure books until 1948. See Philadelphia General Hospital, *Nursing Procedures*, 40. In DeLee's *Obstetrics for Nurses*, p. 116, a nurse is shown taking the blood pressure. Blood pressure technique is not described at all in, for example, Barbara A. Thompson, *Nursing Procedures: A Manual Used in the Teaching of the Principles and Practice of Nursing in the Associated Hospitals in the University of Minnesota School of Nursing* (Minneapolis: The University of Minnesota Press, 1929); and Mary C. Wheeler and Arnalia Metzker, *Nursing Technic* (Philadelphia: J. B. Lippincott, 1930).

70.   Evans, "Losing Touch," 784–807.

71.   Smith, "The Observation of Symptoms," 53.

72.   For more on media images of nurses and physicians, see, for example, Daniel M. Fox and Christopher Lawrence, *Photographing Medicine: Images and Power in Britain and America Since 1840* (New York: Greenwood Press, 1988); and N. J. Krantzler, "Media Images of Physicians and Nurses in the United States," *Social Science & Medicine* 22 (1986): 933–52.

73.   See, for example, Howell, *Technology in the Hospital*; Reiser, *Medicine and the Reign of Technology*; and Stanley J. Reiser, "The Test Tube As Oracle: The

Domination of Diagnostics by Laboratory Analysis," in *History of Diagnostics*, ed. Yosio Kawakita (Proceedings of the 9th International Symposium on the Comparative History of Medicine—East and West, (Osaka, Japan: The Taniguchi Foundation, 1987), 175–85.

74.   See, for example, Stevens, *In Sickness and in Wealth*, 105–31.

75.   See, for example, P. C. Remondino, "The Trained Nurse in Private Practice," *Trained Nurse* 32, no. 2 (1904): 77–82; and Weeks, *Textbook*, 173.

76.   See, for example, Annual Report of the Watts Hospital for the Year Ending 30 November 1922, NCC, Durham, NC., p. 41; and "Suggestions for National Hospital Day Publicity," *Bulletin of the American Hospital Association* 1, no. 1 (1927): 3–23.

77.   For the varied duties and education of the nurse in these fields, see, for example, Charlotte A. Aikens, *Clinical Studies for Nurses*, 2nd ed. (Philadelphia: W. B. Saunders, 1912), 37; Sister Alma, *Clinical Laboratory Manual for Nurses and Technicians* (St. Louis: C. V. Mosby, 1932); Louise B. D'Arby, "The Hospital X-ray Nurse," AJN 17, no. 6 (1917): 488–90; Louise B. D'Arby, "Suggestions for the X-ray Room, II: Fluoroscopic Work and Record Keeping," TNHR 70, no. 5 (1923): 416–17; Henry J. Goeckel, "A Plan for the Laboratory Training of Nurses," *Modern Hospital* 12 (1919, June): 422–23; A. Hazelwood, "The Nurse and the Clinical Laboratory," AJN 27, no. 4 (1927): 259–61; R. M. L. "My Experience in X-ray Work," AJN 20, no. 8 (1920): 626–27; Rose M. Lorish, "The Development of the X-ray Negative," AJN 21, no. 4 (1921): 234–36; Margaret Ossenback, "Training School for Nurses," in the Annual Report of the Watts Hospital for the Year Ending 30 November 1921, NCC, Durham, N.C., pp. 22–27; Olive B. Sweet, "A Hospital Nurse's Day," *U. S. Veterans' Bureau Medical Bulletin* 1, no. 4 (1925): 57–61; Catherine B. Washburn, "Assisting With Diagnostic Tests," AJN 29, no. 6 (1929): 645–48; Edith L. Weart, "The Nurse as Laboratory Technician," AJN 32, no. 12 (1912): 1251–54; and, John B. Zingrone, "Mercy Hospital X-ray Laboratory," *Hospital Progress* 1, no. 3 (1920): 104–7. See also the series by Henry J. Goeckel, "The Laboratory: Its Relation to the Nursing Service," TNHR 70, nos. 1–6 (1923): 44–45, 115–16, 226–27, 320–21, 413–15, and 509–11.

78.   See, for example, Nora D. Dean, "The Roentgenological Field for Nurses," AJN 21, no. 3 (1920): 159–61; E. Blanche Seyfert, "Opportunities for the Nurse in the X-ray Diagnostic Laboratory," TNHR 68 (February 1922): 136–37. Quote on p. 136.

79.   J. M. Parrott, response to Edmundson S. Boice, "The Interne Problem of the Small Hospital," Transactions of the North Carolina Hospital Association, NCC, Pinehurst, N.C., pp. 14–19, quote on p. 19.

80.   See, for example, Seyfert, "Opportunities for the Nurse"; M. Warwick "The Nurse As Laboratory Technician," AJN 27, no. 2 (1927): 95–97; and, Weart, "Nurse as Laboratory Technician."

81.   Seyfert, "Opportunities for the Nurse," 137.

82.   Seyfert, "Opportunities for the Nurse," 137.

83.   Boice, "Interne Problem," 18.

84.   Boice, "Interne Problem," 18.

85.   Boice, "Interne Problem," 18.

86.   I have as yet found no means to determine exactly how many nurses assumed these roles. A nurse is listed as a laboratory technician in the Annual

Report of the Watts Hospital for the Year Ending 30 November 1921, NCC, Durham, N.C., p. 7.

87. Weart, "Nurse as Laboratory Technician," 1251.

88. Seyfert, "Opportunities for the Nurse," 137.

89. D'Arby, "Hospital X-ray Nurse," 488; Dean, "Roentgenological Field," 159; and Seyfert, "Opportunities for the Nurse," 138.

90. Warwick, "Nurse as Laboratory Technician," 97.

91. Mabel McVicker, "The Importance of Understanding Medical Laboratory Tests," AJN 23, no. 1 (1922): 14–16. On p. 14, McVicker wrote that too often, nurses looked on a "test" as something that had to be done because a doctor ordered it and felt relief when it was over because the "routine" work of the ward could then proceed without further interference. However, according to McVicker, nurses would do this work with interest, enthusiasm, and accuracy if they knew the significance of the test and the importance of nurses in assisting with diagnosis.

92. Maud Banfield, "The Cleaning," in *On the Administrative Frontier of Medicine: The First Ten Years of the American Hospital Association. 1899–1908*, ed. Morris J. Vogel (New York: Garland, 1989), 59–62. On p. 61, she uses this phrase in a different context to refer to the superintendent of nurses who tries to "keep an eye" on cleaning.

93. Ethel Johns and Blanche Pfefferkorn, *An Activity Analysis of Nursing* (New York: Committee on the Grading of Nursing Schools, 1934), 83.

94. Harmer, *Textbook*, xi.

95. Bertha Harmer and Virginia Henderson, *Textbook of the Principles and Practice of Nursing*, 4th ed. (New York: Macmillan, 1939), ix.

96. See, for example, Charlotte A. Aikens, *Studies in Ethics for Nurses* (Philadelphia: W. B. Saunders, 1916), 112–13; George H. Hoxie, *Practice of Medicine for Nurses: A Textbook for Nurses and Students of Domestic Science, and a Handbook for All Those Who Care for the Sick* (Philadelphia: W. B. Saunders, 1980), preface; Kilduffe, "The Nurse and Her Relation to Symptomatology," 498.

97. Smith, "The Observation of Symptoms," 54.

98. See, for example, Goodnow, *First-Year Nursing*, 197; and Solis-Cohen, "How to Observe Symptoms," 8.

99. Johns and Pfefferkorn, *Activity Analysis*, 21.

100. Wunderlich, *On the Temperature in Diseases*, 74.

101. Seguin, *Medical Thermometry*, 281.

102. Seguin, *Medical Thermometry*, 281.

103. Wunderlich, *On the Temperature in Diseases*, 75.

104. Seguin, *Medical Thermometry*, 281.

105. Wunderlich, *On the Temperature in Diseases*, 75.

106. Reiser, "Test Tube as Oracle," and "Technology and the Eclipse of Individualism." On the use and abuse of laboratory diagnosis (with an emphasis on the debate in North Carolina), see also, for example, Richard C. Cabot, "The Historical Development and Relative Value of Laboratory and Clinical Methods of Diagnosis," *Boston Medical and Surgical Journal* 157, no. 5 (1907): 150–53 (hereafter referred to as BMSJ); Robert H. Lafferty, "The Importance of Chemistry and Physiology to the General Practitioner," *Transactions of the Medical Society of*

the State of North Carolina 59 (1912): 498–501 (hereafter referred to as TMSNC); Paul H. Ringer, "Abuse of the Laboratory From the Viewpoint of the Laboratory Worker," TMSNC 57 (1910): 377–81; John H. Tucker, "What Aid is the Laboratory in Diagnosis?" TMSNC 58 (1911): 532–36; S. A. Stevens, "The Relation of the Specialist to the General Practitioner," TMSNC 58 (1911): 172–77; W. H. Prioleau, "What Laboratory Work Should Be Done By The Physician Himself?" TMSNC 51 (1904): 324–27.

107. Elizabeth Connolly, "The Nurse and the Fractional Ewald Meal by the Rehfus Method," in Transactions of the Sixth Annual Meeting of the North Carolina Hospital Association, NCC, Asheville, N.C., pp. 80–84.

108. See, for example, J. M. Davis, "Teaching Bacteriology in School [sic] of Nursing," in Official Proceedings of the 32nd Annual Convention of the North Carolina State Nurses' Association, 25–27 October 1934, NCC, Fayetteville, N.C., pp. 59–63; Kilduffe, "The Nurse and Her Relation to Symptomatology"; Smith, "The Observation of Symptoms"; Solis Cohen, "How to Observe Symptoms."

109. Dr. Billings quoted in Ethel Johns and Blanche Pfefferkorn, *The Johns Hopkins Hospital School of Nursing, 1889–1949* (Baltimore: Johns Hopkins Press, 1954), 13.

110. See, for example, W. Gilman Thompson, "The Overtrained Nurse," *New York Medical Journal* 83, no. 17 (1906): 845–49.

111. Thompson, "Overtrained Nurse," 846.

112. See, for example, Richard O. Beard, "The Education of the Nurse in America," *Transactions of the American Hospital Association* 12 (1910): 345–59; Richard C. Cabot, "Suggestions for the Improvement of Training Schools for Nurses," BMSJ 145, no. 21 (1901): 567–69; Thelma Ingles, "The Physicians' View of the Evolving Nursing Profession," *Nursing Forum* 15, no. 2 (1976): 123–64; and "Nursing as a Profession," BMSJ 149, no. 5 (1903): 133–34; John H. Packard, "On the Training of Nurses for the Sick," BMSJ XCV, no. 20 (1876): 573–79; and "The Reciprocal Relations of the Nurse and the Physician," BMSJ 121, no. 17 (1889): 417–18; G. H. M. Rowe, "The Training of Nurses," BMSJ 109, no. 1 (1883): 1–4.

113. See, for example, President's Address, in Transactions of the North Carolina Hospital Association, 20 April 1920, NCC, Charlotte, N.C., p. 8. A physician is quoted as saying: "Don't make a poor doctor and spoil a good nurse."

114. Thompson, "Overtrained Nurse," 848.

115. Packard, "On the Training of Nurses," 577.

116. Carl Mitcham, *Thinking Through Technology: The Path Between Engineering and Philosophy* (Chicago: University of Chicago Press, 1994), 209. What is often forgotten is that most physicians also did not bring technologies into existence but, rather, put them to use. We tend to valorize invention over application and to see physicians (males) as inventors and nurses (females) as only users.

117. Eva Gamarnikow, "Nurse or Woman: Gender and Professionalism in Reformed Nursing, 1860–1923," in *Anthropology and Nursing*, eds. Pat Holden and Jenny Littlewood (London: Routledge, 1986), 110–29. Quote on p. 119. Gamarnikow studied British nursing.

118. Toby Gelfand, "The History of the Medical Profession," in *Companion Encyclopedia*, 1119–50.

119. The lack of evidence here may be more a consequence of the serious

lack of data available to researchers concerning actual nursing practice than a reflection of nurses' nonuse of such technological information as the results of x-ray and laboratory tests. Yet, even textbooks of the period emphasize the nurses' role in acquiring the information for physicians as opposed to using the information themselves in nursing practice.

120. Blanche Pfefferkorn and Marian Rottman, *Clinical Education in Nursing* (New York: Macmillan, 1932). In the section "Extra-Nursing Functions and the Nursing Load," 51–52, these nurses noted that:

> An idea frequently expressed is that technical and medical functions are being steadily transferred to the nursing staff, with encroachment on nursing duties and greatly increased nursing load. This may be true in so far as graduate nurses elect work of that type. Findings from the Bellevue Study reveal an almost negligible amount of time given to activities, other than those of a purely nursing nature. . . . If the assignment, taking and recording of blood pressure, to the nursing staff, adds two hours to a daily load of 100 hours, the increase is not sufficient to burden the nursing service or to affect the quality of the nursing. It seems likely that the time emphasis placed upon new responsibilities outside the immediate field of nursing has been due to the fact that in most institutions, the required nursing load hours exceed the provided nursing hours, and, as a result, any addition to the already existing load is apt to be considered out of its right proportion.

121. Davina Allen, "The Nursing-Medical Boundary: A Negotiated Order?" *Sociology of Health & Illness* 19, no. 4 (1997): 498–520.

122. Mitcham, *Thinking Through Technology*, 152.

123. Leonard Stein, "The Doctor-Nurse Game," *Archives of General Psychiatry* 16 (June 1967): 699–703.

124. Marjory Gordon, *Nursing Diagnosis: Process and Application*, 3rd ed. (St. Louis, Mo.: Mosby, 1994).

125. Gamarnikow, "Nurse or Woman," 123.

126. Rosalind Gill and Keith Grint, "The Gender-Technology Relation: Contemporary Theory and Research," in *The Gender-Technology Relation: Contemporary Theory and Research*, ed. Keith Grint and Rosalind Gill (London: Taylor & Francis, 1995), 1–28. Quote on p. 9.

SECTION 4

THE NATURE OF NURSING KNOWLEDGE

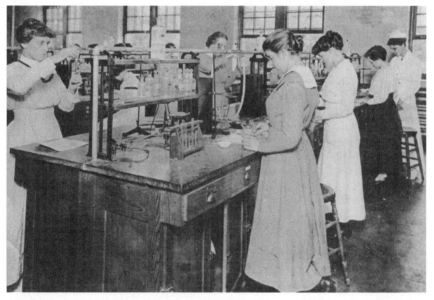

Vassar Training Camp for Nurses, 1918. Courtesy of Agnes Smith Collection, Center for the Study of the History of Nursing, University of Pennsylvania.

Introduction

Joan E. Lynaugh

What do nurses know and how do they know it? Several interlocking elements combine to fuel these perennial questions: the fact that nursing was and is a woman's field, the fact that nursing is a practice profession, the mundane and domestic character of much of nursing's work, and the eccentric history of nursing's educational system. When nursing was invented, the very idea of higher education for women was controversial and even most nurses thought nursing best taught by example and imitation. Good domestic skills, the ability to read and write and do simple arithmetic, willingness to learn and follow rules, and respect for persons in authority—these were the sought after attributes in young women entering the field.

Moreover, even if nursing had not been "women's work" most people saw nursing as a practice profession where skills were learned in action and where knowledge was demonstrated, not explained. Indeed, at the time, it was rare for any career to require classroom education past high school. What turn-of-the-century nurses *should* know was an extension of what every well-instructed young woman would have already learned at home, supplemented by the special routines of the training school. Rather soon, however, nurses began to find that more systematic and detailed learning was badly needed. In fact, the uncertain and inadequate intellectual preparation of the novice nurse became the most intractable problem of 20th century nursing. As historians Hamilton and Reverby make clear, nurse thinkers such as Annie Goodrich, Adelaide Nutting, Lavinia Dock, Lillian Wald, and later Isabel Stewart all deplored what Nutting called the humiliating weakness of the nurse educational system. All disciples of Progressive Era philosopher John Dewey, they understood that knowledge was the power that could transform their world.

Diane Hamilton offers us a tour of the thinking of Dock, Goodrich and Wald. Set on detaching nursing from its religious and benevolent fetters they espoused an ideal of compassion based on commitment to humane authority and the idea of social progress. The key ideas here were secularism, progress and independence for the nurse. But an institutional framework for transforming nurses to meet this vision did not then exist and was very slow to appear. Nurses could not gain a place in America's universities for their subject and, in fact, it took several decades for nurses to debate and decide exactly what would constitute nursing knowledge.

Carole Estabrooks' account of Lavinia Dock's years at the Henry Street Settlement is instructive in this regard. Dock, certainly one of the most intellectually able of nursing's founders, was primarily interested in social reform. Women's suffrage, labor equity, control of vice and venereal disease, and organizing nursing to gain nurses' rights fully occupied her time. Dock's contribution was to urge nurses to develop their social knowledge, to see the world beyond their everyday clinical concerns. Her own personal development at Henry Street is instructive. Estabrooks rightly points out the crippling absence of an intellectual support system, i.e., a college or university, where nurses could think and experiment. The crucial importance of a sheltered and encouraging environment such as the one created by Lillian Wald allowed Dock to expand and explain her vision for nurses.

But, in terms of developing new nursing knowledge, the argument about content really got under way in the late 1920s and 1930s. Susan Reverby describes the limitations of nurses' training and the difficulties of making even small changes in the curriculum of hospital-run schools. She also calls our attention to the prevailing idea that womanly nurses needed no science but, instead, needed high character and better moral values. The university program at Teacher's College in New York City offered hope. It nurtured ideas about science that later were actively injected into the nursing dialogue by Isabel Stewart. Reverby argues that educator Stewart envisioned science mostly as a tool for improving teaching, not as a way to test new knowledge for nursing. Still, by 1929, others were calling on nurses to investigate clinical practice. Teacher's College faculty Martha Ruth Smith and Virginia Henderson sought to make science serve the art of nursing. They wanted to find and name the scientific principles underlying nursing practice. Decades of struggle left the matter of the actual content of nursing still at issue in the years immediately following World War II. As Reverby notes, science proved a difficult intellectual ladder for nursing to climb as we sought to escape from hospital control of our educational system. It would take massive infusions of post World War II federal money for training faculty, building colleges of nursing, and supporting higher education for nurses before the knowledge-building ideas of 1929 could be effected.

Finally, Julie Fairman re-frames the question of nursing knowledge in its relation to medical knowledge by revealing the person to person negotiations between doctors and nurses at work. Her article explores the "travel" of clinical knowledge among practitioners. Re-thinking nursing practice in the years after World War II was stimulated by demands from society for more and better service from physicians and nurses. This new practice and its knowledge requirements revolutionized the content of higher education in nursing. Calls for more and better-quality health care, better access to higher education for nurses, and a new view of women's place in society combined to vastly expand our intellectual expectations for nursing.

Now understood as a specialized field of knowledge, nursing adopted many of the trappings of a science-based field but still struggles to bridge the modern gap between science and the humanities. Clearly, nurses need intimate understanding of the discipline of nursing and need to grasp the social context in which they function. Nurses need to appreciate the social relevance and value orientations of their field; they need to know how to relate to other disciplines and how our heritage influences our perspective. But, what exactly do nurses know and how do they know it? These are questions to visit and answer anew every day.

11

Constructing the Mind of Nursing

Diane Hamilton

Revisionist historical scholars have lately expanded the explanations of nursing's conception beyond "the great woman theory" of Nightingale's genius to suggest that American nursing's roots emanate from a blending of the ideology of domesticity with that of medical science (O'Brien 1987; Lynaugh and Fagin 1988); that nursing is a story of women workers' rationalizing the service industry (Melosh 1982); that nursing is the product of a group of enlightened leaders intent on reform and professionalization (Christy 1969); that nursing developed from the growth of paternalistic hospitals eager to manipulate females and to profit from nurses' work (Ashley 1976); that nursing emerged from interacting social and economic needs related to the care of the ill (Rosenberg 1987); that nursing became visible when philanthropic women and physicians demanded that hospitals employ "lady" nurses (Mottus 1981); and that nursing gained its social and moral justification from its obligation to care (Reverby 1987).[1] Historical inquiry fuels an interpretive argument about the past; each perspective generates new insights to, and another link in, the great chain of explanation and understanding of nursing's history. At the same time we are reminded of unanswered, tantalizing questions.

One genre of unasked questions concerns the ideas on which nurses built their work. What could we discover by conceptualizing nurses' *thinking* as the object of historical research? What were the thoughts and the thinking patterns of the leaders who designed nursing as a vocation for women? And what are the epistemological and ontological assumptions rooted in the history of nurses' thinking?

We know that during the nineteenth century nursing began to distinguish itself from other groups, to organize its activities, and to seek

Note: This chapter was originally published in *Nursing History Review* 2 (1994): 3–28. Copyright © by The American Association for the History of Nursing. Reprinted with permission.

credibility and legitimacy within society. The nurse inventors believed that nurses offered an esoteric service to the public based on some special conception of knowledge. As emerging professionals, nurses professed "to know." Yet the intellectual terrain of nursing remains unexplored. While giving Florence Nightingale credit as nursing's first "theorist," many writers seem to assume that "nursing theory and knowledge development have a short history."[2] This leaves us with a mental picture of a great wasteland of unthinking nurses stretching from Nightingale to mid-twentieth-century nurse thinkers such as Hildegarde Peplau, Faye G. Abdellah, and Ernestine Weidenbach. The apex of thinking, according to this ahistorical view, occurs with the nurse theorists of the late twentieth century. This notion that sophisticated thinking and theorizing began only recently presumes that "modern" ideas are innately superior to earlier ones. It denies that the nurse inventors and nurses who followed were bright, articulate women. These women directed health- and illness-related institutions, and they were fully capable of generating concepts, ideas, and meanings. To view late twentieth-century nursing knowledge as "new" denies the probability that ideas emigrated and immigrated over multiple generations of nurses and nurse-institutions in a social context that perpetually sculpted ideas and thinking.

This chapter reexamines and reflects on a small "thought collective" (a term I explain below) of nurses Lillian Wald, Annie Goodrich, and Lavinia Dock. In it I argue that the institution of nursing includes an intellectual history as much as an economic, social, and political one. Moreover, I will show that, while Wald, Goodrich, and Dock believed their ideas to be "modern" and secular, their conceptualization of nursing rested on religious and spiritual ideas of earlier eras. From these ideas, they selected compassion to be one of the basic guiding principles and virtues of nursing.

Toward the end of the nineteenth century, an amalgam of many ideas coalesced to transform nursing from a servile occupation into a paid vocation. The training school movement, from a slow beginning in mid-century, began to flourish—growing from thirty-five schools in 1890 to 432 schools by the close of the century. Although nursing leaders at the World's Fair in Chicago in 1893 protested against the overwhelming lack of uniformity of instruction in schools of nursing, successful training programs, boasting of both educational standards and strong nursing leadership, were established at several teaching hospitals, including The Johns Hopkins, Bellevue, Boston City, Massachusetts General, New York Hospital, and Connecticut Training School at the New Haven Hospital. Moreover, the American Society of Superintendents of Training Schools for Nurses, later called the National League for Nursing Education, had organized in 1894, and the Nurses' Associated Alumnae of the United States and

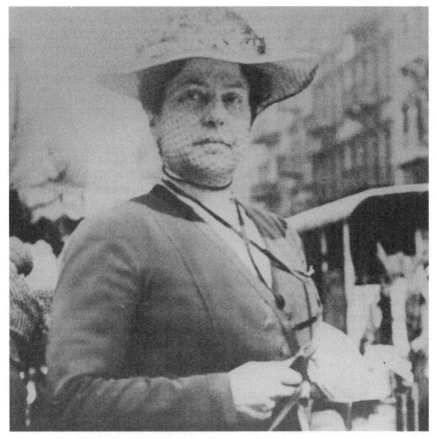

Lillian D. Wald. (Courtesy of the Visiting Nurses Service of New York)

Canada, which became the American Nurses' Association, formed two years later.[3]

This flurry of organizing, in retrospect, was not surprising. Historians generally agree that in the late nineteenth century, Americans from every class organized, usually by occupation, in an effort to adapt to a changing society and economy.[4] The professions, in general, shifted their intellectual orientation from an individualistic and voluntary approach to a collective one in order to function more effectively and thus obtain status, legitimacy, and profit. Nurses, following the footsteps of the more established professions, such as medicine and law, began to form organizations, to standardize educational requirements, to establish journals, and to persuade state legislatures to pass registration and licensing laws.

INTELLECTUAL HISTORY: UNEARTH THE THINKING

Nurse inventors needed an intellectual framework to guide their process of legitimizing nursing. To solidify the concept "nurse," to construct the phenomenon called "professional nursing," to fashion the boundaries of rightness and wrongness of nurse behavior, and to effectively negotiate acceptance of the validity of the trained nurse necessitated both competing ideas and some degree of "sameness of thinking" among the nurse inventors. Yet the exact nature of the nurse inventors' intellectual schema for constructing the "mind of nursing" remains unarticulated.

Ian Hacking, analyzing the relationship between reality and labels, called this legitimating process "making people up" and suggested that the proliferation of labels in the nineteenth century engendered more kinds of people than ever before.[5] As new institutions created new labels, people came forward to accept the labels and to construct their lives accordingly. While nursing had always been part of women's "natural" work, by midcentury nursing had evolved into an occupation with women willing to perform the work for wages, to organize nursing's structure and function, and to profess ideas about nursing in the marketplace.

As new ideas emerge, they carry the marks of their social origins. Classifications, logical thinking, and guiding metaphors are socially constructed, linking ideas and cognition to political, economic, and social problems. What is considered of value or "true" varies across time, for society's perspective is determined by dominant opinions and directed perceptions, popularly labeled the dominant "paradigm" (Kuhn 1962) or "thought style" (Fleck 1979). And although thought styles function as a prism in which reality is refracted, individuals, needing to build a meaningful world, choose from the thought style's smorgasbord of ideas through the groups in which they live. According to philosopher Ludwig Fleck (1979), a group of persons, working and exchanging ideas within institutions, constitutes a thought collective.[6] Thus, thought collectives, functioning within the era's thought style, become the distributors and brokers of institutions' ideas.[7]

Of course, the effect of accepting both the individual and the social context as sculptors of ideas highlights the thorny issue of the relationship between the individual mind and social influences on cognition, between the subjective perceptions and social context, and between the subjective (inside) and the objective (outside) reality of the lived human experience.[8] These dilemmas cannot be ignored by historians studying thinking as a historical event. As historian Dominick LaCapra pointed out, while the social context may, in part, explain how social problems influence the origin of ideas, the social context may neither directly *cause* the ideas nor elucidate the authors' intentions or *meaning* of the ideas.[9] Describing an idea's origin and understanding the meaning of authors' thinking are different. To disclose meaning and offer interpretation, the historian must search for the relationship between the author's intentions and the text, the relationship between the author's life and the text, and the interaction between the culture and its institution and the text, while maintaining the awareness that these relationships will include multiple forms of tensions, incongruities, and contradictions. A good historical interpretation of ideas does not simply impose coherence on what seem to be "scattered" thoughts, but rather stimulates further investigation into seemingly incompatible ideas and beliefs.

An analysis of nurse inventors' thinking cannot suggest that their ideas simply mirrored the pragmatist, the progressive, or the populist thoughts of the historical era that midwived nursing. The notions of nursing are strongly influenced by, but not necessarily caused by, intellectual trends. Nursing was not discovered as a completed product, but rather was constructed by a multitude of persons, in multiple settings, and within more than one context.

Nursing history is not only a story of what happened to whom and when; it is also an analysis of who we are, why we think the way we do, and how the ideas of "what nursing *should* be" and "what nursing is" changed over time. In the process of envisioning and bonding to the identity, the thinking, and the mission of nursing, the nurse inventors fashioned a core of ideas within their social context. They selected ideas that seemed good and true and right for nursing practice, for society, and, maybe more importantly, for themselves. Nursing foremothers such as Lillian Wald, Isabel Hampton Robb, Lavinia Dock, Annie Goodrich, Lillian Clayton, Mary Lent, Ella Crandall, Mary Gardner, Adelaide Nutting, Sophia Palmer, Isabel McIsaac, Mary E. P. Davis, and Louise Darche engaged in, and in many ways formulated, the precedent of "nurse thinking and nursing practice" during what historian Teresa Christy called "the fateful decade" (1890–1900).[10]

THE FATEFUL DECADE

By 1890, just a hundred years after the founding of the Republic, the American promise of egalitarian life was becoming an illusion. The extremes of wealth and poverty were as great as those in the Old World. The structure of American industry had changed dramatically from widespread small-town shopkeeping into centralized, large-scale manufacturing, with national market corporations in a few cities. Small towns shrank in political and economic significance while the complexity and density of industrial and seaport cities increased, with millions of immigrants crowding into the slums of American cities, constituting a proletariat that was not only impoverished but alien.

Despite these social and economic threats to continuity, America was in a hurry to be great. Americans had convinced themselves that their country was predestined for superiority by accepting the doctrine of social Darwinism that promised success to the strong and envisioned progress as an ever accelerating movement. That freedom and democracy would eventually create a pure, rational society seemed obvious to Americans. Moreover, it seemed self-evident that the accumulation of knowledge would catapult society into a promising future. The last decade of the nineteenth century did produce a large body of new thinking, such as James's *Psychology*; Veblen's *Theory of the Leisure Class*; Wine's *Report on Crime and Pauperism*; Boas's *Development of the Culture of Northwest America*; and Dewey's *The School and Society*. But despite idealistic attitudes and an accumulation of knowledge, utopia always seemed just around the corner. As Henry Commager noted, "never had men known so many facts and been masters of so few principles."[11]

Surrounded by the often dismal conditions of a shifting society, Americans could not deny the physical and spiritual reality of the disenfranchised poor. As historian Robert Wiebe notes, late-nineteenth-century America had to acknowledge that society had lost its core and sense of community. As this sobering awareness permeated society, the crises of the communities surfaced as a syndrome that included lack of confidence in the powers of the community, anxiety about self-determination, a search for order, and an enthusiasm for reform.[12]

Harsh urban realities demanded reform. With labor rioting, child mortality rates increasing, and diseases like tuberculosis and syphilis running rampant across class lines, reformers approached the problems with a mood of excited urgency. While some reformers reordered government, child labor laws, or prisons, others entered the city slums to live among the poor. Settlement houses, as outposts of education and culture within depraved cities, were intended to bridge the gulf between the classes, to lessen suspicion and hostility between diverse cultural groups, and to do more than just "hand out" charity. The educated, the cultured, and the privileged "settled" among the poor in order to, as Jane Addams described the movement, "equalize opportunity," not from a motive of philanthropy nor benevolence but from a "sense of humanity."[13]

As a comprehensive institution within the communities, the settlement house, which Jane Addams compared to a university, stood for the application of knowledge, as opposed to research; for emotion and humanity, in contrast to intellectualization; and for equalizing life experiences and opportunities among classes. One natural link to this civic humanism was the public health movement, which, as all nurses know, capitalized on visiting nurses. Equalizing opportunity for the poor and dedication to social welfare in the broadest sense had to include sanitation, hygiene, and regulation of the environments that produced disease. Middle-class reformers found it difficult to enlighten the mind and the spirit without feeding, clothing, sheltering, and caring for the body. Thus, the public health reformers found an easy alliance between the institutions of visiting nurses and settlement houses. The public health movement, designed to be broad in scope, concerned itself with almost every aspect of life: the promotion of health, the prevention of disease, and the maintenance of a standard of living necessary for health. The settlement house movement juxtaposed with the public health movement addressed human welfare in the very broadest sense.[14]

Women, as keepers of the culture's mores, played a major role in these humanistic civic movements. For many of the women serving the settlement house cause, the movement offered opportunities for companionship, intimacy, and self-development, and a purpose for their life. With few employment opportunities open to them, settlement houses became for women a viable option, enabling them to live and work interdependently. Historian William O'Neill coined the phrase "social feminism" as an explanation for women's strong dedication to ideas of social justice and solidarity, while Ellen Lagemann suggests that women's "natural" maternal instinct obligated them to make America a kinder place. Barbara Welter argued that these women moved into the corrupt and unjust cities to transfer the cultural assumptions of women's innate piety, purity, and domesticity onto the urban landscape. Caroll Smith-Rosenberg labeled the woman associated with the settlement house movement "the New Woman," in that she was unmarried, rejected social conventions, and asserted her right to visible power and a public voice. Susan Armeny argued that an older complex of attitudes, called the "sanitary ideal," which loathed individualism and waste but admired order and discipline, provided the motivation and sustaining energy of the settlement house women.[15]

The society of the "fateful decade" resonated to an anxious but hopeful rhythm in which ideas of reform, progress, democracy, idealism, good women, and justice harmonized. Cultural presumptions of the nineteenth century imbued the reformers with a belief that social progress brought democracy and that personal independence conferred personhood and citizenship. They assumed that nothing was beyond their power because they believed that social, economic, and political equity would eventually lead to a less chaotic and fragmented world capable of human perfectability.

A NURSING THOUGHT COLLECTIVE

Ideas of reform, progress, womanhood, justice, and the public's health influenced, enabled, and restricted the nurse inventors' possibilities of thought and focused the mental lens through which they experienced and interpreted reality. The institutions in which the nurse inventors worked and lived provided a second layer of framing. Hospitals, settlement houses, and instructive nursing associations, each with distinctive cultures and politics, provided different institutional contexts for nursing ideas. Moreover, each nurse inventor had personal motivations that influenced her thinking. Thus, society, institutions, and personhood homogenized to create complex contexts in which nurse inventors shaped nursing, created the classification of "trained nurse," and attempted to sculpt reality to validate their ideal.

Although the list of eminent nursing inventors is lengthy, three well-known nurses seem to form a coterie of thinkers.[16] Born within the same decade, their paths crossed at Henry Street Settlement House in New York City, an institution that became agent and counteragent for the ideas that they hoped to broker. Lillian Wald, Lavinia Dock, and Annie Goodrich were very different women whose life journeys became indelibly interconnected, yet their ideas, beliefs, and classifications coalesced to form a foundation for generations of nurses who followed. Wald, Dock, and Goodrich believed they represented a new enlightened era for nursing. And, when thinkers agree that their present day is like no other period, and that a great gulf divides them from the past, philosopher Ludwig Fleck suggests that a thought collective is identifiable.[17] Clearly, Wald, Dock, and Goodrich set themselves apart and relished "modern" nursing's distinctiveness from previous eras of nursing.

Lavinia Dock, addressing the Nurses' Associated Alumnae in 1907, remarked that ancient nursing represented crude ministrations of healing, but that "modern" nursing had finally grasped the essential idea that health was related to social responsibility, social progress, and moral obligation.[18] Dock held that "modern" nursing must be a force in reversing the pathology of human misery and in triumphantly unifying mankind through the spirit of progress. The notion of progress also appealed to Goodrich, who suggested that the "promise of the period upon which nursing has now entered" was self-evident, with the "ills to which man was prey for centuries tracked down and destroyed."[19] Modern nursing was ordained to participate in rearranging life and in transforming society to greater heights. Remarking that "nursing is no longer the handmaiden of the physician, the official wife of medicine, nor the younger sister of the medical family," Wald promoted an independent nursing profession—one that would transfuse hope to the miserable experiences of the masses.[20] And as authors of classic texts, these women, individually and collectively, hoped that their gospels would influence a great awakening within nursing, with individual nurses collectively responsible for the birth of civic righteousness and for the transformation of a troubled society.[21]

Born in the mid-1880s into upper-middle-class families, Dock (1858–1956), Wald (1867–1940), and Goodrich (1866–1955) describe a restlessness in their early lives. Their writings exude a longing to find an opportunity for intellectual self-fulfillment and to have an autonomous role outside their nuclear families. From a practical viewpoint, both Dock and Goodrich reluctantly admitted that their families' financial reversals stimulated their need to earn a wage through nursing; Wald, on the other hand, considered nursing as a life work after her rejection of admission to Vassar College. Yet each woman's written memoir, laced with hesitancy, portrays nursing as much more than a mere wage-earning endeavor. "Nursing work" was for them an opportunity to gain emotional satisfaction by understanding the kinship of mankind. Careful to tread between pure emotion and objective reason, they suggest a commitment to the ideal of nursing as paramount, while denying that nursing was an innate calling.[22]

Dock recalled that some years after sympathetically caring for her dying mother, she responded to a magazine clipping about Isabel Hampton Robb, as if drawn to a "familiar force of healing."[23] Goodrich remembered that she felt nursing to be a perfect outlet for her keen sense of responsibility and independence, even though "she hated sickness and had a horror of death."[24] Wald maintained that her exposure to a Bellevue graduate during her sister's pregnancy "awakened" her interest in nursing.[25]

The personal motivations of these women suggest that their choice of and commitment to nursing reflect a deeper sense of nursing than cognition alone would give. Subtly, their memoirs reveal that nursing provided them with an opportunity for a personal relationship with others, a way of encountering humanity in a face-to-face relationship, and a way of doing good works through the care of needy persons. Goodrich, with the most grandiloquent style of the three women, enthused that "the life of a nurse is indeed transfused with meaning who has by an iota furthered the end of those she serves."[26] More pragmatically, Wald wrote that "contact with ordinary people is a pleasurable satisfaction, for to keep the poor in your consciousness insures the power to transmit faith in a cause, to stir a response, and to change indifference."[27] Dock, expressing regrets, lamented that she lacked the "compassion and warm personal care" essential to good nursing.[28]

Although their transcendental idea of nursing can easily be dismissed as romantic or submissive, too cavalier an attitude toward the nurse inventors' compassionate attitude may obscure understanding. Encountering the underworld of the poor stimulated the nurse inventors to respond with compassion to human pain and misery. Compassion, in turn, became an expected attitude as nurse inventors created nursing practice within the context of Henry Street Settlement House. Their compassionate practice of nursing also served to quell personal restlessness, to offer individual creativity, and to create a purpose and a personal sense of meaning to their lives. Ideal nursing practice was tied to the causes of humanity and to the needs of the collective, which were larger than the individual nurse. And nursing was a means of reaching the goal of an improved society. As Wald wrote, "the nurse makes her contribution to human welfare unified and harmonized with those powers which aim at care and prevention."[29] Nursing, as an ideal, would accept a commitment to social causes and to the development of mankind's mind, body, and spirit.

Nursing legend and nursing history promote the idea that the nineteenth-century nurse was an extension of the pure, obedient, submissive Victorian woman who, as historian Susan Reverby notes, had "an obligation to care."[30] This view suggests that nursing's altruism manifested itself as an obsession with the behavior, the character, and the "being" of the individual nurse, while the "doing" of nursing, it is argued, was rigidly dictated by nurse leaders. The long history of hospital nursing's protracted focus on both the "character of the nurse" and on technique, which historian Ellen Baer calls the "procedure manual of nursing," supports the argument that goodness resided in the nurse who compliantly followed the procedures set by her superiors.[31]

In direct opposition to this traditional distinction, however, Wald, Dock, and Goodrich seemed to be contouring the ideal nature or virtue of nursing *practice*, which required some balanced union and synthesis of being and doing in order to care for others.[32] For the nurse inventors, societal and patient needs, rather than ordained procedures, determined the practice of nursing; the "being" of nursing was a group achievement and a group identity rather than a characteristic of an individual nurse. Nursing *practice* was not, according to Wald, Dock, and Goodrich, synonymous with "doing." Technical training was simply a component of the greater "nursing work," which concerned itself with human beings, relationships, and environment.[33] A bedbath was not a practice, but nursing was.[34] And the "being" of nursing belonged not to the individual nurse, but to the collective group called Nursing. This group identity, which Wald called the "spirit of nursing," was a virtue of nursing that enabled the profession, as a collective, to achieve the needed outcomes of nursing practice. The ideal outcome was conceptualized as a perfected humanity.

Prophetically, Wald feared the loss of the spirit of nursing. In 1908, fifteen years after the establishment of Henry Street Settlement House, Wald, confronted with Metropolitan Life Insurance Company's technocratic focus on money and efficient outcomes, lamented that "the lovely spirit of nursing" might be eroded if nursing colluded with the marketing scams of business.[35] Wald seemed to feel that the high ideals of improving humanity and the reality of bureaucracy would be at odds.

While the nurse inventors subscribed to the spirit of nursing as a virtue, they denied nursing *qua* religion. Goodrich's biographer, Harriet Koch, says that the elder Goodrich wanted her daughter to apply to St. Luke's Hospital (New York), but Annie proudly rebelled stating, "I will not go to a place where they ask if you belong to the Church."[36] And while careful to point out that she was raised in the Episcopal Church, Dock was equally vociferous in her rejection of religion and her acceptance of social justice:

> When I began to reflect, I saw that I had always had certain inarticulate instincts that were sound: a strong sympathy for the oppressed classes, a lively sense of justice, and a keen love of what we mean by freedom and liberty. . . . I had no religious beliefs and I felt no need of them. . . . The flash went through my mind: "there is not a good God." Instantly all regard for and belief in the Church as an institution fell from my mind as stone sinks in water, and never came back.[37]

Dock maintained that the old nursing sisters of the religious order, "closely confined in shackles of mental subjugation and social renunciation," held no hopes of creating a social order, but rather "gave their lives to an unquestioning service of devotion."[38] The key phrase for the nurse inventors was "unquestioning." Proponents of "purposeful and rational obedience" for worker nurses, Dock, Wald, and Goodrich shared an antipathy toward the authority of the church, while admiring, even finding solice within, "religious sentiment."[39] To these nurse inventors, the church's requirement of blind obedience negated emancipation for womanhood, diminished the hope of a better life for humans, and threatened Wald's ideal of nursing having a voice of its own.[40] Yet their zeal, bordering on dogmatic reverence, toward the attributes of compassion, respect, care, devotion, loyalty, harmony, essential dignity, and love seemed to accord them a commitment to some transcendent "other," to give them a feeling of personal importance and inferiority, and to reveal to them the essential questions of human destiny. They created a conceptual boundary between secular and religious nursing and sought to justify its existence. Dock noted that:

> We belong to an age which is learning . . . the thrill of discovery that the human race is capable of improvement; that human society can be voluntarily and consciously built into a nobler and fairer form than those of the past. If now we have secured the freedom which was denied to the sister of the religious orders, we shirk its responsibilities and ignore its duties, but deliberately clothe ourselves again in her narrow-mindedness but without her holy zeal and self-consecration.[41]

The spirit of nursing, to the nurse inventors, was not the spark of organized religion, nor martyrdom, but a compassionate commitment to the
human condition and to the rectification of the beautiful garbage of daily
life. Iconoclastic at their core, the nurse inventors used the argument of
nursing's social value as a battleground for their own doubts about wealth
as a sign of worth, the meaning of human suffering, and their relationship with nature and the universe. In what seems to be an unveiling of
her own wonderment with the nurse's role, Wald relayed a story of an
ignorant, poor, suffering immigrant woman who was bewildered with the
procedures of visiting a maternity center. Wald commented that the role
of the nurse "can be perplexing to these women," but noted, with great
relief and bemusement, that she knew an understanding had been gained
when the immigrant woman commented, "I know what they are—sisters
without religion."[42]

While religious sisters rejected the world and committed themselves
to the spirit of God through caring, the nurse inventors, with secular
superiority, rejected formal religion and committed themselves to reforming the world through the spirit of nursing. While the two sects
approached their task from different perspectives, both nurses and sisters adopted a volitional attitude, dedicating themselves to the relief of
others' pain. Yet to relieve pain, one must be drawn into it, to see it, to
touch it, and to experience it. Nurses and sisters alike could not relieve
pain through the safety of sentiment, but had to descend *into* the patients'
lives so as to encounter the primal awesomeness of the human condition. Raw exposure to the beauty and the tragedy of lives promoted the
hope that something—God and belief, or nursing and reform—gave life
meaning. Thus, despite the nurse inventors' crafted conceptual boundaries to reject the religious nature of nursing, the irony is that both paths
led all the sisters, nuns, and nurses alike deeper into the suffering world
and, thereby, closer to a universal core that yearns to believe that life has
meaning and purpose.

BELIEF AND UNBELIEF

To rebuff religion, while espousing an exalting faith in civic humanism,
progressivism, and the spirit of nursing, did not seem out of the ordinary for the nurse inventors. Before the middle of the nineteenth century, agnosticism and secularization in America seemed almost absurd,
but soon unbelief emerged as an option within the general contours of
society. According to James Turner, the urban landscape, coupled with
advances in technology and science, disrupted society's relationship with
nature and God.[43] While the clergy, by virtue of their office, traditionally
served to explain the mysteries of life and reassure people about the

unknowable, improved newspaper communication and increased travel allowed nineteenth-century Americans to choose points of view that differed from those of their village ministers and priests. Moreover, when universities such as Harvard replaced clerical presidents with professionals, the church's longstanding grip over education declined.

Although science and technology had begun to displace religion as an object of interest by the late 1860s, many "guardians of belief," particularly in the Northeast, sought to harmonize religion and science.[44] Advocates of using practical scientific knowledge to improve society, the moral guardians generated an avalanche of social reforms to reconcile human progress with divine sovereignty. And while "true" knowledge, that is, scientific knowledge, had to be verified by experience or experimentation, the idea that science complemented religion became popular. Science disclosed the laws of nature and being, and the discovery of a law presumed a lawgiver, namely God. Armed with such theories as Herbert Spencer's evolutionism and Auguste Comte's knowledge development, the idea that knowledge grows throughout history supported a belief of a supreme knower—a designer behind the design.[45] For a time it seemed possible that science and religion, bridged by reform, could cohabit and complement one another.

Yet, the conflict between science and religion was not resolved. Darwin's *On the Origin of the Species* applied an ax to even the strongest ties that bound science and religion. And while Darwin's treatise was published in 1859, the significance of the work, which historians continue to argue, affected the worldview for decades. Darwin showed how, through natural selection, organisms developed from the very simple to the extremely complex. The argument of design and, more important, the *Designer* of nature collapsed. Of course, it was still possible to believe in a god, but Darwin offered a plausible alternative explanation to the design theology. As Turner noted, without design, God did not vanish, but would have to be explained by faith rather than by reason and science.[46]

The raging arguments regarding Darwin and the relationship between science and religion threw some believers back to the source of knowledge that they knew—intuition. The believers argued that God remained impervious to human probing, and not even science could penetrate the essence of things that belonged to the Almighty. Still, as science principles became articulate and diffused into the culture, knowledge became associated with the practical, the touchable, and the measurable; God remained in the realm of belief and faith.[47]

By the Gilded Age, religion swelled with Gothic spires rising over American cities and church membership grew to new heights. Although doubters did not acquiesce to religion, they could not relinquish their grip on God without a replacement. Even for doubters, existence demanded some meaning and, thus, "morality" filled the void. Secularized morality, couched in the language of Leslie Stephen's *The Science of Ethics* (1882), argued that "we must love and serve one another."[48] Religious faith and intuition had nothing to do with morality, which, according to the doubters, was obviously based in reason and science. At the heart of this agnostic belief lay two principles—the nobility of the pursuit of truth and the commitment to human progress. As Turner says, progress did for unbelievers what faith did for believers.[49] One could feel that at death one's upright strivings did not evaporate into nothingness but had some moral worth in helping humanity toward higher limits. Truth and meaning, born of faith in God or belief in progress, became sacred.

VIRTUE AS COMPASSION OR ETHICS?

The nurse inventors, born and raised in a social context that praised the morality of service to *Truth* (versus truths), human need, and progress, embraced those ideas from society that made them feel confident in transforming themselves and others. While denying the religious nature of nursing, they selected ideas from the social context that created sense of their lived experience. For Lillian Wald, the reality of life was an immersion in connectedness with the poor immigrants of New York's lower Fast Side. Remembering the window of opportunity that Henry Street Settlement House had given her life, she wrote years later:

> *The East side called up a vague alarming picture of something strange and alien, a vast crowded area, a foreign city within our own for whose conditions we had no concern. Like the rest of the world, I had known little of it. . . . Past odorous fish stands, unregulated, uncovered garbage, and where children played lending themselves inevitably to all forms of inducing. All the maladjustments of our social and economic relations seemed epitomized in this brief journey.*[50]

Assaulted by the lack of essential dignity of the conditions, but awestruck by the interdependence of mankind, she decided to bridge the gap. Living briefly at the College Settlement on Rivington Street, then at the top floor of a flat on Jefferson Street, and finally at the house at Henry Street, Wald and her colleagues lived and worked with the poor for nearly four decades. Outside established hospitals, "free from every form of control, without the benefit of managers, committees, medical encouragement, or police approval, there to do what we could do, to see what we could see, and to publicize all that was wrong and remediable by making the findings known," Wald professed herself a practical idealist who fashioned the spirit of nursing from ideas of "fellowship, harmony, and helping each other to the highest level."[51]

The virtues of what Wald hoped nursing to embody—morality, service, integrity, kinship of mankind, justice, and the art of humanity—effectively denied religion while promoting a differentiated connectedness, a basic oneness, with humankind. The settlement house milieu fostered such a connection. As Dock observed, "Henry Street was perhaps like the pleasantest type of family life—a family to be sure, composed only of women, each one absorbed in busy interests, but in no sense . . . an institution."[52] Each nurse managed patients according "to her best judgment," and nursing practice problems were settled during evening conversation and consultation, "free of any kind of restrictive regulation."[53]

The spirit of nursing for Wald seemed to be akin to the Hebrew notion of *zedakah*, which literally means righteousness, but which usually is translated as compassion.[54] Compassion was not sentiment, but making justice and doing works of mercy. Compassion was not a favor to the poor, but something to which patients had a right, and for the nurse, an opportunity. Compassion was not pity, but celebration of the kinship of the human spirit. Compassion was not private, but public service. Compassion was not simply knowing about the suffering of others, but entering into it, sharing it, and understanding it. Compassion was not anti-intellectual, but sought to know and to understand the interconnections of all things. Compassion was not a commandment, but a spirituality that treated all creation with respect. Compassion was not an organized religion, but it was, for the nurse inventors, a way of life.[55]

Historian Susan Reverby noted that nursing lacked a "conception of nursing as an occupational sisterhood built on caring and the demand for rights" and instead adopted the "need to accept obligations, duties," and thus, exploitation.[56] Yet, this particular thought collective, connected with Henry Street Settlement House, had a vision of nursing as a sisterhood with a core value of compassionate care of humanity *without* the self-sacrifice demanded by organized religion. The terms humanity, progress, fellowship, civic righteousness, unfailing goodness, and ethics—language distinctive of the era—supported the view that the "spirit of nursing" was compassion.

Writing in 1900, Dock noted that she had once advocated establishing a code of ethics as one of the first duties for organizing an association of nurses, but after consideration she withdrew that claim.[57] With a newfound insight that a codified set of ethics was restrictive, Dock proposed that if nurses lived in an ethical manner, consistent with the norms of nursing practice, they would not need a code. Ethical life was more than maxims, just as an intellectual life was more than booklearning. Moreover, Dock, referring to expected nurse behavior within hospitals, indignantly maintained that ethics encompassed more than etiquette. An ethical life was a comprehensive approach to human beings. "If nurses

walked in the spirit of truth and justice principles, the slavishness of obedience and moral cowardice of subordination would be unecessary."[58]
Dock, using the terms *truth and justice,* urged that nurses become internally motivated and identify with nursing's commitment to compassion
rather than follow a set of rules called ethics. She maintained that obedience for either the sake of obedience or for a worthless cause deteri-
orated character, "preventing initiative, independent thought, and
self-reliant action."[59] Only when obedience became a symbol of an understanding that all humans were connected and that "the slave stands on
the level with himself" could a nurse make a contribution to the goal of
unified human welfare.[60]

Echoing Dock's beliefs, Goodrich argued that the ethical significance
of nursing "is indeed its vitalizing force," so much so that "it is consistent
to assert that the terms *good* and *ethical* as applied to nursing practice are
synonymous."[61] The nurse, according to the dramatic Goodrich, "stood
at the gateway of life and death," and it was this critical position that
demanded "the fullest understanding of all that pertains to the creative
task to which she has aspired."[62] Goodrich also denounced etiquette as a
synonym of ethics, pointing out that producing a better world, rather than
politeness, was life's overall ethical objective. The nurse, as an interpreter
of life, ministered to the sick, and these acts of compassion verified that
"the calling, vocation, profession, what you will, is in itself intrinsically
ethical."[63] Nursing, as an exemplification of compassion toward human
suffering, hoped to "heal the body with perchance to save the soul."[64]

The three nurse inventors, exposed to life, death, and the tragedies
of human existence on the New York City streets, could neither tran-
quilize themselves with the trivial nor live wholly in the dimension of the
visible. Like many humans, they sought meaning in their lives. Hoping
to transcend human vulnerability and yearning to be part of a greater
and higher whole, they did not search upward to heaven and organized
religion, but embraced earthly ideas of reform, compassion, and progress
as a means to redeem humanity—and to construct nursing. Yet all true
religions embrace the words *humanity* and *compassion* as an expression of
the commitment to a transcendent other who integrates one's life. Thus,
both nursing and religion, if pursued compassionately, healed wounded
minds, bodies, and spirits. Although the nurse inventors intended an
unyielding boundary between religion and nursing, the kindred missions
of religion and nursing rendered the boundary translucent.

CONCLUSIONS

Early in the twentieth century a thought collective of nursing espoused
the idea that compassion toward humanity was the core value within nurs-

ing. While they denied nursing as a manifestation of conventional religion, Dock, Wald, and Goodrich promoted the notion that compassion was a necessary condition to the "being" of a nurse. They envisioned that secular nursing would emulate the values of the religious sisters without accepting their rules, regulations, and cloistered life. Compassion, once associated with God's authority, would, according to the nurse inventors, be replaced with compassion based on commitment to the authority of humanity and its social progress.

As in most historical research, this is not the end of the story, but rather the beginning. While the idea of compassion as a nursing virtue can be identified within the thought collective of Dock, Wald, and Goodrich, there is plentiful evidence that diversity of thinking among nurses exists through time. Other leaders, such as Harriet Lounsbery (1899), Isabel Hampton Robb (1900), S. Lillian Clayton (1916), and Eva Allerton (1898), writing on the topic of ethics, suggest that the intimacy inherent in nursing practice required religious goodness, trust, the idea of discipline, and obedience. Confronted with the reality of pupil nurses who did not demonstrate the necessary goodness, compassion metamorphosed into ethics, which, in turn, became a set of "rules" of conduct. With these shifts in thinking, the conceptual boundaries between compassion and ethics, between behavior and character, between being a nurse and acting like a nurse, between spiritual development and compliance, between excellence and submission, between commitment to mankind and veneration of leaders, between individuality and perfection, and between teaching and controlling became diffuse and riddled with angst.[65] As Susan Reverby observed, the "theoretical and moral power of nursing," which this article argues was compassion, became devalued and mutated, reduced to a rather rigid rule orientation of nurse leaders.[66] Compassion became compulsion.

And while Reverby analyzes how this "character as ideology" emerged, nurses want to believe that compassion, as a core of nursing, lay dormant (or not so dormant) throughout the decades. The history of nurses' diverse thinking patterns, as well as the social, economic, political, and intellectual factors that influenced changes in thought, is yet to be written. As the century draws to a close, nurses are seeking to reexamine, reframe, and clarify the heritage and tradition of nursing. And once again, the idea of compassion and caring as a central virtue in nursing appeals to the core of nurses. The traditional tenet that "nursing was born in the church . . ." may well be a truism. Or as Matthew Fox notes, "you may call God love, you may call God goodness, but God is best described as compassion."[67]

Acknowledgments

Grateful acknowledgment is made to Lillian Brunner and Joan Lynaugh for their significant contributions to this study. The research was supported by The Lillian Sholtis Brunner Summer Fellowship for Historical Research in Nursing offered by the Center for the Study of the History of Nursing at the University of Pennsylvania.

NOTES

1.   Teresa Christy, *Cornerstone for Nursing Education: A History of the Division of Nursing Education of Teachers College, Columbia University, 1899–1947* (New York: Teachers College Press, 1969); Joanne Ashley, *Hospitals, Paternalism and the Role of the Nurse* (New York: Teachers College Press, 1976); Janet Mottus, *New York Nightingales: The Emergence of the Nursing Profession at Bellevue and New York Hospital, 1850–1920* (Ann Arbor, Mich.: UMI Research Press, 1981); Barbara Melosh, *The Physicians' Hand: Work, Culture, and Conflict in American Nursing* (Philadelphia: Temple University Press, 1982); Patricia O'Brien, "All a Woman's Life Can Bring: the Domestic Roots of Nursing In Philadelphia," *Nursing Research* 36, no. 1 (January/February 1987): 12–17; Susan Reverby, *Ordered to Care: The Dilemma of American Nursing, 1850–1945* (Cambridge, Mass.: Cambridge University Press, 1987); Charles Rosenberg, *The Care of Strangers: The Rise of America's Hospital System* (New York: Basic Books, 1987); Joan Lynaugh and Claire Fagin, "Coming of Age or Coming Apart: Nursing in the 20th Century," *Image 20*, no. 4, (Winter 1988): 184–88.

2.   H. S. Kim, *The Nature of Theoretical Thinking in Nursing* (Norwalk, Conn.: Appleton-Century-Crofts, 1983), 9; Afaf Meleis, *Theoretical Nursing: Development and Progress* (Philadelphia, Pa.: J. B. Lippincott, 1985), 37.

3.   U.S. Department of Commerce, Bureau of Census, *Historical Statistics of the United States: Colonial Times to 1957* (Washington, D.C., 1960), 34; Lavinia Dock and Isabel Stewart, *A Short History of Nursing* (New York: G. P. Putnam's Sons, 1920), 162–66.

4.   The history of the concept and emergence of professions is well documented. See Robert Wiebe, *The Search for Order, 1877–1920* (New York: Hill and Wang, 1967); Magali Sarfatti Larson, *The Rise of Professionalism: A Sociological Analysis* (Berkeley: University of California Press, 1977); Roy Lubove, *The Professional Altruist: The Emergence of Social Work as a Career, 1880–1930* (New York: Atheneum, 1972); Alexander Oleson and John Voss, eds., *The Organization of Knowledge in Modern America* (Baltimore, Md.: The Johns Hopkins University Press, 1979); Thomas Haskell, *The Emergence of Professional Social Science: The American Social Science Association and the Nineteenth-Century Crises of Authority* (Urbana: University of Illinois Press, 1977); Burton Bledstein, *The Culture of Professionalism: The Middle Class and the Development of Higher Education in America* (New York: W. W. Norton and Co., 1979).

5.   Ian Hacking, *Reconstructing Individualism* (Stanford, Calif.: Stanford University Press, 1985).

6.   Ludwig Fleck, *The Genesis and Development of a Scientific Fact* (Chicago: University of Chicago Press, 1979), 25, 38–51.

7.   The literature of the sociology of knowledge is a large body of work. For a beginning discussion, See Emile Durkheirn, *De la División du Travail Social: Etude sur l'Organisation des Sociétés Supérieures,* translated by George Simpson (Paris: Alcan, 1893) [Translation, 1933]; Fleck, *Genesis and Development of a Scientific Fact;* Thomas Kuhn, *The Structure of Scientific Revolutions* (Chicago: University of Chicago Press, 1975); Mary Douglas, *Implicit Meanings* (London: Routledge and Kegan Paul, 1975); Mary Douglas, *How Institutions Think* (Syracuse, N.Y.: Syracuse University Press, 1986).

8.   It is beyond not only the scope but the ability of the author to solve the problem of dualistic thinking. Currently, it is a topic of many articles, seminars, conferences, and think tanks within many disciplines. For a discussion of the dilemma as it relates to history of ideas, see John Toews, "Intellectual History after the Linguistic Turn," *American Historical Review* 92, no. 4 (October 1987): 879–907; Eric Fuhrman, *A Sociology of Knowledge in America, 1883–1915* (Charlottesville: University of Virginia Press, 1980); David Hollinger, *In the American Province* (Baltimore, Md.: The Johns Hopkins University Press, 1985); Dominick LaCapra, *Rethinking Intellectual History: Text, Contexts, Language* (Ithaca, N.Y.: Cornell University Press, 1983); Henrika Kuklick, "The Sociology of Knowledge: Retrospect and Prospect," *Annals Reviews of Sociology* 9 (1983): 287–310.

9.   LaCapra, *Rethinking Intellectual History,* 36.

10.   Christy, *Cornerstone for Nursing Education,* 3–29.

11.   Henry Commager, *The American Mind* (New Haven, Conn.: Yale University, 1952), 212.

12.   Wiebe, *Search for Order,* 3–21.

13.   Jane Addams, *Twenty Years at Hull House* (New York: Macmillan Co., 1938), 90–101.

14.   Public health has a rich history of its own. The orientation of public health has experienced changes, which to some authors is a commentary on social, political, economic, and intellectual shifts within the American social system. See Allen Davis, *Spearheads of Reform: The Social Settlements and the Progressive Movement, 1890–1914* (New York: Oxford University Press, 1967); Barbara Rosencrantz, *Public Health and the State: Changing Views in Massachusetts, 1842–1936* (Cambridge, Mass.: Harvard University Press, 1972); John Duffy, *A History of Public Health in New York City, 1866–1966* (New York: Russell Sage Foundation, 1974); George Rosen, *Preventive Medicine in the United States: 1900–1975* (New York: Prodist, 1977); Karen Buhler-Wilkerson, *False Dawn: The Rise and Decline of Public Health Nursing, 1900–1930* (PhD diss., University of Pennsylvania, 1984).

15.   William O'Neill, *Everyone Was Brave: A History of Feminism in America* (New York: Quandrangle, 1971), 77–106; Ellen Condliffe Lagemann, *A Generation of Women: Social Feminism in the 1920's* (Cambridge, Mass.: Harvard University Press), 154–59; Barbara Welter, "The Cult of True Womanhood: 1800–1860," *American Quarterly* 18 (Summer 1966); Caroll Smith-Rosenberg, *Disorderly Conduct: Visions of Gender in Victorian America* (New York: Oxford University Press, 1985), 77–89, 167–77; Susan Armeny, "Organized Nurses, Women Philanthropists, and the

Intellectual Bases for Cooperation Among Women, 1898–1920," in *The New Nursing History*, ed. Ellen Lagemann (New York: Teachers College, Columbia University, 1983), 13–35.

16. For an overview of nurses who contributed to nursing between the years 1890–1900, see Vern Bullough, Olga Church, and Alice Stein, *American Nursing: A Biographical Dictionary*, vol. 1 (New York: Garland Publishing, 1988) and Vern Bullough, Lilli Sentz, and Alice Stein, *America Nursing: A Biographical Dictionary*, vol. 2 (New York: Garland Press, 1992).

17. Fleck, *Genesis of a Scientific Fact*, 192.

18. Lavinia Dock, "Some Urgent Social Claims," *American Journal of Nursing 1* (January 1907): 895–905.

19. Annie Goodrich, "The Nurse and the University," *The Social and Ethical Significance of Nursing* (New York: MacMillan, 1932), 334.

20. Lillian Wald, *Windows on Henry Street* (Boston, Mass.: Little and Brown, 1934), 75–78.

21. Although Mary Roberts, longtime editor of the *American Journal of Nursing*, called Goodrich, Wald, and M. Adelaide Nutting the "Triumvirate," the Henry Street tie, which eluded Nutting, may be important in terms of how a certain set of nursing ideas formed. Moreover, Dock, Goodrich, and Wald did produce a collection of ideas in book form. While Nutting published articles and certainly wrote two chapters of Nutting and Dock's classic history, *A History of Nursing*, Dock's ideas predominate in both the four volume and the short version of her treatise. In addition to Dock's two works, Goodrich's classic, *Social and Ethical Significance of Nursing*, and Wald's two works on Henry Street Settlement House, *House on Henry Street* and *Windows on Henry Street*, form a grouping of nursing "texts" that are a reasonable starting point for ideas on history of nursing. Of course, the choice of Wald, Dock, and Goodrich as a thought collective is not sacrosanct. Dock and Stewart, *A Short History of Nursing*; Lavinia Dock and M. Adelaide Nutting, *A History of Nursing*, vols. 1–4 (New York: Putnam, 1912); Annie Goodrich, *The Social and Ethical Significance of Nursing* (New York: MacMillan, 1932); Lillian Wald, *House on Henry Street* (New York: Henry Holt and Co., 1915); Wald, *Windows on Henry Street*.

22. Ibid.

23. Lavinia Dock, "Lavinia L. Dock: Self-Portrait," *Nursing Outlook* 25 (January 1977): 23–26.

24. Harriet Berger Koch, *Militant Angle* (New York: MacMillan, 1951) 14.

25. Wald, *House on Henry Street*, 12–16.

26. Goodrich, *Social and Ethical Significance of Nursing*, 10.

27. Wald, *House on Henry Street*, 10.

28. Dock, "Lavinia L. Dock: Self-Portrait," 24.

29. Wald, *House on Henry Street*, 60.

30. Nurse historians, for the most part, cite this argument. See Reverby, *Ordered to Care*.

31. Dr. Ellen D. Baer, telephone conversation with author, 10 February 1992.

32. The term nursing practice was called "nursing work" by the nurse inventors. Anne Bishop and John Scuder, *The Practical, Moral, and Personal Sense of*

Nursing: A Phenomenological Philosophy of Practice (Albany, N.Y.: State University Press, 1990), 173.

33.   The nurse inventors were clear that the mechanics of nursing and the profession of nursing were distinctly different. Goodrich, quoting public health Professor C. E. A. Winslow, liked to say that a nurse must not be "simply an empirically trained upper bedside servant, but understand the 'laws and principles' of science." See Goodrich, *The Social and Ethical Significance of Nursing*, 34. They believed that every nurse needed a broad education so as to grasp the responsibility of their life work: namely, moving the human race toward essential dignity, health, and well-being. Dock used the dualistic language "technical training versus theoretical teaching, nursing versus routine hospital work, details of work versus the spirit of nursing." See Lavinia Dock, "Nursing Organization in Germany and England," "The Nurses' Settlement in New York," and "Ethics or a Code of Ethics?" *Short Papers On Nursing, Subjects, in A Lavinia Dock Reader*, ed. Janet James (1900; reprint, New York: Garland Press, 1985), 16–26, 27–30, 37–40. Also, see Lavinia Dock, "Hospital Organization," *National Hospital Record* 6 (1903): 10–14. In Goodrich's language, "the complete nurse implied attainments in special knowledge as distinguished from mere skill. To effectively interpret life, neither a liberal education nor a high degree of technical skill will suffice. She must be a master of two tongues: of science and of the people." See Goodrich, *The Social and Ethical Significance of Nursing*, 14, 38, 70. And Wald was also clear that the service of the nurse's mind, heart, and hands led to the social betterment of mankind. See: Wald, *House on Henry Street*, 336.

34.   Alasdair MacIntyre, *After Virtue* (Notre Dame, Ind.: University of Notre Dame Press, 1984), 187; Bishop and Scuder, *Practical, Moral, and Personal Sense of Nursing*, 13–28.

35.   Diane Hamilton, "Cost of Caring," *Bulletin of the History of Medicine* 63 (Spring 1989): 414–34.

36.   Koch, *Militant Angel*, 14.

37.   Dock, "Lavinia L. Dock: Self-Portrait," 15.

38.   Dock, "Some Urgent Social Claims," 895–905.

39.   Dock, "Ethics or a Code of Ethics?," 56–57; Mary Roberts, "Lavinia Lloyd Dock, Nurse, Feminist, Internationalist," *American Journal of Nursing* 56 (February 1956): 176–79; Goodrich, *Social and Ethical Significance of Nursing*, 8–9; Wald, *House on Henry Street*, 117.

40.   Wald, *Windows on Henry Street*, 75.

41.   Roberts, "Lavinia Lloyd Dock, Nurse, Feminist, Internationalist," 176–79.

42.   Wald, *Windows on Henry Street*, 92–95.

43.   James Turner, *Without God, Without Creed: The Origins of Unbelief in America* (Baltimore, Md.: The Johns Hopkins University Press, 1985), 116.

44.   Tumer, *Without God, Without Creed*, 124.

45.   Lavinia Dock was a reader, if not admirer, of Herbert Spencer, as was Annie Goodrich, who also had a particular fondness for Tolstoy. For a discussion of the whole controversy, which included Spencer, Darwin, and Aggisiz, see Turner, *Without God, Without Creed*, 150–72; John Hedley Brooke, *Science and Religion* (New York: Cambridge University Press, 1991).

46. The arguments regarding Darwin and the relationship between science and religion are numerous and varied. See Richard Hofstader, *Social Darwinism in American Thought* (Boston, Mass.: Boston University, 1955); Charles Rosenberg, *No Other Gods: On Science and American Social Thought* (Baltimore, Md.: The Johns Hopkins University Press, 1976); Herbert Hovenkamp, *Science and Religion in America: 1800–1860* (Philadelphia: University of Pennsylvania Press, 1978); Bernard Lightman, *The Origins of Agnosticism, Victorian Unbelief and the Limits of Knowledge* (Baltimore, Md.: The Johns Hopkins University Press, 1978); John Cerello, *The Secularization of the Soul* (Philadelphia: University of Pennsylvania Press, 1982); Brooke, *Science and Religion.*

47. Tumer, *Without God, Without Creed,* 202.

48. Leslie Stephen, *The Science of Ethics* (New York: MacMillan, 1882), 32–36.

49. Turner, *Without God, Without Creed,* 217–20.

50. Wald, *Windows on Henry Street,* 3–6.

51. Lillian Wald to unknown person, 31 May 1922, Welfare Division Files, Metropolitan Life Insurance Company Archives, New York City; Wald, *Windows on Henry Street,* 118.

52. Dock, "The Nurses' Settlement in New York," 27–36.

53. Ibid.

54. William Eckhardt, *Compassion: Toward a Science of Value* (Toronto: CPRI Press, 1973), 258.

55. Matthew Fox, *A Spirituality Named Compassion* (San Francisco, Calif.: Harper, 1979).

56. Susan Reverby notes that character as skill became the ideology of the nursing discipline and argues that if the conception of nursing had been based on rights and caring rather than obligation and duty, nursing would have had the ideological material necessary to guard against exploitation. I am arguing that within this particular thought collective the idea of caring and compassion was indeed the ideological base, but do agree with Reverby that it slowly (or not so slowly) mutated, maybe within the contexts of institutional bureaucracy compliance or an "obligation to care." See Reverby, *Ordered to Care,* 58.

57. Dock, "Ethics or a Code of Ethics?" 37–57.

58. Ibid.

59. Ibid.

60. Ibid.

61. Goodrich, *The Social and Ethical Significance of Nursing,* 3–5.

62. Ibid.

63. Ibid., 1–15.

64. Ibid.

65. For a very nice collection of nurse authorship on the topic of ethics, see Nettie Birnbach and Sandra Lewenson, eds., *First Words: Selected Addresses from the National League for Nursing, 1894–1933* (New York: National League for Nursing, 1992), 197–234. Also see Isabel Hampton Robb, *Nursing Ethics For Hospital and Private Use* (Cleveland, Ohio: E. C. Koeckert, 1990), and Harriet Lounsbery, *Nursing Ethics* (New York: Appleton, 1889).

66. Reverby, *Ordered to Care,* 58–59.

67. Fox, *A Spirituality Named Compassion,* 34.

12

A Legitimate Relationship: Nursing, Hospitals, and Science in the Twentieth Century

Susan M. Reverby

At an American Hospital Association (AHA) meeting in 1932, president Paul Keller argued against a nursing report that criticized hospitals for exploiting their student nurses. Searching for language that might really explain the hospital-nursing relationship, Keller declared that nursing was "the one and only legitimate daughter of hospitals."[1] While we might debate this view of nursing's lineage (it could be argued that nursing's legitimate daughter is the hospital), legitimacy in this relationship has been a crucial issue. Over much of the twentieth century American nurses have sought, through professional associations and informal work groups, to establish a basis for their authority separate from physician and hospital control. In attempting to legitimate their right to autonomy as individual workers or as a profession, nurses have struggled against both health-care institutions and the cultural meaning of nursing itself.[2]

This article examines the efforts of a group of twentieth-century nursing educators to lay claim to a transformed definition of nursing and a new kind of nursing education. I argue that these educators appealed to

Note: This chapter was originally published in *The American General Hospital: Communities and Social Context,* eds. Diana E. Long and Janet Golden, 135–156. Ithaca, NY and London: Cornell University Press, 1989. Reprinted with permission.

I am grateful for the interviews granted by Ellen Baer, Florence Downs, Ellen Fuller, and above all, Virginia Henderson. Susan Bell, Joan Lynaugh, and Karen Buhler-Wilkerson were more than helpful in guiding me through the material and answering my endless questions. Russell Maulitz and Joel Howell shared clues to the medical parallels. Allan Brandt, Janet Golden, Diana Long, and Ellen More provided criticism of an earlier draft.

differing conceptions of science in an attempt to legitimate nursing's struggle for freedom from hospital control. But in the general culture it was assumed that the nurse's enduring authority should come from gender, not science; her place of work the bedside or hospital, not the laboratory.[3] Hospitals, in turn, demanded that nursing provide them with a workforce, not a research team. Physicians primarily wanted assistants, not colleagues. Working nurses often wanted reasonable hours, not more education, and nursing educators believed in science, but could not agree on its meaning.[4] Establishing a relationship to science thus became a complicated, yet necessary, task for nursing. It also proved to be a troubling basis for either legitimacy or a change in "daughter" status.

The difficulties began with Florence Nightingale and her model for nursing reform. Nightingale envisioned nursing as an art, rather than a science, which required systematic education and structured practical work. Her ideas for a transformed nursing linked medical and public health notions to her class and religious beliefs. Her mid-nineteenth-century sanitarian's genius served "moral understandings of disease causation," and notions of disease specificity and germ theory did not fit her moral categories.[5] Disease was, for her, a sign of personal disorder; filth and "excrementitious matter," the dangers that kept the patient from recovery. Thus the proper "hospital morale" had to be created in institutions to allow for the natural restorative processes to occur. The creation of such morale—broadly defined as clean drains, sewers, and proper ventilation as well as appropriately fed, cleaned, and disciplined patients—was to be the task of the trained nurse.[6]

Accepting the Victorian idea of separate spheres, she thought women had to be trained to nurse through a disciplined honing of their womanly virtues. She stressed character development, the laws of health, and strict adherence to orders passed through the female hierarchy. Medical therapeutics and "curing" seemed of less importance, and she willingly gave this realm to the physicians. Character and caring, the arenas she did think of great import, were assigned to the trained nurse.[7]

Unwittingly, Nightingale's sanitarian ideas and her beliefs about womanhood provided some of the ideological justification for many of the dilemmas that faced American nursing by 1900. Having fought physician and trustee prejudice against the training of nurses in hospitals in the last quarter of the nineteenth century, American nursing reformers succeeded only too well in the early twentieth. Between 1890 and 1920 the number of nursing schools jumped from 35 to 1,775 and the number of trained nurses from 16 per 100,000 population to 141.[8] Administrators quickly discovered that the opening of a nursing school provided their hospitals, with a young, disciplined, and cheap labor force in exchange for "training." The exigencies of nursing acutely ill or surgical patients continually required, however, the sacrifice of a coherent educational program.

The emphasis on statistical data, comparative mortality rates, and objective testing so central to Nightingale's powerful reformer's outlook are absent from early American nursing education and its textbooks. The "too-muchness," as one nursing educator labeled it, of nursing texts and the "old haphazard way of acquiring instruction by note-taking" thwarted the curious nursing student's critical thinking.[9] Didactic, repetitive, watered-down medical lectures by physicians or older nurses were often provided to the nursing students after they finished ten to twelve hours of ward work.

Ushered onto the wards as timid probationers, students had little time to learn either an objective testing of alternative procedures or the scientific theories underlying nursing care. Training focused on the "one right way" of doing procedures in hopes that following specific rules would cause the least damage to patients from ill-prepared students. Particular adherence to the historically enshrined methods of each nursing school was emphasized. If a student's interest survived her texts and lectures, it was surely rebuked on the wards by student head nurses or the superintendent bent on getting the work done.

Students were not encouraged or even allowed to think objectively about procedures. Few schools gave even a basic science course before the beginning of ward work. Such preliminary or preparatory studies were first introduced at the training school at Waltham in 1895, then at Johns Hopkins in 1901. Ten years later only eighty-six schools had some version of a basic course in their curriculum. Standards varied widely and often did not even reach the level of a high school science course.[10]

The emphasis on discipline, order, and practical skills thus underlay the rationalization and abuse of student labor. Because the workforce was almost entirely women, altruism, sacrifice, and submission were expected, indeed demanded. Exploitation was inevitable in a field where, until the early 1900s, there were no accepted standards for how much work an average student should do, how many patients she could successfully care for, or the mechanisms through which to enforce such standards. In this kind of environment nurses were trained, but they were not educated.

Believing that educational reform was central to professionalizing efforts and clinical improvements, a small group of elite reformers attempted to broaden nursing's scientific content and social outlook. In arguing for an increase in the scientific knowledge necessary for nursing, such leaders first had to fight against deep-seated cultural assumptions about male and female "natural" characteristics as embodied in the doctor and nurse. Such sentiments were articulated in the routine platitudes about female sympathy, caring, and subjectivity (and male objectivity) that graced what one nursing leader described as the "doctor homilies" at graduation exercises.[11] Not unexpectedly, such beliefs were professed more frequently whenever nursing groups pushed for higher educational standards or hospitals experienced nursing shortages.

Even small attempts to improve the students' education met resistance. By the early 1900s the training school at the Massachusetts General Hospital (MGH) had introduced some laboratory and basic science courses. In 1906, when a training school committee sought comments on the program, Dr. James G. Mumford stated the widely held physician opinion that "the nurse in the MGH is being overtrained, in the sense that she is a product of the laboratory, the lecture room and the clinic; with an exaggerated idea of the importance of *science* as compared with the art of nursing."[12] As one nursing educator noted, "the clamor for a cheap worker of the old servant-nurse type" was a recurring theme.[13]

Yet many nurses shared the belief that nursing was the embodiment of womanly virtue and the antithesis of objective science. American nursing educator Annette Fiske, for example, although she authored two science books for nurses and had an M.A. in classics from Radcliffe College before she entered training, spent her professional career in the 1920s arguing against increasing the educational standards. Rather, she called for a reinfusion into nursing of spirituality and service. For a nurse like Annette Fiske, science was but a minor sidelight to the art of caring on nursing's center stage.[14] Nursing was for her and many others still a womanly art requiring inherent character in its practitioners and training in practical skills and moral values in its schools.

The professionalizing elite in nursing had to contend with these understandings of nursing, yet still press their claims for increased status and autonomy. Defining a role for science in nursing became an essential part of this endeavor. But in so doing the leadership had to tread lightly around the Fiskes in their own ranks who rankled at the demands of more courses, the physicians who feared that nurses really wanted to be doctors, and the hospital administrators who didn't want to pay for more nursing education.

These constraints shaped the writings and teachings that emerged from the nursing educators and students at Teachers College (TC), Columbia University, in New York. In 1899 the Society of Superintendents for Nurses arranged for a course in Hospital Economics for nurses at TC. Under the initial leadership of M. Adelaide Nutting, a Johns Hopkins graduate and former superintendent of their nursing school, the course grew into a nursing department, then a division that offered courses, then a certificate program, a bachelor's degree program, and later a graduate program. While a baccalaureate degree in nursing was still primarily a dream, and many nursing schools did not even require a high school diploma for either student entry or a faculty position, TC became what one historian labeled "the cornerstone for nursing education."[15]

From its inception the TC program was under enormous pressure to provide nursing with skilled and well-trained educators and administrators. "It is primarily for the benefit of the training schools that the department exists," Nutting wrote in her annual report in 1910–11.[16] She clearly felt that this program would shape nursing's destiny and provide the basis for its acceptance as a profession. In turn, the program's curriculum, as well as the reports and surveys prepared by individual faculty members, continually reflected the demands placed on it by the national nursing community.[17] At the same time the program could not escape the necessity of making the teaching seem "practical" to its students. A Columbia physicist, for example, when brought in to teach, first went to St. Luke's Hospital to ask the nurses to show him what they did that required a knowledge of physics. He used their answers to structure his course around their specific problems in a clinical setting.[18]

Keenly aware of TC's critical position in nursing, Nutting strove to provide the most relevant and informed teachers possible. Distinguished practitioners like Haven Emerson in public health, S. Josephine Baker in municipal health nursing, C. E. A. Winslow in sanitary science, and Edward Thorndike in psychology, gave TC its reputation for having the most advanced and solid education available for nurses. Away from the relentless pressures of nursing practice that controlled hospital-based training, the TC educators stressed underlying scientific principles in each of their courses. Nutting and the other faculty members thus hoped the teaching would be intellectual as well as practical, linking the art of nursing to a scientific base.

In establishing the TC program these educators espoused a belief in the liberating power of science's seeming objectivity and commitment to truth. In emotional tones, Nutting declared that a "foundation in science or principles" would make possible a "worthier and freer" system of nursing, almost a nursing reformation.[19] Harkening back to the ideas of the "New Learning" of Frances Bacon and other seventeenth-century Puritan reformers, and reformulated in the language of the Progressive Era, was the belief that science could be harnessed to social and political reform. "Pedagogic idealism" and "antiauthoritarianism," central to the scientific vision of the Baconians, was part of this nursing vision.[20]

This understanding of the role of science was clearest in the writing and teaching of Isabel Maitland Stewart, the Canadian-born nurse who was Nutting's protégé and successor at TC. Stewart had been an elementary school teacher in Winnipeg, then retrained as a nurse and practiced primarily in private duty for four and a half years before coming to

TC as a student in 1908. She spent the rest of her life as a nursing educator at TC. Critical of the abuse and rigidity in hospital-based training, Stewart's ideas about transforming nursing were shaped by her close relationship to Nutting and her contact with John Dewey and his beliefs in the democratization that comes with liberal education.[21]

Stewart's concern about a science for nursing was both pragmatic and political. Influenced by her friendship with the efficiency engineers Frank and Lillian Gilbreth and the general concern in the hospital community for standardization and efficiency, Stewart wrote enthusiastically about the promise of scientific management. She hoped that efficiency studies of nursing procedures and tasks, not unlike those being attempted in industry, would validate different nursing procedures and provide the facts on exploitation and inefficiency that could be used to break the hospital's hold on nursing education. With such studies, she believed nursing's base in sentiment could move on to one in science.

Aware of the disdain towards "industrial" models in the healthcare world, Stewart argued for the appropriate modification of such models for measuring both nursing procedures and patient outcome. Her pleas for efficiency and standardization were made judiciously to avoid the charge that she was selling out nursing's soul. American jingoism after World War I also provided Stewart's critics with the argument that she was introducing "German efficiency . . . something heartless and brutal."[22] In a carefully worded 1919 article on standardization, Stewart called for the establishment of "experimental laboratories" to begin the organized study of nursing work.[23] Thus, she hoped to create the infrastructure needed to institutionalize nursing's more scientific stance and ultimately liberate it from hospital control.

As an educator rather than a clinician, Stewart saw science primarily as a methodology for examining a series of problems and an ideology for demanding change. Her emphasis on careful inquiry rather than clinical investigation, and her definition of scientific nursing research was extremely broad. When the call for efficiency studies carried less cultural weight she shifted the ground of her argument, but not its basic outline. In a 1929 article titled "The Science and Art of Nursing," she admitted "that the scientific content of nursing is little more than a thin veneer covering a larger body of traditional material and practice gained largely through experience." Calling for an end to "empiric" nursing, she argued once again for a "scientific inquiry" into nursing procedures. By this she now meant the need for "not only bacteriological and physiological and chemical tests . . . but economic and psychological and sociological measurements also."[24]

In 1930 she tried again to institutionalize these ideas by suggesting a nursing research unit for TC. But the beginning of the depression was hardly an auspicious time to launch a search for funding or to convince the increasingly large numbers of unemployed nurses that such an effort was worthwhile. Even among the TC graduates there seemed to be little understanding or support for such an undertaking. Once back in the hospital they thought the emphasis on underlying principles, much less a research program, was merely an educator's luxury. An alumnae questionnaire revealed that the graduates wanted more "scientific spirit" (as they labeled it) in nursing, but thought that the TC program should have stressed more practical work.[25] Sally Johnson, a superintendent of nurses at MGH and a TC alumna, criticized the distance of the TC faculty from the realities of the training schools: "Where there are three nurses, two orderlies, and a ward helper on, and all but one are en route to the operating room, the front door, the out-patient department, and the electrocardiogram, there is no time for teaching. These are the features of the ward situation over which the faculty at TC have little conception."[26]

The concern of Sally Johnson and the other TC alumnae was, in part, a response to the growing intensity of nursing in the interwar years. Not only was there more to do, but there were more patients. Gone was the almost leisurely nineteenth-century form of caring for semichronically ill patients who lived in the hospital for months at a time. Expanding hospital usage coupled with earlier ambulation meant that more acutely ill patients occupied each hospital bed in a given year. The increasing number of clinical labs and X-ray departments placed new demands on the nurse's time.[27] By the early 1930s, for example, a nurse caring for a diabetic patient had a complicated set of routines that included preparing trays for blood samples, coordinating food intake with insulin injections, and teaching patients how to give their own hypodermics and regulate their diets. The explosion in new equipment and regulations also forced the nurse to monitor an ever more intricate system of requisitions and forms.[28]

Most of this was still being done by students who were supposed to be in training, although they typically worked twelve-hour days, six and a half days a week, and were expected to float from ward to ward when needed.[29] As the TC alumnae noted, as long as students worked, there was only time for a smattering of "scientific spirit" in the typical nursing school. Few in the hospital world were ready to acknowledge that a separation of the nursing service from nursing education would be needed to prepare a nurse who evinced more than a mere spirit of science.

Stewart worked to raise nursing's educational standards and to push for the creation of collegiate programs to solve the dilemma of the hospital's use of student labor. She devoted almost all her energy during the 1930s to an extensive revision of the recommended nursing school curriculum for the National League for Nursing Education, as well as on internal reorganization at TC. Graduate students with an interest in or talent for research were often drafted to work on curriculum projects rather than directed toward advanced clinical work or the laboratory. By 1941, while Stewart continued to call for more nursing research, she clearly meant social science curricular studies.[30] For her, science was increasingly a question of research methods and a political language with which to demand a new form of education. As a faculty member of an education school and one concerned about nursing's continuing problems with its hospital-based training system, she could hardly have been expected to see things in any other way.

Not everyone at TC thought nursing's research focus should take such an educational direction or had this kind of politicized hope for science. By the late 1920s others began to see that science for nursing would have to be based in clinical studies of nursing practice. In 1929, Martha Ruth Smith, a nurse trained at the Peter Bent Brigham Hospital in Boston and at TC, became supervisor of instruction at TC. Facing classes of graduate nurses, Smith and her colleagues discovered that their students almost came to blows over their "fierce and unquestioning loyalties" to the particular methods and nursing practices of their training schools.[31] In hopes that such allegiances would be based on a therapeutic rather than a loyalty standard, Smith and her colleagues began to teach a course in 1930 for graduate students titled "Comparative Nursing Practice." As Smith wrote, the course was intended to "make science serve the art of nursing."[32]

Building on Stewart's earlier dictums about efficiency and standardization, the course taught students to investigate specific nursing problems in the clinical setting. Control groups were set up to investigate differing procedures and their effectiveness. "Scientific facts" underlying the procedures were enumerated and discussed.[33] As a result, some students and faculty were encouraged to evaluate different nursing procedures through the use of standard laboratory methods. TC's *Nursing Education Bulletin* published the results of their work on such topics as "medical and surgical asepsis," "thermometer techniques," and control of bacteriological contamination.[34]

After Smith left TC in 1931 for a faculty position at Simmons College in Boston and later the first deanship in nursing at Boston University, her course was taught by Virginia Henderson. As both a TC student and faculty member from 1931 to 1948, Henderson became increasingly concerned with the failure of nursing to establish a research program in a clinical setting. It was Henderson who, over the years, trained hundreds of nurses in comparative scientific procedures and became the champion of science in nursing practice.

Henderson was a southerner from a respectable and established Virginia family. She trained under the progressive nursing educator Annie

Goodrich at the Army School of Nursing in Washington, D.C. in the early 1920s. From a close personal as well as academic bond with Goodrich, Henderson gained an idealistic and social perspective on nursing that, she recalled, "bore little relevance to the day to day nursing of doing a series of unrelated tasks."[35] After ten years as a public health nurse, a hospital training-school educational director, and a clinical instructor in a hospital outpatient department, she came to TC to obtain her bachelor's degree. Increasingly censorious of hospital-centered care and nursing that focused on tasks rather than the patient's particular problems and needs, she brought to TC a critical view of nursing as it was then taught and practiced.[36]

Isabel Stewart, recognizing Henderson's research interests and intellectual talents early in her TC career, put her to work on the national curriculum study. Fascinated more by the sciences than by educational theory, however, Henderson enrolled in the bacteriology and physiology courses offered in the nursing division. Her scientific bent was further nurtured by Stewart, who encouraged her to take anatomy, physiology, neuroanatomy, and other such courses at Columbia University's medical school.

Henderson's understanding of a science-nursing relationship soon went beyond Stewart's concern with method and Smith's hopes that science might contribute to the nursing arts. With her training, Henderson began to see the possibility of, in her metaphor, a "complete marriage between nursing and science." She has spent the rest of her career trying to implement the terms of this nuptial contract. In her course "Comparative Nursing Practice," Henderson built upon Smith's model. Her students went to the library to investigate the underlying theories of particular nursing problems. When no scientific theory appeared to help explain a situation, Henderson had her students "list the unanswered questions needing further research." This was an unusually innovative approach to nursing education, where the focus was still on the functional division of tasks and the rote learning of procedures. Henderson thus hoped to teach her students to begin to think like questioning researchers.

Henderson saw herself as an outsider at TC, continually arguing for "more advanced clinical teaching than they were doing." Except in the obstetrical nursing-midwifery section, Henderson believed there was very little understanding of the special way nursing could use the underlying basic sciences to change clinical practice. "They really couldn't envision the content," she claimed. "Because the way advanced clinical courses had been taught, with the exception of midwifery, was just a watered-down course or two in a hospital, really an imitation of what physicians do."[37]

Stewart had argued continually that nursing was not medicine and had something very different to offer. As she noted, nurses were not interested "in duplicating, but in complementing and rounding out the efforts of [physicians] and in filling in some of the gaps in the care of patients."[38] But she failed to grasp that to do so would require the development of a clinical science research and educational program, not merely university-based research institutes committed to studying the nursing role and curriculum.

It was Henderson who had a differing vision of what science could mean, and do, for nursing. The physiological approach of her TC professor, Caroline Stackpole, influenced Henderson's evolving ideas on nursing. Focused upon Claude Bernard's notions that health depended upon "the constancy of intercellular fluids" and physiological balance, Henderson sought to apply these concepts to the link between a patient's behavior and physical state. In some ways Henderson's evolving ideas restated nineteenth-century notions of the body as a closed energy system and combined them with the contemporary understanding of physiology's lessons for patient treatment. At a time when many doctors remained skeptical of experimental physiology's ability to solve any clinical problem, Henderson sought a way to use physiological theory to define a scientific base for nursing.[39] In language that sounded much like that of Harvard physiologist Walter Cannon, Henderson wrote "that emotional balance is inseparable from physiological balance" and "an emotion is actually our interpretation of cellular response to fluctuations in the chemical composition of the intercellular fluids."[40] Henderson was attempting to resolve in nursing's clinical practice what one historian has labeled a "common" problem of twentieth-century medicine, "the tension between the cognitive nature of laboratory science and the practical imperatives of clinical practice."[41]

Henderson was not merely concerned with individual body reactions. Influenced by Edward Thorndike's teaching on psychology, she focused on social and cultural environments as much as on individuals. Experiences with the patient focus of rehabilitation medicine further refined her thinking. She was thus beginning to search for a way to use this approach to restoring health as the basis for a nursing education and research program.

By the mid-1940s Henderson began to formulate a perspective for advanced clinical nursing that had "content that was different from medicine's." In a course for advanced students in medical-surgical nursing, Henderson and a small number of like-minded instructors developed an approach that was "unique because it was patient-centered and organized around major nursing problems rather than medical diagnoses and diseases of the body systems."[42] It was the beginning of teaching nurses to care for a whole patient, not just to perform a series of tasks.

However, much of this work remained undeveloped. Henderson, like the other nursing division faculty, was overburdened by work and was expected to teach a variety of subjects. Another nursing educator, recalling her grueling years on the TC faculty, commented: "We taught everything. We were said not to occupy chairs but benches."[43] Furthermore, few of the TC faculty, as in nursing in general, had doctorates, and even fewer had doctorates in fields other than education. They therefore had neither the time nor the training to do systematic clinical research.

In the hospital-based nursing schools the situation was even worse. Although the hours devoted to basic science teaching increased in the early twentieth century, much of it consisted of lectures on countless facts, leading to what one critic called "mental indigestion." In 1932 less than a third of the schools had instructors with a college degree, and the typical school gave over 10 percent of its teaching time to theory and go percent to practice (See Tables 12.1 and 12.2). Over a fifth of the schools had no full-time instructors.[44]

Nor was it clear where advanced, clinically trained nurses would have practiced, or done research, once they completed their education. With the battle to gain acceptance for a baccalaureate education for nurses still to be won, the idea that a nurse might be either a specially skilled clinician or a researcher garnered little support. Advancement in nursing meant administrative or teaching positions, not a career in clinical or laboratory research. Neither the hospitals nor the universities would create a place for such a nurse. Even when the Rockefeller Foundation supported the showcase collegiate nursing program at Yale, their contribution was penurious compared to the funds lavished on the medical school.[45] Clinical science research and advanced training were reserved for physicians or basic scientists.

The nursing and medical cultures had by the 1940s made very different places for research in clinical science. In the early 1920s numerous clinicians and medical school faculty still refused to bow before what one physician labeled "the false gods of the German physiological school" that assume "a man [sic] gropes darkly at the bedside but sees clearly in the laboratory."[46] But by the late 1920s medicine had differentiated the clinical teacher and researcher from the practitioner as foundation largesse and university support paid most of the costs, and the creation of the teaching hospital provided the site and necessary patients. Clinical scientist-physicians with an interest in "disease and therapeutics" found a place on the medical school faculties.[47] Ironically, nursing always had the link to hospitals that medicine had to create, but it lacked the political power and societal approval to transform it into a clinical research base.

Table 12.1 Medical and nursing school curricula, 1928–29

| | Hours for selected subjects[a] | | |
Subjects	Nursing[b] highest	Medicine[c] highest	Medicine lowest
Anatomy	90	1267	480
Biochemistry	30	363	99
Physiology	—	612	224
Pathology	15	473	220
Bacteriology	28	432	124
Pharmacology/ Materia Medica	50	279	104
Obstetrics/gynecology	37	368	168

Sources: Committee on the Grading of Nursing Schools, *The Second Grading* (New York: The Committee, 1932), 157, and *Final Report of the Commission on Medical Education* (New York: Association of American Medical Colleges, 1932), Appendix tables 111–12.
[a] Total required median hours: 631 for nursing, 3,914 for medicine.
[b] Figures for 1,397 nursing schools responding to survey.
[c] Figures from 13 medical schools selected by random.

In this context, Henderson found it increasingly difficult to gain support for the kind of teaching and research she was attempting to create. Emphasis on correct methods or curriculum vastly overshadowed any clinical research. In 1944 Annie Goodrich wrote to her disciple, encouraging her to keep her clinical focus and applauding her work. When it appeared that Henderson had been passed over for a promotion at TC, Goodrich reminded her that "Stewart . . . I fear with many others do[es] not interpret the art and science of nursing as the *Practice* of nursing."[48] In a more recent interview Henderson noted: "I was always more interested in the substance than the method—while so many others were so afraid to be criticized for not doing it correctly that they focused on the method, not the substance."[49]

Goodrich could sustain Henderson as an individual and friend, but she could not change the educational climate at TC or the attitude toward nursing research in the hospital. When another nursing educator, R. Louise McManus, replaced Stewart as head of the TC division in 1947, it became clear that Henderson's approach was not being supported. When McManus asked Henderson to stop teaching both the classroom and in-hospital clinical aspects of her course and to concentrate only on the classroom, Henderson resigned.[50]

Table 12.2 Percentage of nursing schools planning to give at least as many hours as recommended by the National League of Nursing Education in selected subjects

Subject	1929	1932
Anatomy	51	68
Bacteriology	22	38
Chemistry	29	46
Materia Medica	51	69
Principles and Practice of Nursing	49	59
Pathology	52	58
Gynecology	92	91
Obsterics	49	65

Source: Committee on the Grading of Nursing Schools, *The Second Grading* (New York: The Committee, 1932), 158.

During her TC years, Henderson began to formulate a theory of nursing that would become more fully stated in her 1966 publication, *The Nature of Nursing*. Building upon her personal experience in nursing and her understanding of physiology, she tried to place nursing in a continuum with medicine, while providing it with its own explanatory model for practice. With her clinician's understanding, Henderson argued that the nurse had to place herself figuratively "inside" patients in order to become their "counterpart, alter ego, or helper."[51]

Henderson's vision linked research in the basic sciences and the testing of procedures for effectiveness with the patient's needs in order to strengthen the nurse's clinical stance. Even in 1966 her reviewers and admirers noted how necessary and farseeing her concept of nursing was.[52] Bedside nursing and clinical practice remained at the center of her research concerns, but Henderson also remained a maverick and outsider, focusing upon historical-bibliographic work and continually arguing for research on nursing practice.

Science, with its multiple meanings, thus proved a difficult vehicle to harness for nursing's escape from hospital control. When economic and political factors finally made possible the shift from student to staff nursing by World War II, the difficulties of hospital power over nursing and the working lives of nurses remained.[53] In the face of rising nursing shortages and mass discontent over the staff nursing position in the 1950s, nursing research, when it did occur, focused more on the nursing role and the nurse herself than on nursing practice. The lack of support or understanding of the need for any other kind of research, the growing concern with high turnover rates in the hospitals and nurses' dissatisfaction with their work, the cold hand of the education schools, and the assumptions that science in nursing meant methodology or the addition of more courses in the underlying biological sciences, continued to guide nursing higher education. Growing awareness that nursing needed more of a theoretical orientation to justify its demands for more authority led to philosophical studies of nursing as a process and to the development of "grand theory," but not to either more clinical or laboratory research.[54]

The institutional basis for change was created very slowly. In the post-World War II years the number of nurses with both baccalaureate and graduate degrees began to grow. Federal funding for advanced nursing education, coupled with changes in medical therapeutics and technology, helped to generate both the supply and demand for nurses with different kinds of training and orientations to their field.[55] Drawn into the university and away from the hospital's control, nursing education had to meet higher standards for acceptance and to gain support for various types of research.

At TC, Stewart's dream of a nursing research institute was finally realized when the Kellogg and Rockefeller Foundations funded the Institute of Research and Service in Nursing Education in 1953. Seen primarily as an educational research/field service program, however, it focused more on nursing roles and administration than clinical practice.[56] In 1952 a journal titled *Nursing Research* began publication to encourage and report research by nurses. Until quite recently, however, it too was shaped by nursing's commitment to "structure not content," as Henderson labeled it. In a widely read editorial in 1956, Henderson still had to inquire: "Research in nursing practice—When?"[57]

As increasing clinical specialization and the nurse-practitioner movements of the 1960s developed with the help of federal funds, expanding feminist consciousness, and a nursing revolt against the limitations of the administrative track, the importance of Henderson's views were acknowledged and she was resurrected as the grand lady of nursing research. Twenty-one years later, in yet another guest editorial, she could admit that "the emphasis *is* changing." But, she sagely argued: "Nurses are still loathe to take responsibility for designing the methods they use; for undertaking studies that, if the findings were applied, might revolutionize practice. They are, perhaps, less comfortable in collaborating with physiologists and physicians than with social scientists, less likely to expect or ask for a colleague relationship if they work with physicians on questions of health care."[58]

Nursing today is increasingly preoccupied with encouraging more research, but is still divided over what this means. Nurses no longer debate *if* there should be a nursing-science relationship, but rather what that relationship should be. Is nursing a science with a coherent theoretical base and methodology, or an applied science that draws upon the biological and social sciences?[59] However, both sides of this intellectual debate cling to the belief that science—as objective method and/or knowable laws—can save nursing from a professional abyss.

Nursing's creation as gender-appropriate work for women and controlled by the hospitals shaped its founding ideologies, educational structures, professionalizing effort, and place in the health-care hierarchy. In turn, these factors determined the terms the science debate would use. To a Florence Nightingale or an Annette Fiske, science in nursing could not be separated from the conception of woman's role, service, and morality. For an early twentieth-century *science-interested* educator like Isabel Stewart, science was a neutral and objective methodology to harness to nursing's need for a more liberal curriculum, to rationalize its work load, and to improve its professional standing. For a *science-oriented* clinician like Virginia Henderson, however, science drew upon various disciplines that could be used to create an effective clinical nursing practice and theory.[60] Stewart's views were perhaps a more accurate reading of the contemporary possibilities for nursing, but Henderson's were more prescient. Each vision of the science-nursing relationship has continued to contend for the right to define, in Henderson's words, "the nature of nursing."

The hospital's continued pressure on nursing to focus upon patient needs kept a nurse like Virginia Henderson interested in patient-centered clinical study rather than more obscure research. It forced nurses to consider if they have created, or will create, different and effective ways to understand the human reaction to illness. But as our contemporary media headlines about the prevailing nursing shortage suggest, working nurses now have other options and can abandon the hospital when its demands become outrageous or its pay scales too demeaning. Whether science in Stewart's broad vision, or in Henderson's clinical stance, can help to solve this current crisis in the healthcare system remains to be seen. But it is clear that the "legitimate daughter" is seeking new terms for her relationships.

NOTES

1.   Paul Keller, "The Grading Committee and Quality Nursing," *Transactions of the American Hospital Association (1932): 745.*

2.   This chapter is part of my larger work on the evolution of the hospital-nursing relationship; see Susan Reverby, *Ordered to Care: The Dilemma of American Nursing* (New York: Cambridge University Press, 1987). See also Barbara Melosh, *"The Physician's Hand": Work, Culture and Conflict in American Nursing* (Philadelphia: Temple University Press, 1982), and JoAnn Ashley, *Hospitals, Paternalism, and the Role of the Nurse* (New York: Teachers College Press, 1976).

3.   See Melosh, *"The Physician's Hand"*; Leo W. Simmons, "Images of the Nurse: Theory and Studies," in *Nursing Research: A Survey and Assessment,* ed. Leo W. Simmons and Virginia Henderson (New York: Appleton-Century-Crofts, 1964), 167–223, and Anne Hudson Jones, ed., *Images of Nursing in History, Art, and Literature* (Philadelphia: University of Pennsylvania Press, 1986).

4.   For a discussion of the theoretical question of the relationship between "institutional forms and cognitive processes" in the creation of science, see Everett Mendelsohn, "The Social Construction of Scientific Knowledge, " in *The Social Production of Scientific Knowledge,* ed. Everett Mendelsohn, Peter Weingart, and Richard Whitley (Dordrecht, Holland, and Boston: D. Reidel, 1977), 3–26.

5.   Charles Rosenberg, "Florence Nightingale on Contagion: The Hospital as Moral Universe," in *Healing and History,* ed. Charles E. Rosenberg (New York: Science History Publications, 1979), 124.

6.   Florence Nightingale, *Notes on Nursing* (New York: D. Appleton, 1861), 80, and *Notes on Hospitals,* 3d rev. ed. (London: Longmans, Green, 1863), 17.

7.   For further discussion see Reverby, *Ordered to Care,* ch. 3.

8.   Committee on the Grading of Nursing Schools, *Nurses, Patients, and Pocketbooks* (New York: The Committee, 1928), 36–37.

9.   See Florence Nightingale, *Notes on Hospitals and Introductory Notes on Lying-In Institutions: Together with a Proposal for Organising an Institution for Training Midwives and Midwifery Nurses* (London: Longmans, Green, 1871), and Isabel Stewart, *The Education of Nurses* (New York: Macmillan, 1948; reprint, New York: Garland, 1985). On the problem with texts, see Charlotte Aikens, *Primary Studies for Nurses: A Text-book for the First Year Pupil Nurses,* 3d ed. (Philadelphia: W. B. Saunders, 1915).

10.   See M. Adelaide Nutting, *A Sound Economic Basis for Schools of Nursing* (New York: G. P. Putnams, 1926; reprint, New York: Garland, 1984), 73–104. Isabel Stewart does not mention the course at Waltham (probably because she disapproved of the physician control of the school), although it was clearly modeled after the same European courses that influenced Nutting's model at Johns Hopkins. See Annette Fiske, *First Fifty Years of the Waltham Training School for Nurses* (New York: Garland, 1985), 68–78, and Stewart, *Education of Nurses,* 160–61.

11.   Lavinia L. Dock, *A History of Nursing,* vol. 3 (New York: G. P. Putnam's Sons, 1912), 136. See, for example, Henry Fairfield Osborn, *Science and Sentiment* (New York: The Presbyterian Hospital, 1907), 5–6.

12.   Dr. James Mumford to Mrs. Whiteside, December 10, 1906, Box 5, Folder I Ga I, MGH Nursing Records, Rare Books Room, Countway Medical Library, Harvard Medical School, Boston, Mass. See similar complaints from Dr. Joel Goldthwait, William Conant, and Hugh Cabot in the same folder. See also Sylvia Perkins, *A Centennial Review, The Massachusetts General Hospital School of Nursing, 1873–1973* (Boston: School of Nursing Nurses Alumnae Association, 1975), 37–38.

13.   Isabel M. Stewart, "Progress in Nursing Education during 1919," *Modern Hospital* 14 (March 1920): 183.

14.   Annette Fiske, "How Can We Counteract the Prevailing Tendency to Commercialism in Nursing?" *Proceedings of the 17th Annual Meeting of the Massachusetts State Nurses Association,* p. 8, Box 7, Massachusetts Nurses' Association (MNA) Papers, Nursing Archives, Mugar Library, Boston University, Boston, Mass.

15.   Theresa E. Christy, *Cornerstone for Nursing Education* (New York: Teachers College Press, 1969).

16.   TC Department of Nursing and Health, "1910–11 Report of the Department," M. Adelaide Nutting Collection, Box 2, Teachers College (TC) Archives, TC, Columbia University, New York, New York. See also the "1920–21 Report of the Department of Nursing and Health" located in the same box and depository; Isabel M. Stewart, "Twenty-Five Years of Nursing Education in Teachers College, 1899–1925," *Teachers College Bulletin*, 17th ser., no. 3 (February 1926): 7–21, Isabel M. Stewart Papers, Box 4, TC Archives; and Christy, *Cornerstone for Nursing Education*.

17.   Isabel M. Stewart, "The Reminiscences of Isabel M. Stewart," Transcription of taped interviews from the Oral History Research Office, Columbia University, 1916, 325–27, Box 4, Stewart Papers. For a discussion of the continued pressure on the faculty to work for the collective good of nursing, see R. Louise McManus, "Nursing Research—Its Evolution," *American Journal of Nursing* 61 (April 1961): 78.

18.   Christy, *Cornerstone for Nursing Education*, 36, and Stewart, "Reminiscences," 325–29.

19.   Quoted by Stewart, "Twenty-Five Years of Nursing Education," 14.

20.   Wolfgang van den Daele, "The Social Construction of Science: Institutionalisation and Definition of Positive Science in the Latter Half of the Seventeenth Century," in *The Social Production of Scientific Knowledge*, ed. Mendelsohn et al., 32.

21.   See Stewart, *Education of Nurses*; Christy, *Cornerstone for Nursing Education*; and Rosalind Rosenberg, *Beyond Separate Spheres* (New Haven: Yale University Press, 1982) on Dewey's general influence on women in education.

22.   Isabel M. Stewart, "Possibilities of Standardization in Nursing Technique," *Modern Hospital 12* (June 1919): 451–54; Fiske, "How Can We Counteract," 8; Faye G. Abdellah and Virginia Henderson, "Nursing Research," in *Principles and Practice of Nursing*, 6th ed., ed. Virginia Henderson and Gladys Nite (New York: Macmillan, 1978), 1064–66; and Susan Reverby, "Stealing the Golden Eggs: Ernest Amory Codman and the Science and Management of Medicine," *Bulletin of the History of Medicine* 55 (Summer 81): 156–71.

23.   Stewart, "Possibilities of Standardization," 454.

24.   Isabel M. Stewart, "The Science and Art of Nursing," *Nursing Education Bulletin* 2, n.s. (Winter 1929): 1–4.

25.   Response to questionnaires sent to former students in 1923, Box I, Nutting Collection. It is also clear from their annual reports that the department felt on the defensive about not providing totally "practical" courses; see "Report of the Department of Nursing Education for 1923–24," Box I, Nutting Collection.

26.   "Gleanings," n.d., circa 1935, Box 2, Folder 1 D 12, MGH Nursing Collection, Rare Books Room, Countway Medical Library, Harvard Medical School, Boston, Mass.

27.   See each March issue of the *Journal of the American Medical Association* for hospital statistics, and Harry Marks, "Review of Barbara Melosh's 'The Physician's Hand,'" *Technology and Culture* 26 (April 1985): 326–28.

28.   Minnie Goodnow, *The Technic of Nursing*, 2d ed. (Philadelphia: W. B. Saunders, 1931), 354; Marion Elizabeth Derry, "We Can Still Serve, Says Retired

Nurse in Uniform Again," *Hospitals* 18 (February 1944): 32; and Shirley Titus, "The Present Position of Nursing in Hospitals in the United States," *Nosokomeion* 2 (April 1931): 288–97.

29. President of the Alumnae Association of the Capital City School of Nursing, Letter to the Editor, *Washington Post*, February 17, 1933, quoted in Harry Dowling, *City Hospitals: The Undercare of the Underprivileged* (Cambridge: Harvard University Press, 1982), 142.

30. Isabel M. Stewart, "The Responsibility of Nursing Educators for Investigating Their Own Problems," *Nursing Education Bulletin*, n.s. 11 (September 1941): 1–7.

31. Virginia Henderson, "We've 'Come a Long Way,' but What of the Direction?" *Nursing Research* 26 (May–June 1977): 163. See also Martha Ruth Smith, "The Variability in Existing Nursing Practice and Methods of Determining Validity," *Nursing Education Bulletin* 1, n.s. (1930): 10.

32. Martha Ruth Smith, "The Improvement of Nursing Methods," *38th Annual Report of the National League of Nursing Education* (New York: National League of Nursing Education, 1932), 182.

33. Abdellah and Henderson, "Nursing Research," 1064, and Interview by Susan Reverby with Virginia Henderson, New Haven, Conn., March 24, 1984.

34. Smith, "The Variability in Existing Nursing Practice," 10–17; Martha Erdmann and Margaret Welsh, "Studies in Thermometer Technique," *Nursing Education Bulletin* 2, n.s. (Winter 1929): 8–33; and Virginia Henderson, "Medical and Surgical Asepsis," *Nursing Education Bulletin* 3, n.s. (June 1935).

35. Henderson interview; see also Virginia Henderson, "Commencement Address—Grace New Haven Hospital School of Nursing," June 6, 1961, p. 5, Virginia Henderson Papers, Box 1, Folder 6, Nursing Archives, Boston University.

36. Virginia Henderson, *The Nature of Nursing* (New York: Macmillan, 1966), 6–23. The following information and quotations are from the Henderson interview cited in n.33 above, unless otherwise noted.

37. For corroboration of Henderson's contentions see outlines and course descriptions in Box 2, Stewart Papers. For a view of Stewart's interests that stress her clinical concerns, see Christy, *Cornerstone for Nursing Education*, 75–112. Christy's history of the TC division is quite hagiographic and reflects an attempt to show how much the division supported what became important nursing concerns in the 1960s.

38. "Report of Isabel M. Stewart's Trip," draft copy, p. 4, Nutting Collection, Box 9.

39. See John Harley Warner, "Physiology," in *The Education of American Physicians: Historical Essays*, ed. Ronald L. Numbers (Berkeley: University of California Press, 1980), 48–71; Gerald L. Geison, "Divided We Stand: Physiologists and Clinicians in the American Context," in *The Therapeutic Revolution: Essays in the Social History of American Medicine*, ed. Morris Vogel and Charles Rosenberg (Philadelphia: University of Pennsylvania Press, 1979), 67–90; Gerald L. Geison, ea., *Physiology in the American Context, 1850–1940* (Bethesda, Md.: American Physiological Society, 1987); and Saul Benison, A. Clifford Barger, and Elin L. Wolfe, *Walter B. Cannon: The Life and Times of a Young Scientist* (Cambridge: Harvard University Press, 1987).

40.   Henderson, *The Nature of Nursing*, 11. Henderson also contends that some of her thinking was shaped by the physiology courses she took at the Columbia Medical School and the microbiology courses taught at TC by Jean Broadhurst.

41.   Joel D. Howell, "Cardiac Physiology and Clinical Medicine? Two Case Studies," in *Physiology in the American Context*, ed. Geison, 290.

42.   Henderson, *The Nature of Nursing*, 14; Abdellah and Henderson, "Nursing Research," 1965. Around the same time the Yale University School of Nursing was also beginning to use the case method of teaching, rather than the functional method.

43.   Oral History interview with Ruth Sleeper by Mary Ann Garrigan and Lois Monteiro, January 1965, transcript in Box 2, Folder 5, Martha Ruth Smith Papers, Nursing Archives, Boston University.

44.   Margaret Bridgman, *Collegiate Education for Nursing* (New York: Russell Sage Foundation, 1953), 55; Committee on the Grading of Nursing Schools, *The Second Grading* (New York: The Committee, 1932), 55, 155.

45.   Sister Dorothy Sheahan, "The Social Origins of American Nursing and Its Movement into the University" (Ph.D. diss., New York University, 1980), ch. 3. I am grateful to the author for lending me a copy of her thesis.

46.   Dr. Charles Emerson, "Comments—Annual Congress on Medical Education and Licensure," *Journal of the American Medical Association* 74 (March 13, 1920): 757. See also Saul Jarcho, "Medical Education in the United States, 1910–1956," *Journal of the Mt. Sinai Hospital* 26 (July–August 1959): 339–85.

47.   Kenneth M. Ludmerer, *Learning to Heal: The Development of American Medical Education* (New York: Basic Books, 1985), 52, 212, 219–33. See also A. McGehee Harvey, *Science at the Bedside: Clinical Research in American Medicine, 1905–1945* (Baltimore: Johns Hopkins University Press, 1981).

48.   Annie Goodrich to Virginia Henderson, March 3, 1944, Box 3, Henderson Papers. The underlining and capitalization are by Goodrich.

49.   Virginia Henderson to Ellen Baer, telephone conversation, October 10, 1985, and quoted in Baer, "'A Cooperative Venture' in Pursuit of Professional Status: A Research Journal for Nursing," *Nursing Research* 35 (January–February 1987): 21.

50.   Susan Reverby interview with Henderson, March 24, 1984. For a different interpretation of TC's emphasis on clinical content, see Theresa Christy's interview with R. Louise McManus, *Cornerstone for Nursing Education, 105–6.* Not surprisingly, McManus wrote an article titled, "Isabel M. Stewart—Foremost Researcher," *Nursing Researcher* 1 (January 1962): 4–6; see discussion in Baer, "'A Cooperative Venture,'" 18–25.

51.   See both her "Commencement Address," 14, and *The Nature of Nursing.*

52.   See numerous reviews and letters in Box 1, Folder 1, Henderson Papers.

53.   See Reverby, *Ordered to Care*, 180–198, and Melosh, "*The Physician's Hand*," 159–206, for further discussion.

54.   The most influential postwar figure was Martha Rogers at New York University; see her *An Introduction to the Theoretical Basis of Nursing* (Philadelphia: J. P. Lippincott, 1970). For a discussion of the impact of Rogers and her followers on nursing education and theory in the 1950s and 1960s, see Oral History interview with Dean Claire Fagin by Susan Reverby, June and August 1982, School

of Nursing, University of Pennsylvania and Rozella M. Schlotfeldt, "Defining Nursing: A Historic Controversy," *Nursing Research* 35 (January–February 1987): 64–67.

55.   For an overview of the effect of these changes on nursing research and theory development see Susan R. Gortner and Helen Nahm, "An Overview of Nursing Research in the United States," *Nursing Research* 26 (January–February 1977): 10–33.

56.   Helen L. Bunge, "A Review of the First Six Years, 1953–59, with Suggestions for the Future," Institute of Research and Service in Nursing Education Papers, Box I, TC Archives; see also Louice C. Smith, *Helen L. Bunge: Nurse, Teacher, Scholar* (Madison: University of Wisconsin Nursing School, 1979).

57.   See Baer, "'A Cooperative Venture,'" 21, and Virginia Henderson, *Nursing Research* 4 (February 1956): 99.

58.   Virginia Henderson, "We've 'Come a Long Way,'" 163–64.

59.   Susan R. Gortner, "The History and Philosophy of Nursing Science and Research," *Advances in Nursing Science* 5 (January 1983): 1–8, and Jacqueline Fawcett, *Analysis and Evaluation of Conceptual Models of Nursing* (Philadelphia: 1984).

60.   These categories are used by Kathryn Pyne Addelson, "The Man of Professional Wisdom," in *Discovering Reality: Feminist Perspectives on Epistemology, Metaphysics, and Philosophy of Science*, ed. Sandra Harding and Merrill B. Hintikka (Dordrecht, Holland and Boston: Reidel, 1983), 165.

13

Lavinia Lloyd Dock:
The Henry Street Years

Carole A. Estabrooks

Looking back over the past may be much overdone. It may result in an undue veneration for what is behind us in time unless we relate it very clearly to the present and so gain an intelligent certainty of how and where we mean to go in the future.[1]

Lavinia Lloyd Dock (1858–1956) went to work and live at the Henry Street Settlement (HSS) on New York City's Lower East Side in 1896 at thirty-eight years of age.[2] She left in 1915 at the age of fifty-seven. It can be argued that she spent the most productive years of her working life living at the Settlement at 265 Henry Street. While a number of short pieces have been written about Dock, no biography or extensive analyses exist.[3] Material on Dock deals with her historical work, her activity in the International Council of Nurses (ICN), her role in the professionalization of nursing through efforts at organization and registration, and her involvement in the suffrage movement. In an extensive examination of sources, however, I have been unable to locate any material that explicitly discusses Lavinia Dock in the context of the Lower East Side of New York City during the nineteen years she lived and worked there.[4]

I believe that the failure to unravel these years has resulted in misunderstanding about this period of Dock's life and overlooks its singular importance in her development as a leader of international stature. I undertook this project to understand why it was that Dock said "I never began to think until I went to Henry Street and lived with Miss Wald."[5] My thesis is that the Henry Street Settlement provided Dock with the

Note: This chapter was originally published in *Nursing History Review* 3 (1995): 143–72. Copyright © 1995 by The American Association for the History of Nursing. Reprinted with permission.

extensive system of social, political, domestic, and emotional support necessary for her to engage in an unprecedented level of professional and sociopolitical activism over a nineteen-year period. Why she undertook this ambitious agenda is a different matter and beyond the analyses of this article, although insights, where I have had them, are included with the intent that they will cause scholars to rethink this most enigmatic of our early leaders.

THE HENRY STREET SETTLEMENT

The Henry Street Settlement was formally incorporated in 1903.[6] Its 1893 forerunner was founded by Lillian D. Wald and Mary Brewster at 27 Jefferson Street.[7] Two years later, in 1895, they obtained the house at 265 Henry Street, which became known as "The House on Henry Street (HSS)."[8] The HSS is scarcely separable from Lavinia Dock. Dock was Lillian Wald's closest nurse friend for over forty years; being older and having more professional experience than Wald, she was also her mentor—at least during the early years of HSS. Wald called Lavinia Dock "Docky"; to Dock, Wald was "dearest lady."[9] Dock was regarded as one of the "steadies," as a member of Wald's inner circle, the "family."[10] That family was composed of Lavinia Dock, Ysabella Waters, Annie Goodrich, and Florence Kelley.[11]

It is helpful in placing HSS in context to revisit the progressive era, usually taken to include the years from 1890 to 1920. Five problems absorbed reformers of this era: ethical conflict between the values of an agrarian society and an industrialized urban society, the rise of big business, the maldistribution of wealth, the rise of the city, and racism.[12] The forces moving the country were, however, more complex and immediate than such a list suggests. The rise of the city, in particular, had spawned tremendous social problems including overcrowding, inadequate housing, lack of sanitation, sweat shops, child labor, prostitution, and disease.

The Lower East Side

In 1938 Robert Duffus suggested that an appropriate banner over the door of the first tenement house that Lillian Wald visited in 1893 might appropriately have read: "Abandon hope, all ye who enter here."[13] Accounts of the living conditions of the Lower East Side of New York City in the late 1800s and early 1900s bear out Duffus's suggestion.[14] By 1890, as a result of the great waves of immigration that occurred after 1880, the population density of this section of New York City was suffocating.[15]

Families of five to seven typically lived in tenement houses known as "double deckers," often with additional boarders to help pay the exorbitant rents. They lived in one or two rooms, without toilet facilities, water, fresh air, or sunlight. Central airshafts, meant to entrain fresh air into these tall, narrow buildings, served instead as garbage chutes. People often slept on the fire escapes because of the stifling heat; the children played in streets flowing with human and animal refuse, mud, and all manner of filth. Frequently, the home also served as a sweat shop, and it functioned as a sick room when disease was present. In these vermin-filled dwellings children were conceived and born as American citizens—into, for many, a spiral of unrelenting poverty.[16] It is little wonder that for many new immigrants "taking the gas" provided them their only escape from their hopelessness.[17] It was to these urban ills that settlement workers devoted their efforts. Lavinia Dock's life and work during her Henry Street period had several dimensions, extending beyond the boundaries of most of her contemporary settlement colleagues. These dimensions were nursing practice, professionalization, labor activism, the hygiene and morality crusade, and the suffrage crusade. Intertwined with these areas were the complex economic, social, and political forces of American society in the progressive era. The HSS also provided Dock with a separate and special context, without which she would not have achieved or aspired to the same level of accomplishment. What drove Lavinia Dock? Why did she work extensively in so many different areas? Why did she choose to do the things she did? I suspect they needed to be done and that she saw them as each and all part of the unending struggle. I suspect it would never have occurred to her not do them. Lavinia Dock had an intimidating intellect, the social and political conventions of her progressive contemporaries, a fierce determination, and not insignificantly, the support of HSS. She also had the capacity for outrage and the ability to transform that outrage into action. At Henry Street her thinking crystallized; all that remained was the realization of those potentialities.

The Practice of Nursing

The HSS sponsored civic work, social work, country work, and visiting nursing. Visiting nursing distinguished HSS from most other settlements.[18] Civic work included advocating for improved housing, clean streets, better schools, more parks, playgrounds, and garbage disposal. Social work meant organizing boys and girls clubs and domestic classes for immigrant women, and establishing gymnasiums, kindergartens, libraries, and community gathering places where young people could enjoy wholesome entertainment.[19] The country work stemmed from HSS workers' observations that children of the slums did not receive much fresh air and sunshine and from belief that these were essential to healthy childhood development. It may also have stemmed from the settlement workers' upper-middle-class memories of childhood days filled with idyllic country and seaside holidays. By 1911 HSS had seven country places, three of which were open year-round.[20]

Visiting nurses visited and treated the sick in their homes. This aspect of the visiting nurse services was largely concerned with providing direct, hands-on care for people suffering from contagious diseases such as diphtheria, pneumonia, tuberculosis, and typhus. Postpartum care and care of family members injured in accidents also constituted a significant proportion of caseloads. The visiting nurses also ran milk dispensaries for mothers with children,[21] administered first aid at the settlement house or one of its branches, and followed patients from the schools and hospitals. Evidence of the effectiveness of the services rendered by HSS nurses was documented by Wald who ensured that careful records were kept of all of HSS activities. These records show that HSS nurses cared for 3,535 cases of pneumonia in the home in 1914 with a mortality rate of 8.05 percent, compared to a hospital mortality rate of 31.2 percent for 1,612 cases during the same period.[22] Ysabella Waters was largely responsible for the formal statistics that were kept of HSS nursing activities. Her figures indicate remarkable growth in the nursing services from 1902, when nurses made 25,840 visits, to 1913, when they made 188,214 visits.[23]

I have been able to locate few explicit references to Dock's nursing practice while she was at Henry Street. The clinician is, interestingly, the least well understood part of Lavinia Dock. Dock did publish a paper in the *Amencan Journal of Nursing (AJN)* where she discussed the nursing care she gave an elderly man at home in the mountains, thus offering a small insight into her facility with bedside, district-type nursing.[24] It seems reasonable to assume that Dock would have been as particular as Wald at keeping detailed records of her nursing visits while at HSS. Dock left active clinical nursing practice in 1908 at the age of fifty but did not retire from nursing until 1923 at the age of sixty-five.[25]

The lives of the nurses at HSS had a rhythm that was valued. In 1900 Dock wrote what appears to be the only explicit reference she ever made to this daily life at HSS:

> *Breakfast is at half past seven, and unless guests are staying in the house, this is often the only meal at which the members of the family find themselves alone together. The postman comes: letters are opened and read, work and plans for the day are talked over and arranged. Afterwards the rooms are set in order; new cases that have come in are distributed by the head of the family, and the nurses go off on their rounds. The entire day is spent in caring for the sick; and in following out the different lines of work which develop from this, the primary one. The nursing is of course much like the*

work of district nurses in general, except for the entire absence of any kind of restrictive regulation. Each nurse manages her patients and arranges her time according to her best judgement, and all points of interest, knotty problems, and difficult situations are talked over and settled in family council. The calls usually come from the people themselves, though charitable agencies, clergymen, and physicians furnish a certain percentage. Often a nurse is sent for before a doctor is called, and then, if one is needed, she decides whether to apply at the dispensary, or to submit the patient's case to one of the best uptown specialists, or to advise hospital care. . . . As the Settlement family is quite a permanent one, its members entering for indefinite periods and never wishing to leave, the nurses form real friendships with their people, who call upon them in every emergency, year in and year out. In addition to her nursing, each one takes up some special work of her own according to her talent. What this may be will appear after luncheon to which we now return and where one usually finds some visitor or visitors interested and interesting, for no dull or stupid people ever appear at the Settlement. Those who come here have some work or purpose in life and feel a love for it in its various aspects. . . . In the afternoon nursing work is finished, it may be in one or two hours, or not until dinner time, and the specialities are pursued.[26]

Wald kept the bureaucracy of HSS to a minimum; "elastic and uncrystallized" were the terms Dock used.[27] The absence of formalized structures was an asset and was responsible, in part, for the autonomy the nurses experienced. This autonomy naturally attracted well-educated, independent, and spirited young women to HSS—and encouraged them to remain at HSS.

THE PROFESSIONALIZATION OF NURSING

Later described as "the last of the little band of farsighted nurses who ensured a broad and durable foundation for professional nursing,"[28] Dock was a central figure in American and international nursing history in the modern era. She was responsible wholly or in part for several of the initiatives for establishing professional status for American nursing and for bringing nurses throughout the world together. In my opinion her influence has been underestimated. Much of her work on the professionalization of nursing occurred while she was a resident at HSS. This work fell into five general areas: organization, registration, education, history, and communication.

Dock was instrumental in the formal organization of the nursing profession, specifically in the formation of what are known today as the International Council of Nurses (ICN), the American Nurses' Association

(ANA), and the National League for Nursing (NLN).[29] Working with Ethel Gordon Bedford Fenwick she helped found ICN. Dock first met Fenwick in 1892 when Fenwick visited the United States to make arrangements for the British nursing exhibits for the 1893 World's Fair. During that visit Fenwick visited Johns Hopkins where she met Dock, with whom she felt an immediate sense of kindred spirit. It was in 1893 that Fenwick became involved in the International Council of Women, which was to spawn ICN. At the first ICN Congress in 1899, Fenwick was elected president and Dock was elected secretary.[30] Serving as the honorary secretary from 1899 to 1923, Dock traveled at her own expense back and forth across the Atlantic on many occasions, with the ICN papers in a steamer trunk. She wrote the preamble to the ICN constitution, kept the American nurses apprised of news in the AJN, and kept a voluminous correspondence with nurses around the world.[31]

In 1894, after the organizational meetings held at the 1893 Chicago World's Fair, the first convention of the American Society of Superintendents of Training Schools for Nurses was held.[32] This organization became known as the National League for Nursing Education (NLNE) in 1912, and later as NLN. Dock served as its secretary from 1896 to 1901,[33] ably assisting Isabel Hampton Robb in its development. Dock prepared an extensive background paper for the 1896 convention of the Society of Superintendents, recommending a course of action for forming the Nurses' Associated Alumnae of the United States and Canada, later to become ANA.[34]

Dock contributed to the establishment of standards, licensure, and regulation of registries or directories—important initiatives for the Associated Alumnae in its early years.[35] She advocated, when addressing directories, that nurses be able to set their own rates of pay and that there be equality of pay for male and female nurses.[36] She repeatedly advocated minimum standards for the profession,[37] and she spoke on at least three occasions of the need for a code of ethics.[38] Although most of Dock's formal work as an educator occurred before she went to HSS,[39] during her time there she sometimes went to Teacher's College at Columbia University in New York to teach for Adelaide Nutting, and later for Isabel Maitland Stewart.[40] Her contribution to education during her Henry Street years came mostly through her advocacy of standards for the profession.

Lavinia Dock's finest contribution to the professionalization of nursing may have been the history of nursing done in collaboration with Adelaide Nutting.[41] In fact, although Dock was clear that the idea for the history was Nutting's, and although Nutting outlined volumes 1 and 2, Dock wrote all but two of the chapters in the first two volumes and edited and wrote volumes 3 and 4 herself.[42] Of the four-volume history Dock said, "I think I never enjoyed anything more than working with her [Nutting] on that book. It was delightful from beginning to end and all the digging in public libraries, translating, researching and correcting was pure pleasure."[43] As far as I have been able to ascertain this was the first history of nursing. Its contribution to the professionalization of nursing is difficult to estimate, but was surely profound. Mary Roberts has suggested that the four-volume history "brought fame to the authors and added to the prestige of the profession."[44] Later, Dock wrote the widely used *Short History of Nursing* with Isabel Maitland Stewart.[45] That Dock was able to take the time she needed from HSS to travel to Europe to research for the history is illustrative of the flexibility of Wald's administration, of the personal finances of Dock, and of the international contacts that Dock maintained throughout her career.

Janet James argued that Dock became the "communications centre of the professional nursing world" on becoming secretary of ICN.[46] Not only did Dock communicate through her ICN position, but she also wrote prolifically for the AJN. As editor of the Foreign Department from 1900 to 1922, Dock contributed over two hundred columns; she also wrote letters to the editor and contributed many individual articles. In addition, she wrote for nursing journals in other countries. Dock had numerous interests while at HSS, ranging from reporting on HSS initiatives to more rigorous themes.[47] She also maintained an extensive personal correspondence. Nutting retained her letters from Dock, and they survive in the Nutting Papers as testament to Dock's seemingly endless capacity for sharp commentary on current affairs and to the ongoing development of her own thinking.[48]

A WOMAN'S WORLD

The settlement house provided a unique opportunity for the educated American woman in the late 1800s to escape a domestic existence and fulfill herself in meaningful service to society.[49] The HSS provided sources of support to women that were otherwise unavailable as (1) an emotional and economic substitute for traditional family, (2) an effective tie to other women's organizations, (3) an avenue for cooperation with men reformers and their organizations, and (4) a creative setting in which to develop and pursue reform strategy.[50]

In the early years only women worked and lived at HSS. Although this changed, the numbers of men never approached those of women, and an awareness persisted that this was a woman's domain. Doris Daniels devoted an entire chapter to the women's world at HSS, offering the first critical analysis that I found on the nature of this dimension at HSS.[51] Robert Duffus's biography of Wald included a chapter titled "At Home on Henry Street" that superficially explored the notions of family and a female world, but his analysis is less than satisfying.[52] Blanche Cook also explored the nature of the female world at HSS. One of the few open examinations into Lillian Wald's personal relationships, her work is important but lacks in-depth critical analyses.[53] Despite compelling extracts from personal letters, it is difficult to conclude with Cook that the evidence she presents unequivocally demonstrates the lesbian nature of Wald's relationships. Daniels's analysis, however, is more complete. She remains equivocal on the matter of lesbian relationships at HSS, suggesting that Emma Goldman's words about Wald are wise counsel: "service to humanity and her great work of social liberation are such that they can be neither enlarged nor reduced, whatever her sexual habits were."[54] Daniels reminds us, as did Smith-Rosenberg, of the need for caution in using contemporary meanings to interpret the language that these women used in their letters to each other.[55] She also asks whether the question of sexual orientation is relevant. It is clearly not relevant to a judgment of whether an individual or individuals made a contribution to society, or to the nature of such a contribution. It also should not be relevant to an audience's acceptance of a life's work—although throughout history it sometimes has been.

But Dock's sexuality is relevant on two counts. First, it is relevant if one is attempting to offer a full and accurate analysis of a phenomenon such as a settlement house as a separatist female support structure that was essential in providing a level of support that enabled an individual to pursue a lifetime of activism. Second, it is relevant because of the manner in which women-identified women have been denigrated or rendered invisible throughout history and certainly in nursing. The fabrication of invisibility is an insidious and pernicious phenomenon only recently receiving much needed attention by feminist scholars.[56]

Estelle Freedman has argued forcefully that female institution building flourished from 1870 to 1920, and that these separatist institutions (for example, women's clubs, the Women's Christian Temperance Union, the WTUL, settlement houses) were responsible for the major political gains that culminated in the acquisition of woman suffrage.[57] Carroll Smith-Rosenberg cast her analysis in a broader context than that of institution-building and offered us the "new women" who first came to prominence in the late 1800s.[58] These new women, "rejecting conventional female roles and asserting their right to a career, to a public voice, to visible power, laid claim to the rights and privileges customarily accorded bourgeois men."[59] This in combination with the arguments of Kathryn Sklar and John Rousmaniere, and in light of the descriptions Dock has left, convince me that the women's and the nurses' worlds created by Wald and her "family" were fundamental to the achievements of HSS residents. For Lavinia Dock they were of even greater importance given her radical and militant politics.

THE POLITICS

Wald spearheaded the political work of HSS residents, most of whom participated actively in various political actions. Wald's own political style was that of position, influence, and privilege. She was well connected with middle- and upper-class segments of society before she began at Henry Street. Backed by the well-to-do Schiff family throughout her life, she learned many political skills from Jacob Schiff—executive and administrative skills, the value of "right" friends, the art of attending to small matters, and the value of performing little acts of kindness.[60] Most accounts of her character describe a warm and charismatic nature that naturally attracted and frequently charmed people. This was no insignificant asset to an individual who devoted much of her energy to fund raising and fostering the indignation of the public and elected officials regarding conditions in the slums.[61] Wald's personal power was an interesting antithesis to the fiery and often strident nature of Dock, whose influence was of a different nature and whose objectives were accomplished in different ways.[62]

A second domain of political activity was the involvement of the settlement workers in the great "moral issue campaigns"[63] that were conducted at municipal, state, and federal levels. Often Wald took the responsibility for federal work, such as the establishment of the Federal Children's Bureau.[64] While no activity was undertaken that Wald did not support, different members focused on different causes. Dock, although not alone in her support of suffrage, was the militant suffragist of the group. Each member had a cause for which she was uniquely suited. Florence Kelly, a lawyer, was especially involved in legislative activity on behalf of children, the poor, and nearly any disadvantaged group. Lenora O'Reilly, a member of the laity, as the non-nurses were known, was devoted to the labor movement.[65]

Philosophical and political convictions motivated much of the settlement's work. These convictions took the form of anarchism, pacifism, socialism, and strong sympathy for Russia. Wald devoted separate chapters in both of her books on Henry Street to Russia. Dock, the most radical of HSS residents, frequently expressed in her writings, especially her letters, sympathies for Russia. Teresa Christy and Mary Roberts have provided succinct overviews of Dock's political leanings—as socialist, communist, radical, and entirely unorthodox.[66] As an outgrowth of the politics of HSS residents there was an interesting array of visitors to the settlement:

> *Amidst the nursing and regular work that goes on, the social life is one of rare privilege and charm. Not only are interesting people from uptown and elsewhere to be met in the Settlement but all the currents of East Side life run through and across it. Most valued among the family friends are leaders in the world of labor—soldiers of the industrial army—both women and men, who come intimately to the house, and whose work and problems are household words.*[67]

Also visiting the settlement were such individuals as Peter Kropotkin, various friends of the Doukhobors, Tchaikovsky, Gershuni, Marie Sukloff, and Katherine Breshkovsky—all aligned with Russia and the revolution.[68] The Russian anarchist Kropotkin was particularly influential on settlement workers such as Addams, Dock, and Wald.[69]

ORGANIZED LABOR AND THE WOMEN'S MOVEMENT

The labor movement of the progressive era was complex.[70] The women's labor movement was tied closely to the suffrage movement, especially after the formation in 1903 of the Women's Trade Union League (WTUL).[71] In 1886 in the United States the American Federation of Labor (AFL) unionists split from the labor reformists in the Knights of Labor.[72] This split led to the demise of the Knights of Labor, but many women who later formed WTUL were daughters of the reformist Knights of Labor members. Notable among them was Lenora O'Reilly, who was closely associated with HSS and Lavinia Dock.[73] The Knights of Labor and later the WTUL were concerned with labor reform, including legislative action. Labor organization, which was the primary focus of AFL, was but one element of WTUL's activity.[74]

Dock published only one article about the labor movement in the *AJN*.[75] The best evidence for her involvement comes from Wald.[76] I found no evidence that Dock had associations with the labor movement before she went to HSS in 1896. One year after Dock's arrival at HSS, she came into contact with Lenora O'Reilly when the latter directed a garment worker's cooperative at HSS.[77] Dock and the fiery, pragmatic O'Reilly formed a friendship.[78] Although Dock was perhaps more of a theorist than O'Reilly, she was also a serious activist and quite unique among nurses in this way. James implied that the friendship that formed between the two women was influential in helping Dock to formulate her convictions on labor reform.[79] After helping to found WTUL in 1903, Wald made HSS available as a meeting place and Dock organized these events.[80] Dock, herself a member of WTUL, walked in the picket line of the 1909 shirtwaist strike in which 20,000 workers, mostly women, walked out.[81]

Dock's involvement in the labor movement and her extensive efforts toward the professionalization of nursing are not unrelated. I believe that she saw them both as integral parts of "the struggle" for the emancipation of women. The following extract from Dock's 1913 *AJN* paper reflects this:

> *What is our relation to this world of work? I think the answer is: We are morally and honorably bound to do nothing that crushes it down and makes its struggle harder, and we should be glad and thankful to do everything we can to help it upward and onward. . . . How likely is it that workers can secure such legislation and enforcement without the ballot? . . . For the sake of the working woman, whose foothold is less secure than ours, no nurse should be opposed to enfranchisement for women. . . . It seems to me that our status in the working world will always be decided by the attitude that we take toward the needs and problems of the working world. If we are exclusive and shut our minds to all except "professional" subjects, we shall become one-sided specialists and in time lose our usefulness as did the French nuns in hospital work.[82]*

With these words, spoken near the end of her HSS years, Lavinia Dock connected two of the great movements of the progressive era, labor and suffrage.[83]

HYGIENE AND MORALITY

The terms hygiene and morality were in the progressive era euphemisms for venereal diseases and prostitution, and social hygiene was venereal-disease prevention.[84] Throughout the nineteenth century there was a growing awareness of the prevalence of the venereal diseases and their consequences. Prostitution flourished in the large cities, where some suggested that immigrants were supplying large numbers of prostitutes.[85] A New York City investigation in 1913 revealed, however, that immigrant women did not constitute a larger proportion of the prostitute population than nonimmigrants.[86] Feldman describes the nativist/racist attitudes that were prevalent at the time and that in combination with the new science of eugenics caused reformers to focus on the immigrant population congregated in the slums and tenements of cities such as New York.[87]

Concurrently, white slave traffic hysteria spread in the cities. White slave traffic was defined and understood in different ways. At one end of the spectrum it was taken to mean the "normal" sorts of activities that comprised the vice trade, such as prostitution, gambling, and pimping. At the other end of the extreme it was taken to mean a nationally organized, mafia-controlled trade in the procurement and selling of women, connected with systematic pornography and illicit drugs. Egal Feldman and Roy Lubove have suggested that the truth probably fell somewhere in between the two extremes.[88] According to Feldman and Lubove there was enough concern, however, for the passage of the Mann Act prohibiting the transport of women across state lines for immoral purposes; also, settlement workers initiated a special process by which the new female immigrant, especially if she were alone, could be greeted and escorted to safety. Feldman provides several instances of the involvement of settlement workers, in particular Lillian Wald and Jane Addams, in the reform efforts around white slavery and prostitution.[89] The HSS with its focus on nursing and health and its members' concerns for the immigrant woman were involved early in the efforts of the hygiene and morality crusade.[90]

Lavinia Dock was involved in two ways. First, she was an active member of Prince Albert Morrow's American Society for Sanitary and Moral Prophylaxis (ASSMP) formed in 1905.[91] Morrow's society advocated education, an end to the secrecy that led doctors to treat husbands for venereal disease while deliberately keeping their wives ignorant of the problem, and the prevention of prostitution by demanding that men be sexually responsible, eliminating the false notion of the "necessity" of sex for men.[92] As a member she lobbied, for example, for the repeal of the Page Law, which had been passed in June of 1910.[93] Later she published *Hygiene and Morality*. The book grew out of a paper she gave at the 1909 ICN in London. It was a brave venture in a time when people did not talk freely about such things, certainly not respectable women. In a style we recognize as inimitably Dock, she presented a sound, linear description of venereal diseases, of prostitution and white slavery, and of the prevention of venereal diseases. The latter, she argued, could be accomplished by preventing prostitution, by education of the public on sexual matters, and by personal and social prevention.[94]

SUFFRAGE

Overshadowing her other accomplishments, save perhaps her book *History of Nursing*, has been the image of Lavinia Dock as a militant suffragist.[95] The obituary in the *New York Times* on 18 April 1956 read:

LAVINIA L. DOCK
NURSING LEADER
———————————
Noted Settlement Worker Is
Dead at 98—Author Was
a Militant Suffragist

Again, I believe that Dock saw each of the movements to which she devoted her efforts as interconnected and that she saw the overriding goal to be a just society in which all members are meaningfully equal. But if there was one "crusade" to which Dock was spiritually bound, it was suffrage. The women's movement, dated in the United States from the Seneca Falls Convention of 1848, was coming out of a period of inactivity at the turn of the century to begin a final assault on disenfranchisement.[96] The suffrage movement and the labor movement were closely intertwined, especially in light of the reform activities of the settlement workers and of Lavinia Dock in particular. Both movements were flavored by the social and political philosophies of the time and both had radical and sometimes militant elements.[97]

Her suffragism has captured the imagination of historians, would-be historians, students, and others. Perhaps this is because Dock was an exception to the usually conservative, moderate images of historical nursing figures. Probably the most often quoted passages used to illustrate Dock's suffragist zeal were reproduced by Christy, quoting Isabel Maitland Stewart:

> *I was quite young and I'd never seen Miss Dock. . . . I was sure I'd know her when I met her, because she'd be tall and angular and intellectual looking. Who should turn up at the door but this small, short sort of roly poly little person with curly hair. She'd just been at a suffrage meeting, and had "Votes for Women" across her hat and "Votes for Women" across her chest. She said, "Now what am I going to talk about?" I said . . . "you were to talk about nursing on the Continent," "Oh," she said, "very bad. It'll not be any better till they get the suffrage. I'll talk about the suffrage."*
>
> *. . . this suffrage thing—it was the whole thing for her; she wanted not only to work for it but really to suffer for it. . . . She was a member of the advanced wing of the Suffrage Party, and they were having a meeting in Washington at the time that Wilson was beginning to think of the possibility of war. They discussed it, and a friend of mine who was there at the time tells me that Lavinia got up and seized the flag which was there and said, "Youth to the Colors!" and on she marched, out of the door, and they followed her, and she went right to the White House, and they picketed the White House!*
>
> *Anyway, they all went into the cooler for the night. I think it just pleased her to no end.*[98]

The earliest documented suffrage incident in which Dock participated was her arrest in 1896 for attempting to vote.[99] In 1907 she joined the Equality League of Self-Supporting Women,[100] marking the beginning of her most active suffrage years, 1907 to 1923.[101] In 1907 she also made an important speech at the Nurses' Associated Alumnae.[102] Although this speech is most often heralded as the first public beseeching she made to fellow nurses to support woman suffrage, it has implications far beyond suffrage. In this speech Dock, always an eloquent orator, integrated suffrage with the social issues of the day:

> *As the modern nursing movement is emphatically an outcome of the original and general woman movement and as nurses are no longer a dull, uneducated class, but an intelligent army of workers, capable of continuous progress, and fitted to comprehend the idea of social responsibility, it would be a great pity for them to allow one of the most remarkable movements of the day to go on under their eyes without comprehending it. . . . Shall we be an intelligent and enlightened body of citizens, or an inert mass of indifference? . . . I would like to see our national body leave all smaller concerns to the local societies and consciously make itself a moral force on all the great social questions of the day . . . education and educational reforms,—industry and the industrial situation—especially as it relates to women—childlabour . . . prostitution and the white slave traffic with its trail of disease and death, and the recent movement to teach sexual hygiene, to inculcate a single moral standard, and to combat venereal disease of which we make so melancholy an acquaintance. . . . I would like to hear these great social questions discussed in our meetings. I would like to have our journals not afraid to mention the words political equality for women. . . . Unless we possess the ballot we shall not know when we may get up in the morning to find that all we had gained has been taken from us.*[103]

Lavinia Dock wrote Adelaide Nutting sometime between 1909 and 1912, indicating her intent to withdraw from active nursing to work exclusively for suffrage and after suffrage was won, for socialism.[104] Historical work on the suffrage movement, particularly on the National Woman's Party (NWP), which formed as the Congressional Union (CU) in 1913, becoming the NWP in 1917, usually includes mention of Dock.[105] In 1913 Dock joined this new organization led by the charismatic Alice Paul. She quickly became a member of Paul's advisory council and an elder of the party.[106] One of Dock's most well-noted suffrage activities was the 1913 suffrage hike from New York City in which fifteen women dressed as hooded pilgrims and hiked on foot the one hundred and fifty or so miles to Washington.[107]

Dock's most intense suffrage involvement occurred after she left HSS in 1915. Her decision to join NWP has been reputed to be a source of tension between her and nursing colleagues such as Wald and Nutting, because of the militant tactics of NWP. Whether or not this contributed to her departure from HSS is not clear.[108] Some of the activity for which Dock is most famous occurred after 1915, such as her arrests and jail terms. In June 1917 she was one of the first six women arrested and jailed in the United States for the suffrage. In August of that year Dock was sentenced to thirty days in the infamous Occuquan institution, ushering in a more severe phase of punishment. In November of the same year she was again sentenced to Occuquan where treatment of the suffragists was becoming increasingly harsh. This time she received a severe leg injury in a tussle with guards. While Linda Ford does not document the force-feeding of Dock, she does document abhorrently cruel treatment and force-feeding of Dock's comrades in her sixth chapter.[109] Renditions of her suffrage activities and her delight in having been jailed for "the cause" have, in my opinion, done an injustice to Dock's commitment and the grave danger in which she and her comrades placed themselves in the struggle to end the disenfranchisement of women. In defense of militant suffragist tactics Dock wrote in June 1917 at the age of fifty-nine:

> *What is the potent spirit of youth? Is it not the spirit of revolt, of rebellion against senseless and useless and deadening things? Most of all, against injustice, which is of all stupid things the stupidest? . . . Can it be possible that any brain cells not totally crystallized could imagine that giving a stone instead of bread would answer conclusively the demand of the women who, because they are young, fearless, eager and rebellious, are fighting and winning a cause for all women—even for those who are timid, conventional, and inept? . . . Obstructive reactionaries must move on. The young are at the gates!*[110]

"HERE BE DRAGONS"

I have been arguing that the Henry Street Settlement in the Lower East Side of New York City from 1896 to 1915 had a significant influence on Dock. It is difficult to imagine how it could not have influenced a bright, well-educated, spirited, young woman with Quaker blood and an abolitionist tradition.[111] The misery of New York City has been described— hundreds of thousands of people living in conditions that were nearly beyond imagination. Earnest young reformers, many of them middle-class women, breathless with their newly acquired college educations, found the only outlet for their creative energies in the service of the less fortunate. The complexities embodied at 165 Henry Street have been described—anarchists, pacifists, socialists, nurses, labor organizers, suffragists, and educators lived in a female institution where "family" provided the sustaining structure for the work from which they seemed to draw such strength.

The influence of HSS is evident when considered in this passage by Dock in her seventy-fifth year:

> *I never began to think until I went to Henry Street, and lived with Miss Wald. I was then about 38 years old. But as I then began to reflect I saw*

that I had always had certain inarticulate instincts that were sound:—a strong sympathy with oppressed classes, a lively sense of justice and a keen love of what we mean by "freedom" and "liberty"—My first experiments in thinking showed me that I had no religious beliefs and that I felt I had no need of them.[112]

The Henry Street Settlement provided Dock with an extensive support system enabling her to execute an extraordinary program of activism during her nineteen years there. I do not think that Dock had integrated the professional, personal, social, and political spheres prior to arriving at HSS; there, under the protective cloak of the "family" she flourished. While the senior Dock, with her intimidating intellect, was surely Wald's mentor, the younger Wald was also, I believe, Dock's guide—a tempering force, a kindred spirit, "the leading lady" responsible for creating an amazing home. It is difficult to imagine such a home where rules were minimal, intellectual curiosity regularly nourished, practice autonomous, radical politics tolerated and encouraged, freedom to come and go not constrained, and emotional needs met by "bonds of belonging."

Without the constraints of a traditional and paternalistic institution such as a hospital or university, Dock was free to direct her considerable energies to her social and political activism. That sociopolitical influence spilled into her professional activities, enabling her to grasp the whole when her colleagues saw only the part, and contributed to the consistent nature of her activities. Her "self" accepted and nurtured within the family of HSS, she was free to fulfill her potential in a way not permitted most women of her era. She would not have done well in a traditional marriage, a traditional role, or a traditional job. An early intuition regarding marriage and traditional women's roles was revealed as she recalled an episode when she was seventeen:

One day I overheard him say to my hostess, in a casual patronizing tone: "She would make a good wife." Something in his manner conveyed a sense of inferiority. I felt keen mortification—also a sense of alarm. In a flash I seemed to see my freedom gone, myself perhaps a household drudge, and no way out. I said to myself "I never will" and that impression stayed with me all my life.[113]

Regarding traditional jobs, she admitted to having been a failure in a hospital bureaucracy: "At the Cook County I was really a failure. Let me say that, looking back I can confidently assert that my principles, aims, and endeavours were right and sound, but I showed no diplomatic skill in personal relations."[114] Forty-two years later, this wonderfully colorful and deeply radical woman went to prison in the dreaded Occuquan institution for a cause she believed in deeply. Isabel Maitland Stewart described her this way: "You see she was fearless. She would go after anything."[115]

In looking back over the past and attempting to relate it clearly to the present, I realize that I have sought more than understanding from the Henry Street period of Lavinia Dock's life. I have also sought guidance. We live in times not unlike those of the early Henry Street days. Our inner cities—cities within cities—are frightening, bleak places of despair. I am struck by the similarity of issues—poverty, sanitation, prostitution, pornography, child prostitution, child pornography, violence, drugs, communicable diseases, hopelessness. And the issues, each of them, extend beyond the boundaries of our largest cities into the cities, towns, and villages in which each of us live.

Our profession is not dissimilar. We face a time of massive health care reform on this continent. We have before us the challenge to carve out new roles and new ways of doing our work. We have no assurances of our ongoing existence. The status of women, while most would say is undoubtedly improved, is not improved for all women. In many areas it is not improved for most women. Homicide, rape, battery, and abuse are all too commonly committed against women. Children are still the victims of abuse in numbers so staggering one questions whether society does not indeed sanction it. Now, as then, however, we continue to live in a world where we are hopeful that it can and will be better. I see that we might take many lessons from the life of Lavinia Dock during the Henry Street period. These lessons might be found under such titles as leadership, political astuteness and activism, citizenship, commitment, education, global perspectives, health determinants, tenacity, and community.

I found, in studying Lavinia Dock within the tumultuous times of the Henry Street years, three characteristics that stood apart and from which I believe the most urgent lessons must be taken—clear vision, a fearless heart, and passion. In the editorial accompanying Lavinia Dock's "Self-Portrait," Edith Lewis wrote:

> When a cartographer ran out of known world before he ran out of parchment, he inscribed the words "Here be dragons" at the edge of the ominously blank terra incognita, a signal to the voyager that he entered the unknown region at his peril.[116]

A century after the founding of Henry Street, as we search for antidotes to our apathy and our fatigue, as we hope that the young are indeed at the gates, Lewis's metaphor rings loudly: "Bring on the dragons, I say, and some new dragon slayers."[117]

Acknowledgments

The author would like to acknowledge the encouragement of M. Patricia Donahue and Joan E. Lynaugh, and especially Shirley M. Stinson for her assistance and her continued nurturance of the idea of history.

NOTES*

* Notes have been abridged from original article.

1.   Lavinia Dock quoted in Daisy C. Bridges, *A History of the International Council of Nurses, 1899–1964* (Philadelphia: J. B. Lippincott, 1967), 221.

2.   How Dock came to go to the Henry Street Settlement is not documented.

3.   See for example, Peggy L. Chinn, "Historical Roots: Female Nurses and Political Action," *Journal of the New York State Nurses Association* 16 (June 1975): 29–37; Teresa E. Christy, "Portrait of a Leader: Lavinia Lloyd Dock," *Nursing Outlook* 17 (June 1969): 72–75; Idem, "Equal Rights for Women: Voices from the Past," *American Journal of Nursing* 71 (February 1971): 288–93; Janet Wilson James, "Dock, Lavinia Lloyd," in *Notable American Women, The Modern Period*, ed. Barbara Sicherman and Carol Hurd Green (Cambridge, Mass.: Belknap Press of Harvard University Press, 1981); Sally Merideth, "Lavinia Lloyd Dock: Calling Nurses to Support Women's Rights, 1907–1923," *Journal of Nursing History* 3 (November 1987): 70–78; Susan M. Poslysny, "Feminist Friendship: Isabel Hampton Robb, Lavinia Lloyd Dock and Mary Adelaide Nutting," *Image: Journal of Nursing Scholarship* 21 (Summer 1989): 64–68; Mary M. Roberts, "Lavinia Lloyd Dock—Nurse, Feminist, Internationalist," *American Journal of Nursing* 56 (February 1956): 176–79.

4.   Sources for this paper included: (a) the Mary Adelaide Nutting Collection (hereafter called the Nutting Papers) housed on microfiche, University of Alberta Health Sciences Library, (b) nursing journals cited in the CINAHL data base, (c) a manual examination of the first twenty years of the *American Journal of Nursing*, (d) examination of biographical material on Lillian Wald, (e) examination of the New York Public Library Lillian D. Wald papers available on microfilm at the University of Alberta, (f) examination of secondary source material on Lenora O'Reilly, a labor organizer on the Lower East Side during the time Dock lived there and with whom we know Dock was associated and (g) scrutiny of materials pertinent to the various social reform movements in which Dock was involved, e.g., the social hygiene, labor, and suffrage movements. Additionally, discussions were held with archivists at the Pennsylvania State Archives, Harrisburg, Penn.; the Library of Congress, Washington, D.C.; Mugar Memorial Library, Special Collections, Nursing Archives, Boston; and Radcliff College, Schlesinger Library, Cambridge, Massachusetts. Sources not examined were the papers of the National Women's Party (NWP) that exist on microfilm and the oral history of Alice Paul.

5.   Dock, "Self Portrait," 24.

6.   Robert A. Woods and Albert Kennedy, eds., *Handbook of Settlements* (New York: Charities Publication Committee, 1911), 205.

7.   Robert Duffus, *Lillian Wald: Neighbour and Crusader* (New York: Macmillan, 1938), 37–38. In fact, Wald and Brewster spent the summer of 1893 living at the College Settlement House on Rivington Street where women settlement workers taught them about social settlements.

8.   Lillian D. Wald, *The House on Henry Street* (New York: Henry Holt and Company, 1915). In this first-person account Wald vividly describes why she sought to establish a nursing settlement (chap. 1), and describes the first twenty years of her efforts in what is the primary source on the early Henry Street years.

9.   Clare Coss, ed., *Lillian D. Wald: Progressive Activist* (New York: The Feminist Press, 1989), 5–6; Doris Groshen Daniels, *Always a Sister: The Feminism of Lillian D. Wald* (New York: The Feminist Press, 1989), 9, 22–23, 64–65.

10.   Ibid.

11.   Ibid., passim; Blanche Wiesen Cook, "Female Support Networks and Political Activism: Lillian Wald, Crystal Eastman, Emma Goldman," *Chrysalis* 3 (1977): 49. Various reference is made in the literature as to precisely who composed the inner circle at HSS; however, three individuals are always included. These women were not all at HSS at the same time or for the same periods of time; Goodrich, for instance, came in 1916 after Dock had left.

12.   Samuel Eliot Morison, Henry Steele Commager, and William E. Leuchtenburg, *A Concise History of the American Republic*, 2nd ed. (New York: Oxford University Press, 1983), 499–501.

13.   Duffus, *Lillian Wald: Neighbour and Crusader*, 32.

14.   The Lower East Side of New York City is that section of the city bounded on the south by Brooklyn Bridge, on the north by 14th Street, on the west by Broadway, and on the east by the East River.

15.   It has been suggested that in the late 1800s ward eleven in the Lower East Side had a population density greater than that of the infamous Koombarwara district of Bombay at 986 people per acre (Morison et al., *A Concise History*, 500). Kessner in his detailed treatment of immigrants in New York between 1880 and 1915 suggests that during the period 1900–1905, densities on the Lower East Side reached a "choking" 1,700 people per acre in some wards (Thomas Kessner, *The Golden Door, Italian and Jewish Immigrant Mobility in New York City, 1880–1915* (New York: Oxford University Press, 1977),133–34.

16.   Descriptions of tenement housing can be found in Lavinia Dock, "Extracts from the Report of the Tenement House Commission, New York, 1901," *American Journal of Nursing* 1 nos. 8 and 9 (1901): 538–41 and 631–34; Lavinia Dock, "An Experiment in Contagious Nursing," *American Journal of Nursing* 3 no. 12 (1903): 927–33; Dorothy E. Jansen, "The Henry Street Settlement: A Response to the Needs of the Sick Poor," Ph.D. diss., Columbia University, 1979; Kessner, *The Golden Door*; Schoener, *Portal to America*; Lillian D. Wald, *The House on Henry Street*. Dock's 1901 descriptions are particularly vivid accounts of the deplorable housing conditions in New York City at that time.

17.   Kessner, *The Golden Door*, 134.

18.   Jansen, "The Henry Street Settlement," 126. There were other nursing settlements, but none had the wide scope of activities and programs and none reached the level of public prominence and influence that HSS did. See, for example, Woods and Kennedy, *A Handbook of Settlements* for an itemization of the known settlements and their activities in 1911. In addition to Jansen, and Woods and Kennedy, the following are rich sources of data on the activities of HSS and are the sources from which the material in this section is drawn: Barbara A. Backer, "Lillian Wald: Connecting Caring with Activism," *Nursing and Health Care* 14 (March 1993): 122–29; Coss, *Lillian D. Wald Progressive Activist*; Daniels, *Always a Sister*; Allen F. Davis, *Spearheads for Reform: The Social Settlements and the Progressive Movement' 1890–1914* (New York: Oxford University Press, 1967); Lavinia L. Dock, *Short Papers on Nursing Subjects* (New York: M. Louise Longeway, 1900); Duffus, *Lillian Wald: Neighbour and*

Crusader, Norma G. Silverstein, "Lillian Wald at Henry Street, 1893–1895," *Advances in Nursing Science* 7 (January 1975): 1–12; Wald, *The House on Henry Street*; Lillian D. Wald, *Windows on Henry Street* (Boston: Little Brown and Company, 1937). *Windows on Henry Street* is most helpful for the period after 1915.

19. Woods and Kennedy, *A Handbook of Settlements*, identify upwards of 125 clubs in operation by 1911.

20. Woods and Kennedy, *A Handbook of Settlements*, 209; Dock, *Short Papers*, 36, described the country work as "one of the chief joys and satisfactions of the whole work"; Dock ran the HSS Montclaire country home in the summer of 1905: Lavinia Dock to the HSS "family," September 1905, Lillian Wald Papers, New York Public Library collection (NYPL) housed on microfilm at the Health Sciences Library of the University of Alberta, reel #8.

21. In *The House on Henry Street*, 54–57, Wald described the efforts that resulted in some thirty of these milk stations, each run by a nurse, that populated New York City by 1912.

22. Wald, *The House on Henry Street*, 38–39.

23. Jansen, "The Henry Street Settlement," 140. The expansion of HSS beyond 265 Henry Street to include other Lower East Side, citywide, and rural dwellings is also documented in Jansen, and in other sources such as Wald's own accounts.

24. L. L. Dock, "Mountain Medicine," *American Journal of Nursing* 9 (December 1908): 181–83. I was unable to determine in what mountains Dock was working in 1909—she may have been at one of the HSS country homes, although there is nothing in the article to suggest this. A source not available during the writing of this paper was "The HSS Visiting Nurse Files," which are housed at the New York Public Library in New York City. Biographical work on Dock would require accessing these files for more complete data on the Henry Street period. Other unavailable sources were the *Settlement Journal* published sporadically by the HSS from 1904 to 1915.

25. Janet Wilson James, ed., *A Lavinua Dock Reader* (New York: Garland, 1985), xiii, xvi. Although "retired" at sixty-five, Dock remained actively interested in the affairs of the profession, of the women's movement, and of the world in general. Much of the primary source materials available, for example, in the Nutting Papers cover the thirty-three years after her retirement. She continued to be involved in and receive the reports of the New York Visiting Nurse Service that developed from the HSS until, at her own request, at the age of ninety-five, they ceased to send her material (Letter of Lavinia Dock to Marion G. Randall of the Visiting Nurse Service of New York, 28 December 1953, Nutting Papers, microfiche #2634; Roberts, "Lavinia Lloyd Dock," 179; Obituary, "Lavinia Lloyd Dock," *Nursing Outlook* 4 [May 1956]: 298–99).

26. Dock, *Short Papers*, 30–31. The "specialities" that Dock refers to in this passage include teaching English as a second language and teaching home nursing, hygiene, and domestic skills (such as cooking with American food on a frugal budget) in both Yiddish and in English.

27. Dock, *Short Papers*, 35.

28. Obituary, "Lavinia Lloyd Dock," 727.

29. Christy, "The First Fifty Years," *American Journal of Nursing* 71 (September

1971): 1778–84; M. Louise Fitzpatrick, *Prologue to Professionalism: A History of Nursing* (Bowie, Md.: Brady Communications, 1983), chap. 4; James, "Dock, Lavinia Lloyd"; Roberts, "Lavinia Lloyd Dock."

30. Susan McGann, *The Battle of the Nurses* (London: Scutari Press, 1992), chap. 2, 35–57.

31. Mary M. Roberts, "We Honor the Memory of a Citizen of the World," *American Journal of Nursing* 59 (February 1959): 195. Bridges, *A History of the International Council of Nurses* documents the inception and development of ICN. Numerous references to Dock are scattered throughout the book. Bridges does not acknowledge Dock's contribution to the ICN constitution, but Roberts, who knew Dock personally, is quite clear in her 1959 article that Dock ought to be credited with this accomplishment.

32. Christy, "Portrait of a Leader: Isabel Hampton Robb," *Nursing Outlook* 17 (March, 1969): 26–29; Idem, "The First Fifty Years." In both of these articles Christy chronicles the development of NLN and ANA. She also illustrates the tremendous importance of the 1893 World's Fair to nursing. Earlier it was noted (note 2) that Dock and Wald probably met for the first time at the 1893 exhibition and that the 1893 exhibition was important to the formation of the ICN (see note 47). Nursing probably got involved in the World's Fair because Robb was at Johns Hopkins at the time, and the Johns Hopkins doctors had organized an international conference on hospitals in conjunction with the World's Fair (James, *A Lavinia Dock Reader*, ix).

33. James, *A Lavinia Dock Reader*, xi.

34. Christy, "The First Fifty Years," 1778; L. L. Dock, "A National Association for Nurses and Its Legal Organization," in *First Words: Selected Addresses from the National League for Nursing 1894–1933*, ed. Nettie Birnbach and Sandra Lewenson (New York: National League for Nursing Press, 1991), 299–314, (paper presented in 1896 at the Society of Superintendents convention). The Associated Alumnae was formed in 1897; the reference to Canada was dropped when the organization was incorporated in 1901 because New York law prohibited foreign membership.

35. Christy, "The First Fifty Years," 1780–1781.

36. L. L. Dock, "Central Directories and Sliding Scales," *American Journal of Nursing* 7 (October 1906): 10–13; Idem, "Directories for Nurses," in *First Words: Selected Addresses from the National League for Nursing, 87–90,* (paper presented in 897 at the Society of Superintendents convention).

37. L. L. Dock, "What We May Expect from the Law," *American Journal of Nursing* 1 (October 1900): 8–12; Idem, "State Registration for Nurses," *American Journal of Nursing* 2 (September 1902): 979–85; Idem, "The Progress of Registration," *American Journal of Nursing* 6 (February 1906): 297–305; Ibid., "A National Association."

38. L. L. Dock, *Short Papers*, 37–48; Idem, "A National Association"; Idem, "The Duty of Society in Public Work," in *First Words: Selected Addresses from the National League for Nursing*, 319–21. Dock's views on ethics have been largely ignored by scholars. This is unfortunate—her 1900 passage on ethics in nursing in *Short Papers* is provocative, clearly separating her from the nursing educators of her time who taught etiquette in the name of ethics.

39. She was assistant to Isabel Hampton Robb at Johns Hopkins from 1890 to 1893, and Superintendent of Nurses at the Illinois Training School in Chicago from 1893 until 1895: Christy, "Portrait of a Leader," 73; James, *A Lavinia Dock Reader,* ix–x. Roberts has described her as a superb teacher, forthright and fair: Roberts, "Lavinia Lloyd Dock," 177.

40. Christy, "Portrait of a Leader."

41. M. Adelaide Nutting and Lavinia L. Dock, *A History of Nursing,* vols. 1 and 2 (New York: G. P. Putnam's Sons, 1907), and Dock, Lavinia L., *A History of Nursing,* vols. 3 and 4 (New York: G. P. Putnam's Sons, 1912).

42. Dock, "Self Portrait," 26; Roberts, "Lavinia Lloyd Dock," 178.

43. Dock, "Self Portrait," 26.

44. Roberts, "Lavinia Lloyd Dock," 178.

43. Lavinia L. Dock and Isabel M. Stewart, *A Short History of Nursing* (New York: G. P. Putnam's Sons, 1920).

46. James, *A Lavinia Dock Reader,* xii.

47. See for example, Dock, "What We May Expect from the Law"; Lavinia Lloyd Dock, "Some Urgent Social Claims," *American Journal of Nursing* 7 (July 1907): 895–901; Ibid, "The Status of the Nurse in the Working World," *American Journal of Nursing* 13 (September 1913): 971–75. I think these are three of her most important papers, addressing registration, standards, suffrage, and labor issues.

48. In the Nutting Papers and the NYPL Wald Papers, there is little correspondence from Dock for the period 1896 to 1915.

49. Estelle Freedman, "Separatism as Strategy: Female Institution Building and American Feminism, 1870–1930" *Feminist Studies* 3 (Fall 1979): 512–29; John Rousmaniere, "Cultural Hybrid in the Slums: The College Woman and the Settlement House, 1889–1894," *American Quarterly* XXII (Spring 1970): 45–66; Kathryn Kish Sklar, "Hull House in the 1890s: A Community of Women Reformers," *Signs: Journal of Women in Culture and Society* 10 (Summer 1985): 658–77.

50. Sklar, "Hull House in the 1890s," 660.

51. Daniels, *Always a Sister,* chap. 5.

52. Duffus, *Lillian Wald: Neighbour and Crusader.*

53. Cook, "Female Support Networks."

54. Daniels, *Always a Sister,* 74.

55. Daniels, *Always a Sister;* Carroll Smith-Rosenberg, "The Female World of Love and Ritual: Relations between Women in Nineteenth-Century America," *Signs: Journal of Women in Culture and Society* 1 (Autumn, 1975): 1–29.

56. An analysis of the nature of the personal relationships at HSS was not undertaken for this article. Such an analysis would be relevant because there is an undercurrent in many of the writings on Dock that implies she was a man-hater, and hence by default a lesbian, since a commonly held myth about lesbians is that they are all man-haters. Wald's own words in *Windows on Henry Street* were an eloquent repudiation of "charges" against Dock: "Reputed a man-hater, we knew her as a lover of mankind" (p. 47). Further, an analysis of Dock's views, and the views of other of her contemporaries, on physicians would offer an altered perspective with which to view this disparaging charge. While quite different in

their perspectives and their foci, each of the following offers important additions to an understanding of the basis for nurses' opinions of physicians in the collective: Jo Ann Ashley, *Hospitals, Paternalism and the Role of the Nurse* (New York: Teacher's College Press, 1976); Barbara Melosh, *The Physician's Hand: Work, Conflict and Culture in American Nursing* (Philadelphia: Temple University Press, 1982); Susan M. Reverby, *Ordered to Care: The Dilemma of American Nursing, 1850–1945* (Cambridge: Cambridge University Press, 1987).

57.   Freedman, "Separatism as Strategy."

58.   Carroll Smith-Rosenberg, *Disorderly Conduct* (New York: Alfred A. Knopf, 1985), especially pp. 167–81 and 245–96.

59.   Smith-Rosenberg, *Disorderly Conduct,* 176.

60.   Daniels, *Always a Sister,* chap. 3 generally and page 37 in particular.

61.   See for example, Cook, "Female Support Networks," 48–54; Coss, *Lillian D. Wald Progressive Activist,* 1–15; Daniels, *Always a Sister,* 51; Dock cited in Duffus, *Lillian Wald: Neighbour and Crusader,* 344–48.

62.   Wald, unlike Dock, was a recognized political power later in her career, a personal acquaintance of presidents consulted on many matters by all parties, and particularly prudent in timing various of the political tactics in her repertoire, Daniels, *Always a Sister,* 52. This is especially notable given her leftist, socialist political views and is a measure of the public influence that she commanded. Dock, on the other hand, was more likely to attack a problem directly, not uncommonly in a confrontational manner. She, unlike Wald, was apt to intimidate or alienate her adversaries and sometimes her allies.

63.   Woods and Kennedy, *Handbook of Settlements,* 208.

64.   Wald, *The House on Henry Street,* chap. 8.

65.   Wald, *Windows on Henry Street,* 42–44.

66.   Christy, "Portrait of a Leader"; Roberts, "Lavinia Lloyd Dock."

67.   Dock, *Short Papers,* 34.

68.   Wald, *The House on Henry Street,* 234, 238.

69.   James, *A Lavinia Dock Reader,* stated that Dock abandoned social Darwinism for Kropotkin's mutual aid philosophy at HSS (p. x, xi).

70.   There is a large scholarship that has developed around the women's labor movement. The reader is referred to the following sources for some of the frequently cited work that is relevant to this paper: Mary J. Bularzik, "The Bonds of Belonging: Lenora O'Reilly and Social Reform," *Labor History* 24 (Winter 1983): 60–83; Gary Cross and Peter Shergold, "We Think We Are the Oppressed: Gender, White Collar Work, and Grievances of Late Nineteenth-Century Women," *Labor History* 28 (Winter 1987): 23–53; Allen Davis, "The Women's Trade Union League: Origins and Organization," *Labor History* 3 (1964): 3–17; Nancy Schrom Dye, "Feminism or Unionism? The New York Women's Trade Union League and the Labor Movement," *Feminist Studies* 3 (Fall 1975): 111–25; Robin Miller Jacoby, "The Women's Trade Union League and American Feminism," *Feminist Studies* 3 (Fall 1975): 126–40; Alice Kessler-Harris, "Where are the Organized Women Workers?" *Feminist Studies* 3 (Fall 1975): 92–110; Diane Kirkby, "The Wage Earning Woman and the State: The National Women's Trade Union League and Protective Labor Legislation, 1903–1923," *Labor History* 28 (Winter 1987): 54–74.

71. Jacoby, "The Women's Trade Union League"; Kirkby, "The Wage Earning Woman."

72. Kirkby, "The Wage Earning Woman," 67.

73. Bularzik, "The Bonds of Belonging."

74. For WTUL policies and platforms see Kirkby, "The Wage Earning Woman," 70–71.

75. Dock, "Status of the Nurse." There may be other surviving materials by Dock on labor issues in WTUL papers, in WTUL's monthly journal *Life and Labor*, and in the O'Reilly papers, for example, but these were not available.

76. Involvement in the labor movement is not restricted to Dock. Nearly all of the settlement houses were involved in some way. The activities of Lillian Wald, founder and head of HSS, and Jane Addams, founder and head of Hull House in Chicago, were especially intense. Both Addams and Wald published and spoke widely on the matter. It might be speculated that this influenced Dock since she was a lifelong friend of Wald's and since Addams and Wald were also friends for over forty years, Davis, *Spearheads for Reform*, 12.

77. James, *A Lavinia Dock Reader*, x, xi. O'Reilly is considered one of the most important members of WTUL, Davis, *Spearheads for Reform*, 143–44. She figures prominently in any consideration of Dock's activities because she was doubly connected to Dock, first as a resident at HSS during much of Dock's time there, and second as a WTUL member and organizer with Dock of a local unit of the United Garment Workers. There is little material available on the relationship of O'Reilly to Dock. Certainly the only potential primary material of which I am aware is the Lenora O'Reilly papers referred to in note 4.

78. Bularzik, "The Bonds of Belonging"; James, *A Lavinia Dock Reader*.

79. James, *A Lavinia Dock Reader*, x, xi.

80. Daniels, *Always a Sister*, 99–100; Davis, "The Women's Trade Union League," describes WTUL's inception, due in part to Jane Addams's efforts, and its first executive that included both Wald and Addams. The featured speaker of the initial organizing meeting in New York was Lenora O'Reilly.

81. James, *A Lavinia Dock Reader*, xiii; Dye, "Feminism or Unionism," 117.

82. Dock, "Status of the Nurse," 972, 974–75. This paper was a reproduction of the last address she made to a nurses' convention. In it she also indicates (p. 973) that she collected the data for the important study by Josephine Goldmark on *Efficiency and Fatigue*, which examined the effects of long working hours.

83. Jacoby, "The Women's Trade Union League," has provided an important analysis of WTUL as the industrial branch of the women's movement.

84. James, *A Lavinia Dock Reader*, unpaginated section of two pages titled "Hygiene and Morality," prefacing a reproduction of Lavinia L. Dock's, *Hygiene and Morality: A Manual for Nurses and Other's, Giving an Outline of the Medical, Social and Legal Aspects of the Venereal Diseases* (New York: The Knickerbocker Press, 1910).

85. Allan M. Brandt, *No Magic Bullet: A Social History of Venereal Disease in the United States Since 1880* (New York: Oxford University Press, 1987), 21.

86. Egal Feldman, "Prostitution, the Alien Woman and the Progressive Imagination, 1910–1915," *American Quarterly* XIX (Summer 1967): 199.

87. Feldman, "Prostitution, the Alien Woman"; Brandt, *No Magic Bullet*, 19; Dock, *Hygiene and Morality*, 136.

88.   Feldman, "Prostitution, the Alien Woman"; Roy Lubove, "The Progressives and the Prostitute," *The Historian* XXIV (May 1962): 308–30.

89.   Discussions of white slavery can be found in Brandt, *No Magic Bullet*; Dock, *Hygiene and Morality*; Feldman, "Prostitution, the Alien Woman"; James Frank Gardner, "Microbes and Morality: The Social Hygiene Crusade in New York City," Ph.D. diss., Indiana University, 1974; Lubove, "The Progressives and the Prostitute."

90.   Gardner, "Microbes and Morality," 73–74, documents the formation of the first vice commission in New York City, the Committee of Fifteen in late 1900, identifying several of its members as HSS workers or supporters, including Jacob Schiff, long time HSS benefactor.

91.   Brandt, *No Magic Bullet*, 12–24; Gardner, "Microbes and Morality," 10–11, 190–94.

92.   In 1901 Morrow, a dermatologist, had undertaken an important investigation into the incidence of venereal diseases in New York City. He contended that 80 percent of men in the city had been infected with gonorrhea, that 5 to 18 percent had been infected with syphilis, and that one-eighth of all human suffering from disease could be attributed to venereal disease, Brandt, *No Magic Bullet*, 12–13. In an era before chemotherapy this represented a staggering health problem. Further, in the mind of the progressive it represented a significant threat to the integrity of the family—creating sterility among the women (it was estimated that one in seven marriages were infertile because of venereal disease), causing blindness in the children, and creating what they believed would be intergenerational passing on of the disease and the resultant defects.

93.   Gardner, "Microbes and Morality," 190–98, described in some detail the efforts to repeal this law that made it mandatory for prostitutes to be fingerprinted, undergo a physical examination for venereal disease, and if this was positive, be remanded into hospital custody for as long as nine months. The ASSMP protested the law on three grounds: it represented state regulation of prostitution, it represented a double standard of morality, and it was unworkable as a sanitary measure. Gardner details Dock's involvement in the protest, including picketing outside of one of the night courts established for trying the prostitutes, leading a contingent of women to usurp an ASSMP meeting where the 75 percent of women present were not being allowed to speak, and seizing the podium and delivering a diatribe against the Page Law.

94.   Personal prevention really boiled down to preventing masturbation at all ages, requiring all men to produce a clean bill of health prior to marriage, and preventing accidental infection from drinking fountains, toilet seats, and the like. Although these sound quite dated to our ears, they represented the prevailing medical teaching of the time. (Dock, *Hygiene and Morality*, 166).

95.   The term "suffragist" was used to denote someone not aligned with the Pankhursts and the militant British Women's Social and Political Union (WSPU) formed by Mrs. Pankhurst after the British Labour Party failed to deliver the vote to British women. It referred to the more orderly members of the suffrage movement; sometimes the term "constitutionalist" was used. "Suffragette," on the other hand, referred to a supporter of the Pankhursts and their militant tactics: Sidney Roderick Bland, "Techniques of Persuasion: The National Woman's Party and

Woman Suffrage, 1913–1919," Ph.D. diss., The George Washington University, 1972, chap. 1.

96. Eleanor Flexner, *Century of Struggle, The Women's Rights Movement in the United States* (Cambridge, Mass.: Belknap Press of Harvard University Press, 1975), chap. 5.

97. Richard Hofstadter, *Social Darwinism in American Thought*, 2nd ed. (Boston: Beacon Press, 1955) contains an excellent analysis not only of the Social Darwinism movement but also of the trends in social theory from 1890 to 1915 including the influence of anarchism, pragmatism, racism, eugenics, and imperialism. For a contextual discussion of the social forces influencing the settlements see Davis, *Spearheads for Reform*.

98. Christy, "Portrait of a Leader," 74.

99. James, *A Lavinia Dock Reader*, xiv; Linda G. Ford, *Iron Jawed Angels: The Suffrage Militancy of the National Women's Party 1912–1920* (New York: University Press of America, 1991), 97. Dock was not jailed in this instance because Theodore Roosevelt, a sometimes visitor to HSS and friend of Wald, who was New York's Police Commissioner at the time, could not bring himself to incarcerate her.

100. James, *A Lavinia Dock Reader*, xiv–xv; Bland, "Techniques of Persuasion," 27. Bland, "Techniques of Persuasion," 4–42, presented a thorough discussion on the importance of the 1907 formation of the "Equality League" led by Harriette Stanton Thatch, daughter of Elizabeth Cady Stanton, the early suffrage crusader and associate of Susan B. Anthony. Anthony's death in 1906 had left a vacuum in an already stagnant NASWA led by Anna Howard Shaw. Blatch who had lived next door to the Pankhursts for twenty years in England returned to the United States and introduced new life and new tactics into the ailing movement, pulling it out of the "suffrage doldrums."

101. Merideth, "Lavinia L. Dock."

102. Dock, "Some Urgent Social Claims," 895–905.

103. Ibid., passim.

104. Lavinia Dock to Adelaide Nutting, undated, microfiche #2006, Nutting Papers.

105. There is a large volume of scholarship on the women's movement, the suffrage crusade, and the NWP. An extensive itemization of this literature was done in Carole Estabrooks, "LLD: The Life and Times of Lavinia Lloyd Dock 1856 to 1958, Work in Progress," unpublished manuscript, November 1991, University of Alberta. Pertinent to this paper have been the following: Flexner, *Century of Struggle*; Ford, *Iron Jawed Angels*; Inez Hayes Irwin, *The Story of Alice Paul and the National Women's Party* (Fairfax: Denlinger's Publishers, 1964); Christine A. Lunardini, *From Equal Suffrage to Equal Rights, Alice Paul and the National Women's Party, 1910–1978* (New York: New York University Press, 1986); Doris Stevens, *Jailed for Freedom* with an introduction by Janice Law Trecker (New York: Boni and Liveright, 1920; reprint, New York: Schocken, 1976).

106. James, *A Lavinia Dock Reader*, xv. The NWP was made up of predominantly young women; Dock at fifty-five years when she joined was one of the oldest members and was greatly respected as a well-known professional and historian in the nursing field.

107. Bland, "Techniques of Persuasion," 51–52.

108. Two explanations for Dock's departure from HSS have been proposed. In the first of these, individuals such as James, "Dock, Lavinia Lloyd," 197, and Cook, "Female Support Networks," 49, have suggested that it was because of differences in opinion over militant political tactics between Dock and Lillian Wald, the head resident of HSS. Daniels has suggested that it was because of Dock's family obligations (see Daniels, *Always a Sister*, 25, 90).

109. Ford, *Iron Jawed Angels*, 149, 160, 180.

110. Ford, *Iron Jawed Angels*, 154.

111. Estabrooks, "LLD," demonstrated that Dock's maternal grandmother (Mire Lloyd) was a Hicksite Quaker and that her maternal grandfather (Aaron Bombaugh) was an abolitionist who assisted Dorothea Dix in her efforts to improve the plight of the mentally ill. He was also a member of the Unitarian Society and an anti-Mason. Many of the reformers and suffragists had a Quaker heritage, for example Susan B. Anthony and Alice Paul were both Quakers.

112. Dock, "Self-Portrait," 24.

113. Ibid., 25.

114. Ibid., 23–24. It is interesting to speculate what might have been if Dock had not failed at the Cook County supervisory job which she held from 1893 to 1895. In her "Self-Portrait" she discusses this failure as having resulted in her going to Henry Street.

115. Quoted in Christy, "Portrait of a Leader," 75.

116. Edith Lewis, "Editorial: Heroines and Dragons," *Nursing Outlook* 25 (January 1977): 21.

117. Ibid.

14

Delegated by Default or Negotiated by Need?: Physicians, Nurse Practitioners, and the Process of Clinical Thinking

Julie Fairman

Since the mid-1960s, the nurse practitioners (NPs) movement has grown rapidly and has become a source of health care for many of our nation's citizens. By 1997, there were more than 63,000 NPs providing health services to patients of all ages, geographic locations, and socioeconomic levels.[1] After one to two years of clinical and theoretical education at the graduate level, NPs are prepared to practice skills many still consider to be solely in the physician's domain. As one physician recently noted in an article critical of NPs, "For many of us, the use of NPs to supplant physicians goes against the oath we took and our views about the responsibility of practicing medicine. . . . Medicine . . . has been reduced to protocols that can be managed by technology and lesser trained providers. . . . Physicians have lost control of their own profession. We have given up our authority. . . . Hippocrates would not be proud."[2]

The purpose of this paper is to examine the context that supported nurse-physician negotiations during the 1960s concerning the boundaries of nursing and medical knowledge and practice. I will argue that factors such as changes in nursing and medical education and practice, federal entitlement policies, and economics supported changes in knowledge and skill domains through a process of negotiation rather than delegation. This is an important distinction because negotiation implies agency—the ability of all negotiators, even when one party holds greater power, to make choices of some kind—while delegation is characterized by a one-sided process with choices usually ascribed to the party with

---

Note: This chapter was originally published in *Medical Humanities Review*, 13, No. 1 (Spring 1999): 38–58. Reprinted with permission.

most power.[3] Nurses and physicians both made choices about relinquishing traditional tasks and the knowledge embedded in them or about taking on new ones that redefined their immediate work boundaries at the point of patient care. These choices in turn supported the development of the nurse practitioner role.

The negotiation of interest in this paper was centered around an essential part of traditional medical practice, the process of clinical thinking. In this paper, clinical thinking is defined as the skills and knowledge that physicians traditionally used to (1) organize and collect particular patient data (e.g., performing a physical examination, eliciting patient symptoms through the patient history, and, given the symptoms, ordering diagnostic tests), (2) determine what was wrong with the patient (e.g., create a diagnosis), and (3) decide what could be done (formulating treatment options) and what should be done (prescribing treatment and making decisions about prognosis).[4] Clinical thinking is a dynamic process that incorporates technology and the intellectual and experiential part of medicine and is applied within the gendered, social, and political construction of the individual physician and the profession itself.

The negotiations centered on clinical thinking because they occurred at the point of care at the bedside or in the exam room, between individual nurses, physicians, and patients—this is where clinical thinking was used most intensely and the opportunity for dialogue was most likely. At this point, the negotiations were continuous and involved informal and sometimes tacit social interactions framed by the personalities of the individual doctors and nurses and local community needs. They were supported and nourished by the mutual dependency of medical and nursing professionals as they struggled together to provide health care for their clients and meaningful work for themselves. In fact, and perhaps most germane to this argument, negotiations were not mandated "from above" by the edicts of national organizations such as the American Medical Association or the American Nurses' Association, or educational institutions. They happened in a seemingly disconnected way in many different places and only later came together as a movement.

Although imbalances in power existed between the nurse and physician negotiators and each party may have held different perspectives on how the negotiations proceeded, incongruence of power and perspective did not prevent the process from occurring because both physicians and nurses obtained what they needed or wanted from the process.[5] Among other things, physicians received help in their busy practices and the freedom to pursue more interesting cases by teaching nurses to perform various parts (e.g., physical examination, history-taking, decision-making based on the data collected) of the clinical thinking process. Participating nurses, in turn, agreed to the instruction and were eager to take on skills traditionally performed by medical professionals. Nurses received the benefits of status linked to the skills and the ability to practice in new and more meaningful ways that corresponded with their experience and education. They may have also received an unexpected benefit. The negotiations resulted in an artificial segmentation and fragmentation of clinical thinking that exposed the political character and permeability of the legally and socially constructed practice barriers created by physicians' control of the process. These barriers traditionally defined physicians' practice and authority in society and protected their monopoly over health care.

The experiences of nurses and physicians in the 1960s seen through the lens of the nurse practitioner movement provide a broadened historical framework for examining contemporary health care and the complex knowledge claims of the professions. Nursing and medicine, although separate in their professional philosophies, moved in both parallel and intersecting paths to restructure patient care during this time period. Indeed, the changes experienced by both professions were pivotal to the shape of later practices, although the mutual dependency of medicine and nursing in the provision of patient care has long been ignored in the literature.[6] The 1960s were a time of crucial change for American health care, and the ramifications of the strategies devised and decisions made by national leaders and local practitioners to cope with change continue to influence health care provision, contemporary practice, and relationships between nurses and physicians to this day.

CLINICAL THINKING

The process of clinical thinking is a dynamic entity of patient data collection and generation of treatment choices that exists within the social, political, and experiential construction of the individual physician and the profession itself. Physicians have used the process of clinical thinking to define themselves and give coherence and validity to the medical role. Physicians' position—their authority and power—was traditionally predicated on their clinical thinking skills, and, in fact, contemporary health services, including diagnostic tests and procedures, admitting privileges, and collection of patient services, are organized around the clinical thinking process of physicians.[7] Clinical thinking is, then, more than a functional process; it is the foundation upon which physicians legitimize and define their social and professional status and authority and through which they claim "ownership" of the patient.

In general, their sense of ownership has infused physicians with overwhelming personal and professional responsibility for each step of clinical thinking. Relinquishing part of the process, even to colleagues, would have broken its integrity and required physicians to disregard powerful medical school socialization. Even into the 1970s, Barbara Bates wrote, medical school teachers specifically warned against sharing any portion of the physician's traditional role, and most physicians had heard their professors preach that, "Any good consultant does his own history and physical."[8] This sense of individual responsibility (e.g., In order to be responsible for patient care I have to verify the data collected by another physician) extended to a culturally derived suspicion of others' judgment, even colleagues', and especially those not trained at the same institution or in the same profession.

Until the mid-twentieth century, physicians dominated the formal process of and secured responsibility for clinical thinking although many instances can be cited of nurses, in particular, informally and temporarily participating in parts of the process. Nurses, for example, performed various technical skills for data collection, informally engaged in circumspect diagnosing of patients, made treatment decisions during emergencies, or even coached interns and residents through routine treatment decisions.[9] Even so, physicians legally and situationally controlled the process. Despite unacknowledged and informal participation from nurses and other professionals, physicians remained responsible for and made the final decisions about interpretation of data and medical treatment of patients until the health care environment of the 1960s supported loosening of medical control.[10]

NURSING EDUCATION AND PRACTICE

Physicians' domination of clinical thinking was probably not unreasonable before mid-century. Until that time most nurses had neither the education in the basic or applied sciences nor the support of the profession itself to broaden nursing roles by taking on the responsibility of clinical thinking. The process of clinical thinking did not fit the paradigm of nursing care practiced by most nurses who, by the mid-1950s, were educated and employed primarily in hospitals where physicians held jurisdictional dominance.[11]

Isabel Stewart's functional method of nursing, originating in the 1930s, was popular and accepted by most hospital training schools until the late 1960s.[12] The functional method involved training nurses to provide care in hospitals based on technical expertise (e.g., the knowledge of procedures) without a sound intellectual understanding of the principles on which the procedures were based or the goals to which they were directed. As a result, much of nursing practice, no matter where it was applied, was rule-based and activity-oriented and relied heavily on the repetition of skills and procedures rather than the integration of scientific or social science theory into decision-making or planning of care. Of course, by the late 1950s many schools included classes in basic and behavioral sciences, but many of these schools failed to teach students how to integrate this knowledge into their clinical practice.[13] As a result, nursing expertise was judged by the parameters of technical knowledge rather than the intellectual component of patient care.

During the 1950s and 1960s, certain nursing leaders argued that the nursing care needs of patients in contemporary hospitals were not being met by functionally prepared nurses. Acknowledging the discrepancy between nurses' knowledge and patients' needs, leaders and scholars such as sociologist Esther Lucille Brown and nurses Hildegard Peplau and Virginia Henderson developed ideologies of nursing care that were based on the individual needs and problems of patients and framed by theories from the basic and social sciences.[14] After she left Teacher's College in the early 1950s, Virginia Henderson, through her writings and work as a consultant to national and international nursing organizations, refined her scientifically based, patient-oriented philosophy of clinical nursing that continues to influence modern nursing care.[15] Both Brown and Peplau wrote about the connection between patients' emotions and their physical conditions and devised models of interpersonal care supported by applied and basic science theories.[16]

The individualized patient-care concept as designed by these nursing leaders was perhaps idealized but undeniably more germane to the care of patients in hospitals of the time period than the functional method. Patients experienced complex medical problems, typically acute episodes of chronic illnesses, rather than the infectious diseases seen in earlier decades. The nursing care required by patients undergoing new procedures such as mitral valve surgery and large-scale operations for cancer and taking new medications such as mercurial diuretics had to be based upon their physiological and psychosocial needs rather than upon traditional routines or procedures. Patient conditions changed rapidly and required nurses who could make assessments and then make decisions to act.

Based upon the writings of nurses like Henderson and Peplau and stimulated by the clinical realities in health-care institutions and the lack of care in rural and urban clinics, innovative nurses began to conceptualize new practice philosophies and innovative education programs. These initiatives were designed to provide nurses with an intellectual clinical component based on a liberal arts education in universities and colleges and to support a broader role for nurses.[17] Examples include innovative programs such as the clinical nurse graduate curriculum devised by Francis Reiter at New York Medical College.[18] In this program, nurses learned to examine patients' responses to their illnesses (rather than categorize patients by the number and type of procedures needed) and to provide care based on a rational analytical decision-making process similar to clinical thinking—without the medical diagnosis and treatment component—that was applicable to nursing practice. Later, Dorothy Smith, of New York University and then University of Florida, experimented with the idea of a nurse clinician—a nurse with responsibility for a particular patient area, who was on call twenty-four hours a day for consultation with nurses and physicians about decisions concerning nursing care.[19] In Colorado, Loretta Ford helped design a graduate curriculum for pediatric nurses to provide preventive ambulatory health services to poor rural Colorado children. This program included courses rarely found in nurse training schools—pathophysiology, child development, and health promotion. The curriculum prepared students to understand the underlying principles of healthy child care and patient education and to provide preventive nursing services outside of the hospital in collaborative practices with physicians.[20] Laura Simms at Cornell University-New York Hospital School of Nursing developed the clinical nurse specialist role to utilize expert clinicians as consultants to generalist nurses. The concept of an expert clinician (rather than an expert in procedures) developed across nursing specialties and was seen in oncology, nephrology, psychiatry, and the intensive care unit.[21] These experiments did not attempt to make nursing practice more like medicine, but intended a paradigmatic shift in the practice of nursing. Patients, their responses to their illnesses, their families, and their life styles became foci of care. This multi-point focus provided nurses with a broader perspective for formulating patient care questions, making decisions about treatment, and taking action. The diverse geographic origins and the multiple configurations of the programs provide an appreciation of the breadth of changes occurring in American nursing during the 1960s.

Although the movement to patient-focused education and practice began to accelerate in the early 1960s, as seen in the popularity of clinical decision-making texts such as Harmer and Henderson's *Principles and Practices of Nursing*, institutional resistance and reluctance of the profession counter-balanced and even slowed acceptance of these ideas by nurses.[22] Most nurses were socialized in training schools to believe their practice was dependent on the orders of physicians and that there was little they, as nurses, should do independently. Traditional patterns of authority and discipline discouraged many nurses from challenging the status quo and worked to keep most nurses from moving beyond conventional practice patterns.[23] More independent practice patterns also presented a risk to many nurses unprepared to take on the challenges. Fear and misunderstanding by nurses themselves presented a formidable obstacle to a shifting practice paradigm.

The position of nursing within higher education also initially slowed acceptance of the new practice philosophy. Although nursing education had begun to move into colleges and universities in the early twentieth century, there were only a handful of clinically based graduate university programs for nursing in the early 1960s. Most existing programs taught nurses to be educators and supervisors rather than clinical experts and offered courses that focused on educational theories and management styles rather than human development and pathophysiology.

At the same time, the number of clinically based programs began to grow, supported by massive federal investment in nursing education. Numerous reports predicting a nursing shortage, a dawning and generalized understanding by analysts of nursing that the nurses trained in hospital schools were unprepared to care for complex patients, and a growing population of chronically ill patients who needed care outside of hospitals provided the stimulus for federal funding. During the 1960s, federal aid supported the growth of college-based training programs for nurses and the proliferation of community colleges and the associate degree nursing programs based in them. Even so, until the mid-1960s few avenues existed for nurses who wanted to increase their clinical expertise after training.[24] Then, in the mid-60s, Regional Medical Programs began to provide continuing education programs for nurses and doctors, focusing primarily on heart disease, cancer, and strokes and, later, the Great Society programs of the Johnson administration included entitlement programs that provided post-graduate clinical training for both physicians and nurses committed to work with disadvantaged patients. Continuing education programs offered by universities, hospital nursing services, or professional organizations became local cottage industries as nurses tried to keep up with the care requirements of their patients.

Despite these obstacles and in response to the daily realities of clinical practice, critical care nurses, public health nurses, nurse midwives, nurses in urban and rural clinics, and other emerging nursing specialties (such as oncology and nephrology) were developing parallel practice philosophies similar to those generated by leaders in colleges and universities. These settings in particular may have more easily supported broader nursing roles because physicians' jurisdictional boundaries in these areas were more porous due to weak or absent institutional control.[25] Architecturally discrete areas, such as intensive care and dialysis units, limited institutional interference. In urban and rural health clinics, an absence of other physicians or restrictive administrative policies may have offered both nurses and physicians the opportunity to lay aside traditional relationships and ways of communicating.

In these areas, at the bedside, or in the examination room, nurses and physicians negotiated with each other and traded knowledge. In both public clinics and intensive care, nurses spent a great deal of time with their patients and were able to more broadly inform physicians about the patients' emotional and clinical conditions. Physicians, on the other hand, taught individual nurses how to integrate the process of clinical thinking into their practice.[26] As one Arkansas intensive care nurse noted, "doctors and nurses trained each other, and after a year or so, nurses were smarter than the doctors."[27] Another nurse explained, "I taught a million of them [physicians] how to do dialysis . . . and I learned renal disease . . . there was never anything written down, just an unspoken agreement."[28] Physicians also taught nurses to use the *language* of clinical thinking and by doing so gave implicit permission for nurses to engage in the politically important process of communicating more effectively about their patients with those in the higher status group. Nurses in these practice areas developed new ways of thinking and talking about patients that reflected clinical realities and exposed the dangers of a method of nursing practice predicated on a rule-based functional system.

Some nurses whose expertise was derived from experience and who, through their practice, had gained an appreciation of their potential to practice more broadly than the traditional model perpetuated by the training schools, were interested and ready to take on new responsibilities. Perhaps buttressed also by the emerging Women's movement and Civil Rights movement and working with compatible, liberal-minded physicians who were unthreatened by enlarging nurse practice roles, these nurses were ready to enter into negotiations with physicians to integrate their ways of thinking and skills into nursing practice.

MEDICAL EDUCATION AND PRACTICE

By the end of the 1950s, most middle-class Americans considered health care a basic right earned through employer-financed or privately purchased insurance supported by middle-class prosperity. Increased popularity and affordability of hospital insurance supported greater utilization of hospitals and the medical and surgical specialists who practiced there.[29] In contrast, there was also a growing population of citizens in low-paying non-union jobs, especially in urban areas, who were ineligible for federal assistance and could not afford physician fees. This group of clients began to seek care in overburdened city and county health clinics, hospital walk-in clinics, and emergency rooms. Urban hospitals felt the crush as much as rural providers—federal support for medical training programs focused on specialty practice rather than general medical practice and led to fewer professionals, such as medical fellows, to staff emergency rooms and outpatient clinics.[30]

As the public demand for health resources grew, medical leaders warned of a doctor shortage although the number of physicians in active practice was growing, supported also by federal programs that promoted specialty medical and surgical training. In 1950, the total number of active nonfederal physicians was 117 per one hundred thousand population. By 1971, this ratio had increased to 152 per one hundred thousand population.[31] What seemed to be happening in the medical field was a shift of new manpower from lower-paying and lower-prestige areas of practice such as general practice to the medical and surgical subspecialties, a shift which actually started prior to World War II. The number of subspecialists grew as the number of general practitioners dropped from 120,000 in 1931 to 56,000 in 1971.[32] In 1955, forty-four percent of active practicing physicians reported themselves to be full-time specialists. This proportion increased to fifty-five percent in 1960, and to seventy percent in 1965.[33]

Because of the drop in numbers, general practitioners faced enormous demand for their services, especially from growing families with children and older adults. Even the combined force of general practitioners and pediatricians (whose number was growing in tandem with other medical specialists) could not supply the manpower to accommodate the demand for children's services, in particular. As the ratio of pediatricians per thousand children under the age of fifteen rose from seven to sixteen per thousand over a period of twenty-one years from 1940 to 1960, the ratio of the *combination* of pediatricians and general practitioners decreased from 352 to 151 per thousand children.[34] Additionally, most of the growing population of specialists practiced in urban academic or suburban area hospitals, resulting in a growing shortage of primary care physicians in rural and inner city areas.[35] In 1971, the number of physicians per thousand population varied from 195 physicians in the largest metropolitan areas to forty-two in some rural areas. In 1963, 98 counties in the United States were without active physicians, and by 1971 the number of counties had grown to 133.[36] The result was a net loss of care providers during a critical period of increasing demand for primary care services. An expanding population of children produced by the baby boom and a period of relative prosperity that allowed a larger population to afford private pediatric services contributed to the demand. Additionally, a larger number of poorer families won access to health services through President Lyndon Johnson's Great Society programs, the social initiative that produced Medicare, Medicaid, and a system of urban and rural community health clinics.

As primary care physicians at the local level complained about their overwhelming workload, national commissions perpetuated the perceptions of a generalized physician manpower shortage and suggested possible solutions, most of which focused on methods to support physician practice. In 1952, the President's Commission on the Health Needs of the Nation documented a severe technician shortage (the technician category included nurses, as the largest group, along with health aides, and practical nurses) and suggested the development of schools of auxiliary medical services.[37] In 1956, the Report on Paramedical Personnel of the Surgeon-General's Consultant Group on Medical Education also noted a shortage of paramedical personnel (nurses, health aides, technicians, and practical nurses) to meet present or expected needs of chronically ill patients.[38] In 1959, the Bane Committee (part of the Surgeon General's Consultant Group on Medical Education) tied the perceived manpower shortage in medicine to those of other allied health professions. The Committee noted that physicians could not carry out their increasingly complex responsibilities without the collaboration of other health professionals.[39] These results were echoed in the 1965 report of the President's Commission on Heart Disease, Cancer, and Stroke, and the 1965 Coggeshall Report of the Executive Committee of the Association of American Medical Colleges, which also recommended that medical schools assume responsibility for the evaluation and training of allied health professionals.[40] For over ten years, these reports shared common themes: essentially, the health of American citizens was threatened by a physician shortage, and the threat was even more serious because of the shortage of other types of health personnel who supported physicians' practice. All of these reports, in general, perpetuated the primacy of physicians in health care and viewed all others as adjuncts (although necessary adjuncts) to medical practice.

Considering the common themes, it is not surprising that few innovative strategies emerged from the reports. Most of the reports recommended increased funding for physician education in general and strengthening of medicine's control over the training of auxiliary personnel, including nurses. In a sense, however, the reports provided perhaps an unintended opening for other health professionals to broaden their roles by taking on functions traditionally considered within the realm of medicine. Physicians, the reports reminded policy makers and other professional groups, needed relief from the more mundane and less complex portions of practice. The reports also clearly supported physicians' role in the allocation of tasks to other professionals.

More important, however, many of these reports were after-the-fact and merely documented the stresses and complexities general practitioners and pediatricians had been facing for several years and for which they had been devising their own private strategies for relief. By the early 1960s, most of these strategies involved delegation of administrative and clerical tasks, such as completion of insurance forms, stocking of clinics, inventory of supplies, and answering phones, to nurses and allied health professionals.[41] But in some areas, grass-roots physicians, perhaps taking to heart the openings provided by the reports and seeking relief, began to negotiate with nurses and offered to train them to perform certain functional and intellectual skills that were part of clinical thinking.[42] In return, nurses agreed to incorporate new knowledge into their practice and to perform new tasks, with the proviso that physicians were available for support when needed. As one nurse practitioner noted, ". . . He [the physician] taught us to do things that needed to be done when he couldn't get there, like suture lacerations, . . . but he wanted us to do everything we could to help him, but he was always there to make the decision. . . . It was a teaching/learning situation you [had] to go through with each physician, . . . we probably taught them a lot about how to get along with people that they didn't get in their training."[43]

The most formative discussions concerning knowledge claims and skills were played out at the parochial level and occurred informally among individual nurses, physicians, and patients. At the grass roots, in clinics and private practices, individual nurses and physicians negotiated responsibility and authority according to community and practice needs and personal prerogatives. In rural areas, for example, a physician may have had responsibility for several clinics in different counties but was unable to hire or afford a partner—both the practice area and salary may have been uncompetitive with urban or suburban practices. The nurse practitioner may have provided coverage for patients when the physicians could not physically be at the clinic. A nurse practitioner described a similar practice relationship:

> *He [the physician] was in the one clinic one day and another clinic another day. He had a private practice too. But he was always available by phone and always responded immediately. . . . I was with him two and a half days [per week] and really learned an awful lot from him. . . . He didn't have a problem with nurses learning to do this [contraceptive care] and he really taught me to take care of a lot of abnormal patients. . . .[44]*

Even when the numbers of nurse practitioner training programs exploded in the early 1970s, physicians and nurses negotiated practice relationships on an ad hoc basis, one by one by one.

PRACTICE EXPERIMENTS

Breaking the process of clinical thinking into components that could be performed by providers other than physicians, although logical at the time, was an extraordinary power shift, for fragmentation opened the whole clinical thinking process to multiple constituencies vying for a place "at the bedside" in the traditional sense or "at the examination table." Loosening (not relinquishing) control over an almost sacred tradition and trusting others' ability to perform the skills was an inadvertently revolutionary act by physicians. In a very real sense, by shattering the integrity of the whole, even when the individual skills traded during negotiations seemed relatively simple and mundane, physicians provided multiple disciplines the opportunity to question physicians' clinical authority and their complex knowledge claims. If nurses, for example, accurately and intellectually collected patient data from the history and physical assessment, why couldn't they move to the next step to establish diagnoses and treatment plans? Why not optometrists or acupuncturists? Questions such as these created a crescendo of debate in medical and nursing professional organizations during the 1960s and later concerning knowledge domains and practice boundaries, while negotiations continued between individual nurses and physicians.[45]

Some of the questions were later addressed through research studies reported in the literature, although the findings rarely terminated discussion. Long before the seminal 1986 Office of Technology Assessment study determined that nurse practitioners could safely care for over three-fourths of patients presenting to primary care physicians and that multiple patient satisfaction studies rated nurse practitioner services highly, earlier studies made the same points.[46] Among others, Henry Silver, in his 1968 study of nurse practitioners working in an urban Denver neighborhood, noted the lack of patient resistance, and that nurses independently cared for over eighty percent of children in one health station. Only eighteen percent of the children required referrals to physicians or other health facilities.[47]

Vignettes describing the successes of newly negotiated nurse-physician practices began to appear in the professional literature in the early 1960s. By 1967, there were almost 100 examples of nurses and physicians working together in what were then unconventional relationships. It is also quite possible that many more experiences went unreported, by physicians in particular, for fear of investigations and reprisals from members of highly conservative state medical and nursing licensure boards which might have accused them of training and encouraging nurses to practice medicine.[48]

While each experience was unique because it was based on the particular needs of a specific practice, community, or presence of a pre-existing practice relationship between and a nurse and physician(s), there were many similarities in the kinds of work nurses were doing in the practices. Interestingly, many of the tasks nurses agreed to take on in the early experiments were those that encompassed anticipatory guidance and touched quite closely on the services upon which many clients judged the quality of the physician-patient relationship. These services, such as psychosocial care, well-child care, patient education, and dispensing minor medical advice, were part of the medical profession's traditional mission, particularly for pediatricians. From the late 19th century when Abraham Jacobi encouraged physicians to think about the mental hygiene of children when analyzing their physical complaints, to Benjamin Spock's advice book *Baby and Child Care* in 1946, to the "new pediatrics" movement of the 1950s, physicians held the psychosocial component of care to be their own responsibility. In fact, the emphasis on psychosocial practice heightened in the 1950s when developmental research became an accepted form of academic scholarship.[49]

More frequently, however, nurses performed tasks physicians considered less complex, routine, and time consuming, such as well-child examinations, or uncomplicated (the typical cold or flu) sick-child visits. These tasks, in addition to long practice hours, low status and pay, and repetitive patient profiles and routines made primary pediatric practice intellectually unstimulating and boring.[50] For pediatricians, there was a wide discrepancy between their postgraduate education as residents in acute care hospital facilities working with specialized clients and the realities of everyday practice where most patients were similar and healthy. The breach between the educational experiences and practice realities of pediatricians widened in the 1950s as hospitals themselves became more complex and technologically oriented. Office practice proved a weak competitor compared to residency experiences. Some physicians regarded the nurse practitioner as the relief valve to a more stimulating and complex practice, and as a financially attractive alternative to hiring a physician partner.

One of the earliest reported experiments came in 1961, from the Collaborative Study of Prenatal Factors in Cerebral Palsy and Neurological Diseases in Providence, Rhode Island. Specially trained public health nurses conducted screenings of infants to detect physical defects, a task previously performed only by physicians. In this study, public health nurses were found to be as highly effective as pediatricians in screening efforts.[51] In 1963, in Northview Heights, near Pittsburgh, Pennsylvania, a health clinic based in a housing project and supported by funding by the Allegheny County Medical Society and numerous community agencies, employed two nurses to manage routine medical problems and provide immunizations.[52] In the same year, a nursing care clinic was established at the Thomas F. Gailor Out-Patient Clinics, in Memphis, Tennessee, to reduce the excessive workload created by poor, chronically ill patients visiting the hospital outpatient clinics for routine observation and continuation of long-term treatments. Using protocols developed by physicians, the nurses staffed the clinics themselves, independently referred patients to specialists, and provided supervision of patients with chronic, stable conditions.[53]

Charles Lewis and Barbara Resnick reported on a nurse clinic established in 1964 at the University of Kansas Medical Center that was perhaps one of the most progressive early expanded nursing role experiments. All of the nurses in this clinic held graduate degrees or baccalaureate degrees, had considerable clinical experience, and served as the primary source of care for adults with chronic illness. The nurses practiced according to standing orders written for patients in each diagnostic class—each protocol defined the limits within which the nurses might initiate or alter medical care. Lewis and Resnick's analysis indicated significant reduction in the frequency of complaints, a marked reduction in patients seeking out doctors for minor complaints, and a marked shift in the preference of patients for nurses to perform certain functions. The researchers concluded that the nurses provided competent and effective care to uncomplicated chronically ill patients comparable to that of physicians in outpatient clinics and that this care was based on patient need rather than physician prerogative.[54]

Many leaders of physicians' professional organizations and many of their members viewed the NP quite differently, as a health care worker who replicated medical practice models. NPs were not seen as offering a distinct and different kind of health care. Rather, these physicians could only see NPs as less educated pretenders to the medical throne. Nor, it seemed, could the worth of the services provided by NPs be examined without devaluing them in comparison to medical services (e.g., through the use of labels such "non-physician," "paramedical" or "mid-level provider" in the medical media). At the same time, there were constant discussions in the literature by both nurses and physicians as to whether or not NPs were indeed practicing nursing or medicine.[55] The discussions occurring outside of the immediate practice relationships reflected the rhetorical strategies and diverse perspectives of the two professions (in contrast to the individual practitioners) in their attempts to define, authenticate, and control new roles and relationships. Each profession's rhetoric aimed to solidify or challenge existing power structures within the context of the changing health care environment, and as a result there was little national consensus on education, practice, and knowledge domains.

The needs of individual practitioners and the daily clinical realities they faced were quite different from the overarching priorities of national leaders who were more concerned with issues of power and authority. At the site of patient care, at the intersection between the individual nurse, physician, and patient, incongruities of perspective coexisted—they didn't negate the negotiation process. Theoretical differences in perspective were, in a sense, separate from the immediate work each individual performed, and they diffused when put into practice. The different perspectives may not have mattered much because each nurse and physician received something important he or she needed or wanted from the process, and together they were able to provide health care regardless of their perception of the trade.[56]

Parallel conversations of individual practitioners resulting from different perspectives can be seen in the language used to describe the process of negotiation. Nurses, in general, discussed "taking on" skills, which implied the power to make choices, or agency on their part to acquire a different skill or knowledge repertoire. In fact, nurses had to agree to take on new knowledge and skills. Nurses could have chosen to decline the opportunity and in fact some were reluctant, especially at first, to take on certain responsibilities that required knowledge or experience they did not have, or practice without adequate physician supervision.[57] Physicians, on the other hand, spoke of "delegating" skills to nurses.[58] To delegate something implies causation or volition, meaning that one group must decide, because of circumstances such as economics or politics, to convey or cause the movement of ideas or objects to others.[59] A hierarchy is implicit—someone with power decides to empower someone else to do things usually reserved for those higher in the hierarchy. Agency remains with the delegator, and the receiving party remains under the delegator's control, or assumes control only temporarily.

The idea of agency is important when thinking about the emerging relationships developing between NPs and physicians during the 1960s and about how a compatible practice emerged despite competing perspectives. Parallel explanations from two early participants are illustrative. For example, Loretta Ford, who with Henry Silver developed the nurse practitioner program at the University of Colorado in 1965, described the movement as an outgrowth of her work on curriculum development. To Ford, the NP model was clearly a nursing model and nurses merely used the physician shortage as an opportunity for role expansion.[60] In contrast, Henry Silver, her colleague, described the joint efforts as a response to physician shortages and physicians' need to improve preventive health services for children.[61]

From their parallel conversations emerged two models of patient care that were distinctly different in ideology and agency, but which met the needs of both practitioners and patients. To Ford, the NP was a nurse practicing in an expanded role—not a new category of health professional. To this end, NP education belonged in institutions of higher nursing education. To Silver, the NP represented a new subset of medical worker who happened to have basic nursing education. Although the NP worked collaboratively with the physician, Silver believed the physician still controlled the socialization, oversight, and most of the education, which could have occurred anywhere. From these diverse perspectives, Ford and Silver managed to practice collaboratively and educate numerous nurse practitioners who went on to formulate their own practice negotiations.

In the mid to late 1960s, other categories of health care providers, such as physician associates (PA), emerged and contributed to the complexity of the dialogue at many levels surrounding negotiated roles. Many physicians and nurses saw the NP and the PA as part of the same movement to support the shortage of primary care physicians.[62] In fact, many commentators, including nursing authors, tended to refer collectively to the NP and PA, although both were explicit categories with specific ideologies and alliances.[63]

Based on a 1961 conceptualization by Charles Hudson, the first PA program was inaugurated at Duke University in 1965, the same year Ford and Silver developed the NP program in Colorado. The PA program, in contrast, was based on the model of military medical corpsmen training and admitted four ex-corpsmen for the first class. Women were not admitted to the program during its early years, primarily to exclude nurses— Hudson had been unable to successfully negotiate with most of the nursing faculty at the University to accept the new role. In 24 months, students were trained as "data gatherers," to elicit health history data; to perform physical examinations, lumbar punctures, gastric analyses, and pulmonary function tests; and to apply casts.[64] After their training, students were expected to find employment in physicians' offices or busy urban and rural health clinics, as the "extension of the physician's arms, legs, and mind. . ."[65]

Physician assistant students learned many of the same skills nurse practitioners incorporated into their clinical repertoire, but without much of the attendant outcry from the medical professions that surrounded nurses' expanded role. Unlike nurse practitioners, physician associates were conceptualized with clearer authority lines and ideological bent; they were practicing medicine under the supervision of physicians and had few, if any, other professional loyalties. The meanings implicit in the labels, *physician* assistant and *nurse* practitioner, and the common practice boundaries perhaps polarized national debate even further. When nurses were later actively recruited into PA programs, nursing leaders voiced loud concerns, including charges of "controlling male paternalism," and "enslavement" of nurses, and set about actively opposing PAs in both the professional and popular literature.[66] Local negotiations between nurses and physicians for devising new practice patterns became even more critical and essential in order to counteract the potential effects on patient care of battles occurring at the national level.

CONCLUSION

Throughout the 1960s and into later decades, nurse practitioner roles continued to expand and formalize, in part due to progressive changes in nursing education as it continued to move into universities and colleges. More graduate programs began to offer clinical degrees, and more nurses began to take active roles in the training of nurse practitioners in the mid to late 1970s. At the same time, broadened feminist perspectives and changes in the health care arena produced a supportive environment for NPs to develop a professional character that was more pro-active and independent of physician identity, and that politically challenged professional medicine's control of the dialogue surrounding patient interactions.

In the last 20 years, the nurse practitioner movement was also supported by changes in the health care environment that created new categories of chronic diseases and new standards of care based on economics and efficiency. Advances in medicine that lengthened the survival of patients with chronic illnesses also created new management problems as "unintended by-products of technologic change."[67] These problems, which included the long-term effect of chronic hypertension, hypercholesterolemia, and functional disabilities (e.g., difficulty walking, dressing, and writing or sexual dysfunction) caused by treatment complications and side effects, were particularly responsive to care provided by nurse practitioners. In a sense, a whole new category of health problems was created that affected patients' quality of life and provided the framework for questions about jurisdictional boundaries. Who is the most effective health care provider to offer treatment and guidance to patients at risk for complications of chronic illness? Or, from the perspective of modern health care and its assumptions of individual responsibilities and informed choices, what is the most effective *combination* of practitioners to provide the best care for these patients? Can collegiality and negotiation of roles be maintained between two professional groups that now assert some commonality of skills and knowledge but different social status and philosophical foundations?

In many ways parties outside of medicine and nursing have recently directed the discourse, albeit with particular perspectives focused on economics, efficiency, and power. Through this discourse the foundation for negotiations between NPs and physicians was altered as NPs gained autonomy through access to third-party reimbursement no longer tied to physician supervision. Since 1977, with the passage of the Rural Health Clinics Act (P.L. 95–210), NPs (as well as PAs) practicing in free-standing, physician-directed rural clinics located in health professions shortage areas (HPSA) received Medicare reimbursement through payment to their physician employers. Later, the 1997 Balanced Budget Act lifted Medicare restrictions to cover direct reimbursement for NPs and PAs in all nonhospital sites and removed requirements for physician supervision, although NP reimbursement is usually a percentage of physician rates. Health Maintenance Organizations (HMOs) employ nurse practitioners as lower cost providers for healthy populations, as do the Armed Forces. Federal programs such as the Civilian Health and Medical Program of the Uniformed Services directly reimburse nurse practitioners for their services. Nursing schools such as the University of Pennsylvania have begun nurse practitioner-run provider agencies that serve chronically ill indigent and elderly population groups.

Even so, there remains room for negotiations. NPs negotiated prescriptive authority, perhaps the last bastion of physician's control of the clinical thinking process, in some form in forty-eight state professional regulating bodies by 1995. Of these, however, only eleven allowed independent prescription of routine or formulary drugs by nurses.[68] Nurses in states without legal sanction of prescriptive authority rely on negotiations with physician colleagues to provide drug therapy—this involves devices (both legal and not legal depending upon the perspective and state) such as pre-signed or pre-printed prescription forms. This issue has come to symbolize the perceived arbitrariness of physicians' control of the patient, and has served to intensify already hotly contested debates over professional knowledge domains.

The NP movement provides a foundation from which to view the actual work of the delivery of health care and the intellectual framing of knowledge domains. Because of changes in physicians' practice patterns and nursing practice and education, physicians and nurses engaged in negotiations that met the needs and expectations of both groups in different ways. Physicians traded pieces of their traditional power base, components of clinical thinking, to nurses for the opportunity to focus on the more important, satisfying, and less boring aspects of medical practice. Nurses, who were becoming more educated and competent in the care of clinically diverse populations, were willing and even eager to take on broader nursing roles and claim the process of clinical thinking as their own, according to their own ideology. Clinical thinking, even those parts physicians considered mundane, represented competency and political power to nurses. By parceling out parts of clinical thinking, physicians unlocked the door to the process that had been their source of clinical authority and power base for decades. This did not occur by physicians' "default" of these skills and knowledge to nurses but through a conscious, bipartisan process still framing contemporary relationships among nurses, physicians, and patients.

Negotiations continue between nurse practitioners and physicians, but there now seems a limit to what individual practitioners can accomplish and expect because the factor of economic competition has entered into the equation. NPs tend to practice in areas that have the highest concentration of physicians instead of in rural communities that lack access to medical care. This choice of practice environment demands broader contact between greater numbers of nurse practitioners and physicians, thereby creating a foundation for economic and political competition. Physicians, already under siege from shrinking reimbursements and oversight from HMOs are now also faced, perhaps, with the effects of decisions set in process over three decades ago. The number of NPs in practice has grown exponentially. In 1970, there were only 250 NPs practicing in the United States. By 1980, there were 20,000 NPs, and by 1997, 63,000.[69] The rapid growth in numbers of NPs has occurred during a period of physician surplus and a projected twenty-four percent increase in physician supply between 1995 and 2005.[70] One may feel quite confident from the numbers alone that jurisdictional disputes will continue and competition will complicate negotiations between NPs and physicians as they compete for patients.

To seek meaning for contemporary debates occurring within the highly competitive health care environment, it may be instructive to reconsider the last four decades. Although local negotiations between individual physicians and nurses may have been anchored by assumptions about the "good" of the patient at the point of care, on the professional level hierarchical relationships and power were at stake. The practical negotiation of responsibilities achieved by physicians and nurses in response to clinical realities was not replicated at the upper levels of professional organization. Professional, hierarchical interests dissipated when individual physician and nurse turned their clinical attention to patient needs. In this highly volatile time, doctors, nurses and their professional organizations must consider the consequences of their failure to defuse competitive issues in the interest of patient care. The failure to do so will only fuel further competition and compromise both professions' obligation to patients. In this scenario neither Hippocrates nor Nightingale would be proud.

NOTES

1.   Norma Lang, Eileen Sullivan-Marx, and Melinda Jenkins, "Advanced Practice Nurses and Success of Organized Delivery Systems," *The American Journal of Managed Care* II (February 1996): 129–135; Richard A. Cooper, Prakash Laud, and Craig L. Dietrich, "Current and Projected Workforce of Nonphysician Clinicians," *JAMA* 280, no. 9 (2 September 1998): 788–794.

2.   Geraldine Wade, "Hippocrates Beware: Nurse Practitioners Eroding Practice of Medicine," *American College of Physicians Observer* 18, no. 4 (April 1998): 4.

3.   Andrew Abbott, *The System of Professions: An Essay on the Division of Expert Labor* (Chicago: Chicago University Press, 1988), 143–157.

4.   There are many terms used in the literature to describe the process of clinical thinking. Clinical judgment [Alvan R. Feinstein, *Clinical Judgment* (Baltimore: Williams and Wilkins, 1967); H. Tristram Engelhardt, Jr., Stuart F. Spicker, and Bernard Towers, *Clinical Judgment: A Critical Appraisal* (Boston: D. Reidel Publishing Co., 1977)] and diagnostic reasoning are two examples. The terms actually connotate very similar concepts. Feinstein's idea of clinical judgment, however, relies more heavily on symptom grouping and categorization (using mathematical principles) for the purpose of rationalizing treatment decisions and developing an accurate prognosis. I prefer to use clinical thinking as suggested by Barbara Bates, *A Guide to Physical Examination and History Taking*, 6th ed. (Philadelphia: J.B. Lippincott Co, 1995), 635–648. Bates's presentation combines rationalization with flexibility to accommodate patient individuality and social circumstances in treatment decisions.

5.   Many scholars acknowledge the ability for negotiations to occur when parties do not share the same status or power. See Anselm Strauss, Shizuko Fagerhaugh, B. Suczek, and Carolyn Wiener, *Social Organization of Medical Work* (Chicago: University of Chicago Press, 1985); Eliot Friedson, *Professionalism Reborn* (Chicago: University of Chicago Press, 1994). For negotiations in particular settings where power between negotiators is also uneven see Rue Bucher and L. Schatzman, "Negotiating a Division of Labor Among Professionals in the State Mental Hospitals," *Psychiatry* 27 (1964): 266–77; Julie Fairman, "Watchful Vigilance: Nursing Care, Technology, and the Development of Intensive Care Units," *Nursing Research* 41 (January/February 1992): 56–60.

6.   There is also very little historiography pertaining to the nurse practitioner movement in general. Exceptions are Barbara Brush and Elizabeth Capezuti's article "Revisiting 'A Nurse for All Settings': The NP Movement, 1965–1995," *Journal of the American Academy of NPs* 8, no. 1 (January 1996): 5–11.

7.   Eliot Freidson, *Professional Dominance: The Social Structure of Medical Care* (New York: Atherton Press, 1970), xi.

8.   Barbara Bates, "Physician and Nurse Practitioner: Conflict and Reward," *Annals of Internal Medicine* 82 (5 May 1975): 702–706.

9.   For descriptions of nurses involved in informal decision-making see Leonard Stein, "The Doctor-Nurse Game," *Archives of General Psychiatry* 16 (June 1967): 699–703; various chapters in Rose L. Coser, *Life on the Ward* (E. Lansing, Mich.: Michigan State University Press, 1962); Rose L. Coser, Howard Becker, B. Greer, Everett C. Hughes, and Anselm Strauss, *Boys in White: Student Cultures in Medical Schools* (Chicago: University of Chicago Press, 1961).

10.   For a discussion on decision-making authority in intensive care units see Julie Fairman and Joan Lynaugh, *American Critical Care: A History* (Philadelphia: University of Pennsylvania Press, 1998), chap. 4.

11.   U.S. Department of Health, Education, and Welfare, Public Health Service, *Nursing Resources: A Progress Report of the Program of the Division of Nursing Resources*, PHSP # 551, (Washington, D.C.: GPO, 1958), chart 3. For the concept

of jurisdictional dominance and the importance of the workplace in establishing professional exclusivity see Abbott, *The System of Professions*, chap. 5.

12.   Isabel Stewart was an educator at Teacher's College, Columbia University, New York, and also the chair of the Committee on Curriculum of the National League for Nursing Education, which published *A Curriculum Guide For Schools of Nursing* in 1937. The 1937 curriculum was the culmination of a gradual change in nursing education originating at the turn of the century, from a training system based on rudimentary case methods to a functional, rule-based efficiency method. Although there are many definitions of functional method, I have used the perspective drawn from Frances Reiter, "The Nurse-clinician," *International Nursing Review*, 13, no. 4 (1966):63. For a more detailed analysis of Stewart's method and influence on hospital nursing see Julie Fairman, "Thinking About Patients. Nursing Science in the 1950s," *Reflections* 23, no. 3 (3rd/4th Quarter, 1997): 30–32; Susan Reverby, "A Legitimate Relationship: Nursing, Hospitals, and Science in the Twentieth Century," in *The American General Hospital: Communities and Social Contexts*, ed. Diana Long and Janet Golden (Ithaca, N.Y.: Cornell University Press, 1989), 135–156.

13.   National League for Nursing, *Report on Hospital Schools of Nursing*, 1957 (New York: NLN, Inc., 1959), 18.

14.   Esther Lucile Brown, *Nursing for the Future* (New York: Russell Sage Foundation, 1948); Esther Lucile Brown, *Newer Dimensions of Patient Care*, Parts 1–4 (New York: Russell Sage Foundation, 1961); Hildegard Peplau, *Interpersonal Relations in Nursing* (New York: G.P. Putnam's Sons, 1952); and later, Virginia Henderson, "The Nature of Nursing," *American Journal of Nursing*, 64 (1964): 62–68. Henderson began to think about clinically based nursing practice in the 1940s but did not publish many of her thoughts until after she left Teachers College in the 1950s.

15.   Henderson, "The Nature of Nursing." Henderson published many other important articles and texts but this essay is the most often quoted and most representative of the changes occurring in nursing during the time period.

16.   Explication of the models are found in Brown, *Nursing for the Future* and *Newer Dimensions*, and in Peplau, *Interpersonal Relations*.

17.   For a comprehensive overview of nursing education delivered by nurse training schools see Joan Lynaugh and Barbara Bates, *American Nursing: From Hospital to Health Systems* (Cambridge: Blackwood Press, in conj. with the Milbank Memorial Fund, 1996), chap. 1.

18.   Frances Reiter, "The Improvement of Nursing Practice," Speeches presented at the American Nurses' Association Section, Regional Conferences for Professional Nurses (Kansas City, MO: ANA, 1961), 3–11; Reiter, "The Nurse-clinician," 62–71.

19.   For a general view of Smith's philosophy and practice see *The Collected Works of Dorothy M. Smith, 1948–1967* (Gainesville, Fla.: College of Nursing Section, Univ. of Florida Alumni Association, 1968).

20.   Loretta Ford, Marguerite Cobb, and Margaret Taylor, *Defining Clinical Content [of] Graduate Nursing Programs: Community Health Nursing* (Boulder, CO: Western Interstate Commission for Higher Education, 1967); Loretta Ford, and

Henry Silver, "The Expanded Role of the Nurse in Child Care," *Nursing Outlook*, 15 (1967): 43–45.

21. Laura L. Simms, "The Clinical Nursing Specialists," *Journal of the American Medical Association*, 198 (1966): 675–678.

22. Virginia Henderson co-authored *Textbook of the Principles and Practice of Nursing with Bertha Harmer* (who began the series in 1922) in 1929, 1934, 1939 and 1955 (New York: The Macmillan Co). See also Virginia Henderson, *Basic Principles of Nursing Care* (Geneva: International Council of Nurses, 1960).

23. Bonnie Bullough, "Is the Nurse Practitioner Role a Source of Increased Work Satisfaction?" *Nursing Research* 23, no. 1 (January/February 1974): 14–19; Charles Lewis and Barbara Resnik, "Nurse Clinics and Progressive Ambulatory Patient Care," *New England Journal of Medicine* 277, no. 23 (7 December 1967): 1236–1241.

24. For a discussion of federal funding of nursing education see Lynaugh and Brush, *American Nursing*, chap. 1.

25. See Abbott, *The System of Professionals*, 125–135 for a discussion of the influence of workplace in professional jurisdictional differentiation.

26. Fairman, "Thinking About Patients," 30–32.

27. Barbara Rollins, telephone interview with Joan Lynaugh, 23 March 1990 (Origins and Conceptualization of Critical Care Nursing in 20th Century America, Joan Lynaugh, PI).

28. Elizabeth Cameron, oral history interview by Julie Fairman, 16 May 1996, Philadelphia, (Analysis of the Relationship Between Nurses and Physicians During the Development of Dialysis Technology, Julie Fairman, PI).

29. These themes are presented by Rosemary Stevens, *American Medicine and the Public Interest: A History of Specialization*, updated edition with a new introduction, (Berkeley: University of California Press, 1998); Rosemary Stevens, *In Sickness and in Wealth: American Hospitals in the Twentieth Century*, (New York: Basic Books, 1989).

30. This trend changed in the early 1970s. The Health Professions Educational Assistance Program made training funds available to specialties other than psychiatrists and physiatrists, including family practice specialists. See Louis M. Rousselot, "Federal Efforts to Influence Physician Education, Specialization Distribution Projections and Options," *The American Journal of Medicine* 55, no. 2 (August 1973): 123–130.

31. American Medical Association, *Distribution of Physicians in the United States, 1971. Regional, State, County, and Metropolitan Areas* (Chicago, IL.: AMA, 1972), 10–18.

32. Rosemary Stevens, *American Medicine*, 162, table 1; James K. Cooper and Karen Heald, "Is There a Doctor Shortage?" *JAMA* 227, no. 12 (March 25 1974): 1410–1411.

33. Patricia Kendall, "Medical Specialization: Trends and Contributing Factors," in *Psychosocial Aspects of Medical Training*, ed. R. H. Coombs and C. E. Vincent (Springfield, IL.: C. Thomas, 1971), 461.

34. William Stewart and Maryland Pennell, "Pediatric Manpower in the United States and Its Implications'" *Pediatrics* 31 (February 1963): 316–317.

35.   For an overview' see Rashi Fein, *The Doctor Shortage: An Economic Diagnosis* (Washington, D.C.: Brookings Institute, 1967).

36.   American Medical Association, *Distribution of Physicians*, 10–18.

37.   *President's Commission on the Health Needs of the Nation*. Vol. 1 (Washington, D.C.: GPO, 1952).

38.   Surgeon General's Consultant Group, Subcommittee on Paramedical Personnel in Rehabilitation and Care of the Chronically ill, "Mobilization and Health Manpower, Sect. II," (Washington' D.C.: GPO, 1956).

39.   Surgeon General's Consultant Group on Medical Education, "Physicians for a Growing America," Public Health Service Publication # 709 (Washington, D.C.: GPO, 1959).

40.   President's Commission on Heart Disease, Cancer, and Stroke, "Report to the President: A National Program to Conquer Heart Disease, Cancer, and Stroke," Vol. I and II (Washington, D.C.: GPO, 1964–1965); L. T. Coggeshall, "Planning for Medical Progress through Education," The Executive Council of the Association of American Medical Colleges (Evanston, IL.: The Association of American Medical Colleges, 1965).

41.   These strategies are described in numerous articles in the 1950s and 1960s. The best overview of these strategies is found in Alfred Yankauer, John Connelly, and Jacob Feldman, "Allied Health Worker Utilization in Pediatric Practice in Massachusetts and in the United States," *Pediatrics* 42, no. 5 (November 1968): 733–742; Alfred Yankauer, John Connelly, and Jacob Feldman, "Task Performance and Task Delegation in Pediatric Office Practice," *American Journal of Public Health* 59, no. 7 (July 1969): 1104–1117.

42.   See for example, Earl Siegel and Sylvia C. Bryson, "A Redefinition of the Role of the Public Health Nurse in Child Health Supervision," *American Journal of Public Health* 53, no. 7 (July 1963): 1015–1024; Nancy Martin, "Freeing the Doctor From Well-baby Care," *Medical Economics* 44, no. 4 (13 November 1967): 118–124, 127; John P. Connelly, John D. Stoeckle, Edna S. Lepper, and Ruth M. Farrisey, "The Physician and the Nurse—Their Interprofessional Work in Office and Hospital Ambulatory Settings," *The New England Journal of Medicine* 275, no. 14 (6 October 1966): 765–768.

43.   Faye Davis, telephone oral history interview by M.J. Murphy, 14 March 1997 (The Pioneers' Stories: Work Histories of Early Nurse Practitioners in Pennsylvania, Julie Fairman, PI).

44.   Bonita Roche, telephone oral history interview by M.J. Murphy, 4 October 1997 (The Pioneers' Stories: Work Histories of Early Nurse Practitioners in Pennsylvania, Julie Fairman, PI).

45.   Barbara Bates, personal communication with Julie Fairman, 13 November 1997, Bryn Mawr, Pa.; See also Barbara Bates, "Physician and Nurse Practitioner: Conflict and Reward," *Annals of Internal Medicine* 82 (5 May 1975): 702–706; Wayne Mente, "Professional Values in Medical Practice," *New England Journal of Medicine* 280, no. 17 (24 April 1969): 930–936; Robert Kane and Rosalie Kane, "Physicians' Attitudes of Omnipotence in a University Hospital," *Journal of Medical Education*, part 2, 44 (August 1969): 684–689.

46.   Many supporters of nurse practitioners point to the 1986 study as one

of the defining moments of the development of the nurse practitioner role. Office of Technology Assessment, United States Congress, *Nurse Practitioners, Physician Assistants, and Certified Nurse-Midwives: A Policy Analysis*, HAS 37 (Washington, DC: GPO, 1986).

47. Henry Silver, "Use of New Types of Allied Health Professionals in Providing Care for Children," *American Journal of Diseases of Children* 116 (November 1968): 486–490.

48. See for example, Pennsylvania State Board of Medical Education and Licensure, minutes of the Board meetings, 10/22/71, 1/6/72, 12/4/73, Department of Professional and Occupational Affairs, Harrisburg, PA.

49. Sydney Halpern, *American Pediatrics, The Social Dynamics of Professionalism, 1880–1980* (Berkeley: University of California Press, 1988), 128.

50. Ibid., 132; See also various reports in professional journals, e.g., Clifford Taylor, "Medicine's Most Frustrating Specialty," *Medical Economics* 28, no. 20 (1959): 111–115.

51. G. Solomons and M. Hatton, "The Public Health Nurse as an Objective Scientific Observer," *Nursing Outlook* 9 (1961): 486.

52. Kenneth Rogers, Mary Mally, and Florence Marcus, "A General Medical Practice Using Nonphysician Personnel," *JAMA* 206, no. 8 (18 November 1968): 1753–1757. Nurses were also prescribing medications in 4 percent of the cases.

53. Nobel Guthrie, John Runyan, Glenn Clark, and Oscar Marvin, "The Clinical Nursing Conference: A Preliminary Report," *New England Journal of Medicine* 270, no. 26 (25 June 1964): 1411–1413.

54. Charles Lewis and Barbara Resnik, "Nurse Clinics and Progressive Ambulatory Patient Care," *New England Journal of Medicine* 277, no. 23 (7 December 1967): 1236–1241.

55. For an analysis of the American Medical Association and American Nurses' Association perspective on this issue see Natalie Holt, "Confusion's Masterpiece: The Development of the Physician Associate Profession," *Bulletin of the History of Medicine* 72, no. 2 (Summer 1998): 246–278.

56. For a discussion on incompatible perspectives in the division of work and knowledge see Eliot Freidson, *Doctoring Together: A Study of Professional Social Control* (New York: Elsevier, 1976).

57. Roche, interview; Davies interview.

58. See for example, Robert D. Coye and Marc R. Hansen, "The Doctor's Associate," *JAMA* 209, no. 4 (28 July 1969): 529–533; Abraham B. Bergman, Jeffrey L. Probstfield and Ralph J. Wedgwood, "Task Identification in Pediatric Practice," *American Journal of the Diseases of Children* 118 (September 1969): 459–468.

59. *The American Heritage Dictionary of the English Language*, 3rd edition (Boston: Houghton Mifflin Co.), 493.

60. Loretta Ford, "Nurse Practitioners: History of a New Idea and Predictions for the Future," in *Nursing in the 1980s. Crises-Opportunities-Challenges* ed. Linda Aiken (Philadelphia: J.B. Lippincott, 1982), 231–248.

61. Silver, "Use of New Types"; Henry Silver, Loretta Ford, and Lewis Day, "The Pediatric Nurse-Practitioner Program," *JAMA* 204, no. 4 (22 April 1968): 88–92.

62. Holt, "Confusion's Masterpiece," 246–278.

63.   See for example, "The Physician's Assistant Programs," *RN* 33, no. 10 (October 1970): 43–46.

64.   Bernice Shaw, "A Look Inside Three Programs," *RN* 33, no. 10 (October 1970): 36–42.

65.   Charles L. Hudson, "Expansion of Medical Professional Services with Nonprofessional Personnel," *JAMA* 176 (1961): 840.

66.   Martha E. Rogers, "Nursing: To Be or Not to Be?" *Nursing Outlook* 29 (January, 1972):41–44; Eleanor Lambertsen, "Not Quite MD, More Than PA," *Hospitals* 45 (1 December 1971): 70–76, 136.

67.   Charles Rosenberg, "Banishing Risk: Or the More Things Change the More They Remain the Same," *Perspectives in Biology and Medicine*, 39, no. 1 (Autumn 1995): 35.

68.   Linda J. Pearson, "1995 Annual Update of How Each State Stands on Legislative Issues Affecting Advanced Nursing Practice," *Nurse Practitioner* 20, no. 13 (1995): 51.

69.   Cooper, Laud and Dietrich, "Current and Projected Workforce," 789; American Academy of Nurse Practitioners, *Scope of Practice* (Austin, TX: AANP, 1995).

70.   Richard A. Cooper, "Perspectives on the Physician Work-Force to the Year 2020" *JAMA* 274 (1995): 1534–1543.

SECTION 5

CONCLUSION

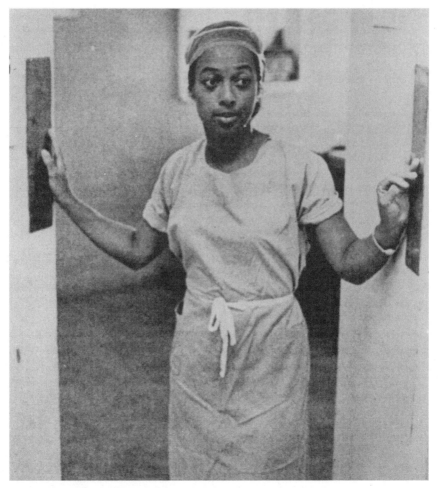

Captain Marian J. Scott in Vietnam, circa 1965. Courtesy of the Center for the Study of the History of Nursing, University of Pennsylvania.

Conclusion

Sylvia D. Rinker

The historical articles gathered in this book reflect significant, fundamental problems in nursing that have resisted simple solutions over the years. The complicated debates surrounding nursing's search for identity, the struggle for authority and power, and designating what counts as nursing knowledge intertwine, creating perplexing problems that continue today to raise controversy and debate in the discipline. Indeed, the very dilemmas inherent in these issues make them of ongoing significance to the discipline.[1]

Identity questions about who is the nurse, what constitutes nursing responsibilities, and what society and the profession can or should expect from nurses are governed by nurses' ever-present desire for power and authority over their work, a yearning that marks every human endeavor. Changing hierarchies within nursing and the social forces that determine nursing's position in society reflect ongoing debates about how the system operates, who changes it, upon whose authority such change is predicated, and ultimately who brings proposed changes to fruition. Nursing's expanding knowledge base raises further questions about what constitutes nursing knowledge, who owns it, who exercises it, and finally, who benefits from it? Thoughtful analyses, such as that offered by authors of the articles included in this book, add new dimensions to our understanding of the origins and meanings of familiar traditions and ongoing predicaments in nursing.

Lending a sense of coherence to past experience, history reveals that issues that have endured across the ages continue to pervade current nursing practice. One of the primary benefits of history is the opportunity to replace familiar myth-making about the past with insightful understanding. However, informing the debate, rather than serving any particular ideology, is the primary purpose of history.[2] As historians accumulate, review, and interpret evidence from the past, pieces of the puzzle are replaced and repositioned, and a necessary and continuous revision is made possible. As D'Antonio points out in the last chapter of the book, "Revisiting and Rethinking the Rewriting of Nursing History," the growing body of historical studies of nursing have begun to move nursing's history beyond the mere description of events. We now have available a more richly textured and nuanced story that provokes a fuller understanding of the meaning and the impact of choices made in the past for the current and future practice of nursing. Just as nurse clinicians gather and interpret data from their own particular perspectives, historians research archival documents, focus on different aspects of the issue, and emphasize different outcomes. For example, in the introductory chapter, Lynaugh discusses the accidental, unintended outcomes of the choices nurses made, while in the concluding chapter, D'Antonio identifies the underlying power held by nurses who made conscious choices for their nursing actions. Neither author claims to possess the full interpretation, but juxtaposing both articles equips the reader with a fuller context for understanding the consequences and opportunities involved in decision-making. Many diverse interpretations are needed because it is impossible, even for the most zealous of investigators, to find an absolutely clean slate of circumstances to explain life experiences. Historical research from a variety of sources is needed to dispel the murkiness that surrounds past events.

The cumulative efforts of historians of differing perspectives create a professional memory essential to illuminate present and future decisions. Current practice was shaped and has evolved directly as a consequence of choices made by our predecessors. As a record of the outcome of choices made—or not made—history can provide a foundation for informed decision-making for the future. But D'Antonio cogently notes that historical research should also focus on the processes through which such decisions were made. Such processes, she argues, may well be more important than the choices themselves, because of what they reveal about nursing, the options available to nurses, and nurses' working and living environments.

It is both comforting and distressing to realize, through the reading of nursing history, that while expressed values in nursing have not changed, as a profession nurses have been consistently ambivalent in the practice of those values. For example, while it would be difficult to find a nurse who does not espouse compassion as an optimum way of relating to patients, our selected readings suggest that issues of the nurse's identity, the ongoing struggle for power and authority, and the search for what counts as nursing knowledge often overshadowed nurses' expression of compassion as they cared for patients. Isabel Hampton and other nurse leaders who participated in the 1893 Chicago World's Fair would surely have been dismayed could they have known that at the end of the twentieth century, as at its outset, society's need for nursing continues to be greater than society's readiness to pay the cost for such services. Moreover, Isabel Hampton's cry in 1893 that a nurse could be any and everything continues to reverberate today, as the debate on the appropriate educational entry level has yet to be resolved. But they (and we) might take heart from the work of historians who have placed the dreams of nursing leaders within the context of the time, place, and custom in which they lived and practiced. If we are to move beyond age-old constraints, we must focus our activism not just on our professional sense of responsibility and agency, but also on the social policies that define nursing practice in the current health care setting. Will we actively create or passively accept the policies that dictate current practice? The choices we make, whether with deliberate intent or by default, will soon become our own historical legacy.

A careful reading of these articles and introductory essays leads to tantalizing questions that remain to be answered or that need further exploration. It is the editors' hope that this book stimulates readers to ask questions for which answers lie in the intellectual pursuit of our past. The complex interrelationships suggested by the discussion of the issues addressed in this book have the potential to guide future historians into rich fields whose insights have heretofore only been suggested. The articles here collected are but some examples of intelligent and scholarly nursing history. Our bibliography contains others that we encourage our readers to ponder. Our plea is that you join us in reading, researching, and writing nursing history, making available to future generations an ever-growing historical interpretation of the enduring issues in nursing.

NOTES

1.   Peggy Chinn. *Developing the Discipline: Critical Studies in Nursing History and Professional Issues,* v. (Gaithersburg, MD: Aspen, 1994.)

2.   John Tosh. *The Pursuit of History,* 21. (London: Longman, 1987.)

15

Revisiting and Rethinking the Rewriting of Nursing History

Patricia D'Antonio

In 1984, Janet Wilson James turned a fairly prosaic request to review a series of recently published books on the history of nursing into an intriguing and influential essay about the current state of scholarship on the subject.[1] That essay, "Writing and Rewriting Nursing History," argued that traditionally descriptive narratives of nursing's past could no longer exist in historiographic isolation from relevant themes in social and women's history. James was not the first to advance this argument: Celia Davies and Ellen Lagemann had previously done so in introductions to works in their respective collections of essays.[2] Davies, concentrating on scholarship by British historians in the late 1970s, and Lagemann, considering American papers presented at the Rockefeller Archive Center's conference on the history of nursing in 1981, paid more attention than did James, in fact, to attempts to ground revisionist nursing history in the "new" social history and its emphasis on the mighty triumvirate of race, class, and gender.

Nevertheless, James had been a colleague and a friend to authors of both the more cautious and uncritical narrations of nursing's historical progress and those attempting newer, more conceptually driven approaches. Hence, her analysis explicitly reached out to both. She respected the works of those who focused on nursing's achievements;

I am indebted to Joan Lynaugh, Susan Reverby, Charles Rosenberg, Eleanor Crowder, and Karen Buhler-Wilkerson for their insightful critiques of an earlier version of this manuscript. I am also grateful to the *Bulletin*'s two anonymous reviewers for their help in contextualizing a later version. The footnotes have been edited in this reprint.

Note: This chapter was originally published in *The Bulletin of the History of Medicine* 73, (1999): 268–290. Reprinted with permission.

these studies were, she explained, "the first investigations of important topics, the product of devoted effort."[3] Yet their wish to "filter out the intractable problems" inherent in their topic had so narrowed their perspective that they had lost the stirring interpretive sweep that their early-twentieth-century nursing predecessors had brought to their own historical narratives.[4] Some other works, however, excited her: Barbara Melosh's emphasis on nursing's workplace culture; Christopher Maggs's attention to issues of demography, social class, and gender stereotyping; and Wanda Heistand's explorations of the implications of family history for nursing's history were "signs," she suggested, "of life and thought reviving."[5] The resuscitation, however, had yet to be declared successful. "Nursing history," James concluded, still looked "something like the elephant as described by the blind men."[6] Some pieces of its past had received intriguing reconsiderations; others were completely ignored. Still, she found promise for the future, particularly in the opening of the "two-way street" between the historical traditions of nursing and those of the liberal arts.

Now, a decade later, it is worth pausing to consider what effect the cross-disciplinary reciprocity that James championed has had on the writing of nursing's history. At first glance, that effect seems profound. Understanding the work of nurses has reshaped historians' sense of the historical hospital, the treatment of disease, the birth of babies, and the role of women in their families and their communities.[7] And there are now few stories told about nurses by nurses without some reference, however fleeting, to the issues of gender, class, race, and the politics of professionalism.[8] There is, to be sure, considerable debate in the field about the ultimate implications of such analyses for nursing's history. Has nursing, for example, been defined by gender, or has its work transcended sex-based stereotypes? Have class and race differences only bred divisiveness, or has the heterogeneity of the nursing work force helped the discipline forge an identity akin to that of those it served? Has the professionalizing agenda devalued nursing's craft traditions, or has it been a vehicle of upward economic mobility and respected social status? The historians dealing with such questions no longer fall into neatly defined categories: those who trained first as clinicians are often as willing to explore the implications of class analysis as are those who trained exclusively in the liberal arts to entertain notions of professionalizing power.

The problem, however, is that the "two-way street" James envisioned has seen much of its meaningful intellectual traffic slow to a crawl. The publication of Barbara Melosh's *The Physician's Hand* in 1982, Susan Reverby's *Ordered to Care* in 1987, and Darlene Clark Hine's *Black Women in White* in 1989 essentially established these debates, and the succeeding years have seen little in the way of conceptual refinement or reconsideration.[9] A certain complacency has, in fact, crept into the field as scholars have left largely unchallenged an overarching paradigm that casts nursing's history as one of socially structured contradictions. Reverby's cogent argument that nurses have been historically "ordered to care in a society that refuses to value caring" has had the most salience with most historians.[10] But nursing has also been conceptualized as having been trapped by the rhetoric of professionalism in labor markets moved only by the tactics of trade unionism;[11] as having been bound (both by intent and by perception) to the social status of medicine, while simultaneously trying to assert its disciplinary independence;[12] or as seeking to transform its patients' place in the social fabric of American life even as nursing care replicated much of America's gendered, class, ethnic, and racial consciousness.[13]

Yet there are works that are beginning to break the "traffic jam" and suggest new ways of thinking about nursing's history. They suggest, on a very concrete level, that the contradictions faced by nurses were neither unnegotiable nor insurmountable.[14] More important, however, they offer a different way of conceptualizing the interconnectedness between the evidence and its implications at a point when the debates about the role of gender, class, race, and mobility in nursing's past still veer uneasily between positions celebrating the discipline's transcendence and those chiding its rigidity. They suggest that rather than being passively defined by socially constructed stereotypes, women actively embraced the gendered meaning of nursing for the ease with which it allowed them to create work identities that remained connected to their personal identities despite their formal relationship to the world of productive work. Culture, community, and consciousness, of course, mediated the workings of such an identity for nurses, as for most working women, and created the boundaries that were, often simultaneously, both a source of their strength and a dam around their ambition. Still, women's commitment to the idea, if not always the reality, of nursing stirred within them the possibility of using a particularly constructed gendered identity to step out of—or, perhaps more important, step up from—the traditional conventions of their particular starting place.

The timing of this reconsideration seems, in keeping with James's gentle urging of reciprocity, quite propitious. For while historians generally acknowledge that women's domestic identity shaped the meaning and place of work in their lives, the material links between the construction of a gendered identity, work, and agency remain elusive. Works to date, in fact, have primarily explored the enduring complexity of these links. We now, for example, more clearly understand that women's culture and experiences can never be completely recounted solely in terms of their relationship with paid labor; that is, situations outside the workplace—

women's places within the social fabric of their communities, their neighborhoods, and their families—have emerged as equally powerful determinants of their consciousness, their roles, and their sense of agency. As a result, we have discovered the almost seamless interconnectedness of women's working and private lives.[15] To turn again to nursing's history, we now know how women such as Martha Ballard, the late-eighteenth-century subject of Laurel Thatcher Ulrich's *Midwife's Tale,* and her early-twentieth-century successors, described by Charlotte Borst in *Catching Babies,* lived their lives enmeshed in the simultaneity of their roles as midwives, mothers, spouses, neighbors, and friends.[16]

Women, like their midwife sisters, still lived much of their lives outside the nexus of wage-based activities. Even so, we are beginning to understand that the idea of work, if not work itself, did hold significant salience for them. That is, non-wage-earning women looked both to their own experiences and to those of their neighbors and kin to construct an enduring idea of themselves as past or potential workers. They drew power from this idea. It could—at times, and under conditions that acknowledged their enduring rights as participatory partisans—spark frank labor activism, either in the form of consumer boycotts or in the form of militant class action.[17] And it worked in more subtle, more conservative ways as well. The status and satisfaction that many women found in their domestic roles, for example, seem to have existed in counterpoint to the drudgery, and often the degradation, they experienced as factory hands, mill workers, or domestic servants.[18]

In all, such studies point to the enduring relationship between consciousness, role, and agency—although now a relationship forged and experienced outside as well as inside the workplace. Yet, questions remain. How can we, for example, both privilege women's work and acknowledge that women rarely secured their identities in relation only to productive employment? And how might we understand women's construction of a gendered identity through work and attend to the ways in which such an identity shaped the meaning and the place of work in their lives? The history of nursing cannot yet lay claim to any groundbreaking answers, but in its rethinking we can construct a window through which we may glimpse the contours of such a terrain.

REVISITING NURSING HISTORY

Perhaps it may be most useful to begin our rethinking (and recontextualizing) of nursing's history by considering a brief portrait of the women who would be nurses. It does seem fairly clear that these women knew exactly what kind of bargain they were striking when they applied to the hospital-run nurses' training schools in the late nineteenth and early twentieth centuries: they expected to trade two (and often three) years of their lives spent in arduous and exploited service for a diploma that promised a seemingly respected and respectable means of making one's way in the world.[19] Yet, these women arrived at their schools with relatively privileged social positions. Some came with solidly middle-class credentials: they had more education, more resources, and more choices available to them then did most other working women. Many more others came from working-class and farm families, but, unlike most of their working-class and farming sisters, they came from financially secure households that needed neither their unpaid labor nor their immediate wages. As the twentieth century progressed, and as sales, secretarial, and other white-collar occupations were opened to women, nursing lost many of its more-promising urban recruits.[20] Still, at a time when most working-class women found themselves more tightly enmeshed than ever in their families' patriarchal wage economies, nursing promised increasingly rural and suburban women almost unprecedented social and economic independence.[21]

Nursing women sought—each class group in its own way—to create new opportunities for themselves. Thus, "making one's way in the world" may more correctly capture the multiple meanings of that nursing diploma. For some women, often termed the "elite" because their middle-class background frequently catapulted them into leadership positions, it meant entry into a female world of almost unparalleled autonomy, control, and professional status. For others, frequently categorized as nursing's rank-and-file workers, it meant entry into a skilled craft that combined the sanctity of a feminine "calling," the promise of economic self-support, and a taste of the freedom of the urban working world.[22] But the nursing diploma meant even more: it also meant the possibility of constructing lives with meaningful, easily accomplished, and socially sanctioned connections between personal responsibilities and professional commitments, and between private interests and public concerns. The careers of most rank-and-file nurses certainly bear this out, if in fairly traditional ways: they followed a relatively conventional life-cycle path in that they chose work whose requisite schooling seemingly enhanced their status, social worth, and marital prospects; they worked until marriage; and, if necessary, they reentered the labor market later in life.[23]

Even more interesting, if less well analyzed, are the ways in which many elite nurses, often deliberately eschewing the bourgeois primacy of marriage and family responsibilities, also used nursing to construct interconnected personal and professional lives that as rarely as those of their rank-and-file sisters presented substantive challenges to prevailing norms about women's prescribed roles. It is hard not to be struck (to cite fairly concrete examples) with the ease with which many moved back and forth between directing a training school and caring for sick kin, or between leading battles for professional prerogatives and recuperating from the strain with extended sojourns in Europe.[24] And one has to be impressed: these women not only forged an alternative life-cycle path for themselves and, perhaps, for other women, but also turned their deeply held notions of bourgeois respectability to their advantage in their quest for autonomy in and control of their lives. It has long been argued that nursing leaders had to assume at least the veneer of "ladylike" behaviors in order to soften their public's perception of their powerful role—but it may be equally true that these behaviors were no veneer, and that the perception that was softened was their own of themselves.[25]

These women were powerful: they collectively transformed America's health-care system. Indeed, they were not just the "foot-soldiers" of reform,[26] they were more the "marines"—they established, maintained, and, to a fair degree, controlled the beachhead from which first hospitals and later scientific medicine launched their final assaults. Their attack seems to have proceeded on several fronts. They heeded Florence Nightingale's injunctions about the critical importance of a healing environment, but they fundamentally changed her emphasis. The good care given by these nurses seemed less the manipulation of the environment to meet patients' needs than the manipulation of patients to meet worksite demands.[27] They may have maintained their power through the manipulation of hierarchical bureaucracies; their tight organizational structure, in fact, seems to have strengthened nurses' position in the often uncharted and treacherous waters of interprofessional relationships.[28] Indeed, while there is merit in Martha Vicinus's argument that the rigid structure of training schools left its pupils unprepared for the collaborative demands of independent practice, she may have overlooked the ways in which it did provide keen administrative and political skills.[29] Yet, in the end, these same skills may have left nursing unprepared for peace. Nurses may well have loathed relinquishing their very real power and control after the war was won. Judith Walzer Leavitt's most recent work on obstetrical nurses, for example, suggests that they held on tenaciously to rigid routines and regimented experiences even as their leaders, their medical colleagues, and birthing women themselves pushed for a more fluid and flexible, patient-centered hospital experience.[30]

Lest we get too carried away, we would do well to remember that these skills in managing the sick brought few material rewards. Nursing remained a sex-stereotyped, segmented, often overcrowded, and always low-paying occupation that significantly restricted the skills of its practitioners. Canadian public health nurses, for example, spread a joke among themselves in the early 1920s that underscores how thoroughly these women understood the absurdity of the position in which they often found themselves: a patient, so the story goes, asked the nurse if she didn't think it was nice weather. I don't know, the nurse replied, you had better ask your physician.[31] In the end, even explicitly acknowledged clinical ability carried with it the weight of significant cultural baggage. At best, the work of nurses exposed profound social ambivalence about the power of women over ill and helpless men; at worst, it provoked outright hostility to their perceived domination.[32]

RETHINKING NURSING HISTORY

It may well seem that we are, at this point, in the midst of yet another contradiction in nursing's history: women with power who are stigmatized because of it. In another take on the relationships among nursing, gender, and power, Reverby, in her enormously influential *Ordered to Care*, argues that because nursing developed within an ideology of "duty" rather than "rights," cultural assumptions simply reaffirmed these women's responsibility to care without giving them the concomitant power to determine how their caring would find its form in actual practice. That is, they would work for love, not money—thus caught in the socially constructed bind of perceiving altruism as the antithesis of autonomy, and trapped there by class divisions that precluded the development of any new ideology based on gender.[33] Reverby's hard-hitting analysis, influenced by contemporaneous arguments about women's "different voices," superbly illustrates the contextual limitations of language and political vision in nursing's historical quest for an independent role in the home and the hospital. But such an analysis works only if we continue to place work within the health-care system at the center of these women's lives. And it works only if we persist in thinking of the rewards of its attendant labor market in fairly conventional terms.

Obviously, it would be foolish to dismiss the importance of stories of nursing women despondent about, and destitute because of, their life and their chosen work.[34] Their experiences, in fact, leave little doubt that those rank-and-file clinicians who, either by choice or by chance, nursed over a lifetime found little value placed on their years of experience, faced profound economic insecurity in sickness and old age, and saw their hopes and aspirations effectively dashed by erstwhile leaders who, in their own quest to induce the "right kind of woman" into nursing, wished only that they would fade quietly away. But their plight may not have been prototypical: the vast majority of nurses left the workforce within ten years of their graduation from training school.[35] That we know so much more about the disaffected minority, however legitimate their issues, may again point to the limitations of placing work at the heart of our approach.

But what if we turn to issues raised in women's history, and reposition identity rather than work at the center of our analysis of the relationships among nursing, gender, and power? Identity is, and has been, a critical (albeit ambiguous) variable in nursing. It is, and perhaps has been, almost an article of faith among nurses that there is something transcendent in their title—that "once a nurse, always a nurse," regardless of what work they may go on to do.[36] This notion does have some historical grounding. In early-twentieth-century America, for example, we can catch glimpses of its quite pragmatic role. The ironic humor that women "fresh from the farm" attached to instructions for more "lady-like" ways to haul mattresses, for example, suggests that they fully understood the social and economic price of a nursing diploma in their quest for bourgeois respectability.[37] And in early-twentieth-century Britain, we can see its more affective workings. There, Henriette Donner argues, the shared experiences of volunteer nurses during World War I helped them transcend the horror of their work and the rigidity of the military structure within which it took place. As important, these experiences created a sense of communality that gave new meaning and satisfaction to their lives, then and (for many) for decades afterward.[38]

These studies do begin to disentangle the relationship between work and consciousness, and they suggest the direction in which we might proceed. If, in fact, nursing women drew as much of their identity from their social place in a particular community—be it farm, training school, or the Red Cross—as they did from their structural place in an occupational labor market, then we must wonder about the worth of their nonmaterial as well as their material rewards. That is, as we find our way out of the seeming contradiction in the relationship between nursing and power, we must wonder whether women bartered transient workplace exploitation and devaluation for the enduring status and prestige that their identity as nurses gave them in their communities.[39]

This bartering did occur on an unequal playing field. Scholars have argued (often from an explicitly feminist framework) that nurses historically experienced both the promise and the problems of a culturally assigned role within the patriarchal structure of the home, the community, and the hospital. To the extent to which they joined with such a structure, they enjoyed the power—to a greater or lesser degree, depending upon one's perspective—to rule their own matriarchal domain. But once they attempted to challenge the underpinnings of gendered roles, to transform accepted notions of "women's proper place," they confronted (and rarely successfully) the far greater power of entrenched masculine prerogatives and sanctified feminine privilege.[40] The fate of nurses in war stands as a case in point. As the "angels of the battlefield," they received the respect and the recognition that had so often eluded them in civilian practice. But once they shed their angel's wings and demanded rank—that is, the official right to issue formal orders to men— they quickly discovered just how ethereal was the support that had kept them aloft.[41]

Yet, nurses essentially agreed to the rules governing play. Despite some historians' portrayal of them as "proto-feminists" engaged in radical change, and in spite of others' conceptual obliqueness about the very meaning of feminism, it now seems that nurses were collectively rather conservative and sought primarily—and this was no insignificant achievement—to create their own influential place within established structures and traditions.[42] They were not alone in this particular quest. Elizabeth Leonard end Jane Schultz argue, in separate works, that white, middle-class, Yankee nursing women appropriated the conventional acceptance of women's unique moral responsibility for the care of the sick and then used it to expand the boundaries of women's proper place both during and after the Civil War.[43] Nor were they, like their sisters, disempowered. As we move through time into the early twentieth century, for example, we can turn to Karen Buhler-Wilkerson's and Diane Hamilton's studies of the relationship between the Metropolitan Life Insurance Company and public health nurses. Here we see a collaboration that took place within a shared paternalistic framework that cast immigrants and the working poor as duty-bound Americans capable (with proper instruction, of course) of choosing the moral imperative of health. Still, public health nurses seized the opportunity and transformed what Met Life considered a fairly narrow role in sickness care and health education into one of such profound social significance that Abraham Flexner, the reformer of medical education and would-be rationalizer of the standards underpinning the privileged concept, considered the possibility that their work might indeed be "professional."[44]

There were, to be sure, moments when some nurses did break free from conservative conventions. For example, Frances Patai describes the collaboration between Jewish and African-American nurses who, linked by a political commitment to democratic values, briefly worked together for the Spanish Republic during that country's Civil War.[45] Moreover, as Carroll Smith-Rosenberg argues, Lillian Wald, a nurse and a prominent Progressive Era public health reformer, worked with other "New Women" both inside and outside nursing to create a coherent and politically powerful alternative to existing social structures.[46] But they could not sustain it. Unlike more mainstream nursing women, their vision of an androgynous community existed apart from conventional sources of institutional power, and isolated from the material resources with which they might have challenged the inevitable reassertion of male prerogatives. Thus it may be quite telling that Wald is best remembered for her achievements as the consummate political insider, skillfully recognizing and seizing opportunities to push but not to destroy the boundaries around acceptable women's work.[47] And it may be as telling that the successes she and her peers did achieve occurred within a re-created community with its own particular construction of the meaning of the boundaries around the enmeshed issues of gender, race, class, and social place.

For nursing, Hine reminds us in *Black Women in White*, took on different meanings for different nurses at different times with different places in their own communities of family, friends, and colleagues. Her study—the most conceptual of what, to date, have been primarily descriptive accounts of the struggles and achievements of women of color—argues that even as African-American nurses contended with their own divisive class issues, they remained joined both by choice and by institutional and social racism to a community beyond that of their hospitals. Their work and their lives were as inextricably intertwined with their particular social and cultural milieu as they were with that of the American health-care system. They gave care, and their community, in turn, rewarded them with the status and prestige that white nurses often found lacking.[48] That community involved other African-American women who, as Vanessa Gamble and Susan Smith remind us in their respective studies of black hospitals and clubwomen, had always drawn support for their health-care activism from a strong tradition of racial self-help.[49] And, as both Susan Reverby (in her more recent study of Eunice Rivers, the African-American nurse involved in the infamous Tuskegee Syphilis Study) and Shula Marks (in her work on South African nursing) argue, it was a community in which the matrix of gender, class, race, and, in particular, the often explosive representations of sexuality created a different understanding of both their experiences and the nature of their links to the wider, white world.[50]

The introduction of race, long overdue, has invigorated the study of nursing's history. But it may also well be that Hine's and her colleagues' enduring contribution to the field will extend beyond that of exploring racial themes. Their achievement may be refocusing our attention on the community as an analytic construct that allows us to move from the self-evident premise that nurses made choices within the boundaries of time, place, race, and social custom, to study the processes through which they made such choices.[51] When we do so, the negotiations between domestic roles, community responsibilities, and work (not surprisingly) loom large. But the focus shifts. Linda Walsh, for example, in her study of midwives in early-twentieth-century Philadelphia, challenges the notion that only men's paid labor structured the rhythms of a family's domestic life. Her work suggests that the most important support for midwifery practice came from husbands who not only saw these women as strong, intelligent, and committed, but who, often on a moment's notice, altered their own work and social schedules to care for their small children and to continue the daily household routines during their wives' absences.[52] The midwives' gendered domestic and social responsibilities, it must be noted, were relevant: Borst's Wisconsin midwives generally did not practice until their children were school-aged, and then they usually restricted their practice to their own immediate, ethnic neighboroods.[53] But neither was their life necessarily conflicted. As Anna Carastro (one midwife "discovered" by Walsh) explained when asked about problems in blending the personal and the professional: "If she has that ambition . . . , it's not going to be hard. Anything you do with all your heart, you don't think of the hardship. You enjoy every moment."[54]

While it probably was harder than Carastro retrospectively admitted, the point is that she and other midwives did seem to live their lives, if not entirely on their own terms, then on terms that made sense to them.[55] But what of other nurses? Or, more correctly, what of others, both trained and untrained, both paid and unpaid, for whom nursing was equally embedded within the context of their social place? Their work, as both Christine Stansell and Emily Abel argue in their respective studies of urban and rural working-class women, was as much linked to the enduring traditions of class, ethnic, and racial neighborliness as it was to their ability to sell their skills in the wage-labor market.[56] Thus, we have no reason to continue to assume that this work ended with their marriages. We might assume that marriage—and, later, children—changed the structure of their work: their domestic responsibilities quite likely precluded the possibility of their spending the sustained days, weeks, and even months with sick patients that they had as private-duty nurses. But the well-documented demand that women maintain their nursing role within the socially gendered division of labor suggests that the work itself continued, even if its form became more episodic. It remained work fraught with ambiguities. It threw them into sustained relationships with family and friends that were characterized as often by tensions and turmoil as by warmth and solicitude; it disrupted the rhythms of their lives, even as it allowed them to develop a role outside their family's domestic economy.[57] But it remained important work. Contemporary commentators' observations that organized nursing ignored the needs of those too poor to afford private-duty nurses yet too rich to qualify for the free care of visiting nurses may have missed this admittedly hidden market.[58] We need to bring it to light. More important, we need to bring to light the meaning of this market to those who participated in it.

Here, new studies of the history of nursing in the South prove particularly instructive. For there, during the nineteenth and early twentieth centuries, nursing was an essentially feminine construct only within the tight confines of one's immediate family. Middle- and upper-class white women rarely nursed those with whom they claimed no blood ties. The nursing of neighboring strangers lay within the domain of elite white men and, to a far greater extent, of slaves and (later) disenfranchised black women.[59] Social place merged with race and gendered attributes. Nursing during yellow-fever epidemics, for example, demanded the courage and the stamina that only heroic, high-status men might provide; the more routine, tedious, and demeaning day-to-day work of nursing needed the patience and persistence of others more accustomed to such menial service.[60] That the South had, by World War I, finally developed the social, economic, and political capital needed to support the construction of hospitals points, again, to a necessary (but not, in and of itself, sufficient) explanation of change. As important, World War I marked the first time the actual work of nursing—that is, the actual care of the sick, not just (as best exemplified by the women of Charleston's Ladies Benevolent Society) organizing others to do that work—became acceptable to the South's elite white women.[61] They took on nursing as their patriotic contribution to the war effort and, as in the North in an earlier time, other white women of other classes followed rather quickly in their wake.

Southern history does remind us that women's wresting the heroic dimensions of nursing from men remains an important, although little-recognized, achievement. But for our purposes, the incorporation of the heroic and the prestigious into this now-complete gendering of nursing's work with strangers as well as with kin suggests the role that a formal nursing identity played in support of women's sense of agency. Touchstones of valor, status, and recognition outside those traditionally available in their families and communities gave women who in marriage returned to the conventions surrounding the socially gendered division of domestic labor, a new base of socially legitimated authority. This base institutionalized age-old traditions of power.[62] For if every woman had indeed been a nurse, the specialized skill, the deep commitment, and the relatively privileged position with respect to the wage-labor market that had allowed a few the opportunity to create a socially valued and valuable place for themselves, independent of one they might claim through the place of their fathers or their husbands, had always had to be individually earned.[63] Now that place could be assumed—by them, by their communities, and by the wider world. This assumption remained inherently gender-affirming. It celebrated the women that these relatively conservative nurses were. But it also celebrated the women that they wanted to become. A formal nursing identity—that is, a gendered identity built around the social salience of a particular kind of work—

enabled these women to create a more coherent, a more generalizable, and, ultimately, a more sustained independent place for themselves within their chosen sphere. It gave already rather privileged women, now as a group rather than as individuals, the power to renegotiate the terms of some of the inequities they experienced and to shape their own sense of the value of work in their lives.

We have now, it must be noted, entered into more speculative terrain. Yet tantalizing (albeit fragmentary) data exist to support such a premise. It helps make sense of the fact, for example, that in Mary Neth's analysis of the family labor system in the Midwest, the early-twentieth-century farm wife who enjoyed the most egalitarian relationship with her husband had as her model a mother who also served as a "nurse" for her community.[64] It helps us understand why, in Shirley Veith's study of baccalaureate nursing education at the University of Kansas in the 1920s, students articulated an alternative sense of professionalism that demanded respect for both their femaleness and the liberal arts education that might give it some coherent form.[65] And, to return again to Borst's *Catching Babies*, we may have yet another explanation for why midwifery practice remained grounded in tightly bounded ethnic communities, even though simple economics suggested the value of expansion.[66] In the end, then, the value that nursing women placed on their work resonated more with their identity as women and less with that as labor-market participants. They thus recast work as a gender-affirming strategy to be honed within, but to be deployed outside, the nexus of wage-based relations.

Nursing women's recasting of the relationship between work and identity did, as has been well established, eschew both workplace activism and formal links with percolating currents of feminist thinking. They largely rejected class consciousness, labor militancy, gendered solidarity, and the repudiation of patriarchy as legitimate coins with which they might buy power at home and at work—and, like other conservative working women, they have therefore been tarred with the brush of consenting to the terms of their own oppression.[67] Yet, as this reconceptualized history suggests, they were neither ideological victims of a "false consciousness" nor pragmatic, but short-sighted, actors responding only to historically specific circumstances. Rather, in their embrace of the social boundaries set by their time, place, and local custom, nursing women—from Civil War examples onward—also allowed themselves to experience and to incorporate into their own identities changing notions about women's "proper" roles. A dialectic, of sorts, existed between them and their more radical sisters both within and outside nursing. The latter, pulling from their own culture, consciousness, place in a recreated community, and

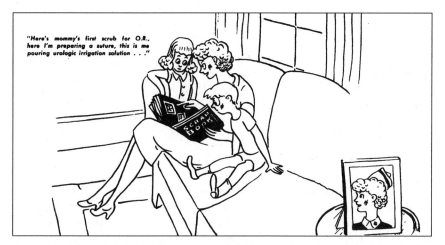

"Here's mommy's first scrub for O.R., here I'm preparing a suture, this is me pouring urologic irrigation solution . . ."

Women maintained their identity as nurses after they withdrew from active labor-market participation. Reprinted with permission from Marguerite J. Holmes, "What's Wrong with Getting Involved," *Nursing Outlook*, 1960, 8:251.

different sense of appropriate activism, articulated the dimensions of change; the former authenticated, solidified, and ultimately sustained the salient pieces of the message.

We can see this again when we leap through time to the decades after World War II. Even at mid-century, we might still argue that women's experience of the new wage-labor market continued to work primarily as a gender-affirming strategy (see Fig. 1).[68] But nursing women had also begun to incorporate into their identity a new sense of the legitimacy of challenges to the deferential expectations of an established hierarchy. By the 1960s, new nursing roles had emerged to meet new demands to care for new kinds of patients in new places.[69] And it should not be surprising that these roles expressed the autonomy, the control, and the self-determination that women—as well as African-Americans and the poor—now felt were due them.

In fact, the next rewriting of nursing's history may well focus on how these most traditional of all working women worked slowly, steadily, yet often tumultously within the boundaries of prevailing social structures, cultural traditions, and gendered assumptions, to eventually legitimate what had earlier been perceived as fairly radical messages. And it may well be, in keeping with James's urging of reciprocity, that in this retelling of their story we will find a new way to redefine and recapture the power inherent in the ways these women chose to define their lives.

NOTES*

*   Notes have been abridged from original article.

1.   Janet Wilson James, "Writing and Rewriting Nursing History: A Review Essay," *Bull. Hist. Med.*, 1984, 58: 568–84.

2.   Celia Davies, ed., *Rewriting Nursing History* (London: Croom Helm, 1980), pp. 11–17; Ellen Condliffe Lagemann, ed., *Nursing History: New Perspectives, New Possibilities* (New York: Teachers College Press, 1983), pp. 1–12.

3.   James, 'Writing and Rewriting" (n. 1), p. 574.

4.   Ibid., p. 569.

5.   Ibid., p. 568; see also. p. 584.

6.   Ibid.

7.   For example, Morris Vogel's very well-received *The Invention of the Modern Hospital: Boston, 1870–1930* (Chicago: University of Chicago Press, 1980) never mentions nursing as a part of the hospital reform movement. However, Charles Rosenberg, *The Care of Strangers: The Rise of America's Hospital System* (New York: Basic Books,1987), casts nurses in the pivotal role of "foot soldiers" in that same reform movement. See also Alan Kraut, *Silent Travelers: Germs, Genes, and the "Immigrant Menace"* (New York: Basic Books, 1994); Barbara Bates, *Bargaining for Life: A Social History of Tuberculosis, 1876–1938* (Philadelphia: University of Pennsylvania Press, 1992); Rosemary Stevens, *In Sickness and in Wealth: American Hospitals in the Twentieth Century* (New York: Basic Books, 1989); Judith Walzer Leavitt, *Brought to Bed: A History of Childbearing in America, 1750 to 1950* (New York: Oxford University Press, 1986).

8.   See, for example, Patricia Haase, *The Origins and Rise of Associate Degree Nursing Education* (Durham, N.C.: Duke University Press, in cooperation with the National League for Nursing, 1990).

9.   Barbara Melosh, *"The Physician's Hand": Work Culture and Conflict in American Nursing* (Philadelphia: Temple University Press, 1982); Susan M. Reverby, *Ordered to Care: The Dilemma of American Nursing, 1850–1945* (New York: Cambridge University Press, 1987); Darlene Clark Hine, *Black Women in White: Racial Conflict and Cooperation in the Nursing Profession, 1890–1950* (Bloomington: University of Indiana Press, 1989).

10.   Reverby, *Ordered to Care* (n. 9), p. 1.

11.   Melosh, *Physician's Hand* (n. 9).

12.   Rosenberg, *Care of Strangers* (n. 7), chap. 9.

13.   Jessica Robbins, "Class Struggles in the Tubercular World: Nurses, Patients, and Physicians, 1903–1915," *Bull. Hist. Med.*, 1997, 71: 412–34; Kraut, *Silent Travelers* (n. 7), chap. 8.

14.   Kathleen Hall Jamieson addresses this theoretical issue for today's working women in *Beyond the Double Bind: Women and Leadership* (New York: Oxford University Press, 1995). For such biographical data on American nurses, see Martin Kaufman, ed., *Dictionary of American Nursing Biography* (New York: Greenwood Press, 1988); Vern Bullough, Olga Maranjian Church, and Alice P. Stein, eds., *American Nursing: A Biographical Dictionary* (New York: Garland Publishing, 1988); Vern Bullough, Lilli Sentz, and Alice P. Stein, eds., *American*

Nursing: A Biographical Dictionary, vol. 2 (New York: Garland Reference Library of the Social Sciences, 1992).

15.   For perceptive reviews of this literature, see Ava Baron, "Gender and Labor History," in *Work Engendered: Toward a New History of American Labor*, ed. idem (Ithaca: Cornell University Press, 1991), pp. 1–46; Mari Jo Buhle, "Gender and Labor History," in *Perspectives on American Labor History: The Problem of Synthesis*, ed. J. Carroll Moody and Alice Kessler-Harris (DeKalb: Northern Illinois University Press, 1989), pp. 55–82.

16.   Laurel Thatcher Ulrich, *A Midwife's Tale: The Life of Martha Ballard, Based on Her Diary, 1785–1812* (New York: Knopf, 1990); Charlotte G. Borst, *Catching Babies: The Professionalization of Childbirth, 1870–1920* (Cambridge: Harvard University Press, 1995).

17.   Addis Cameron, in fact, argues that just such a consciousness mobilized many of Lawrence, Massachusetts' non-wage-earning women in support of its famous textile strike of 1912: see "Bread and Roses Revisited: Women's Culture and Working-Class Activism in the Lawrence Strike of 1912," in *Women, Work, and Protest: A Century of U.S. Women's Labor History*, ed. Ruth Milkman (Boston: Routledge & Kegan Paul, 1985), pp. 42–61. On boycotts, see Dana Frank, "Gender, Consumer Organizing, and the Seattle Labor Movement, 1919–1929," in Ava Baron, *Work Engendered* (n. 15), pp. 273–95.

18.   For examples, see Judy Giles, "A Home of One's Own: Women and Domesticity in England, 1918–1950," *Women's Stud. Internat. Forum*, 1993, 16: 239–53; Sharon Harley, "For the Good of Family and Race: Gender, Work, and Domestic Roles in the Black Community, 1880–1930," *Signs*, 1990, 15: 336–49.

19.   For a vivid description of ways in which women survived the training-school experience, see Douglas Baldwin, "Discipline, Obedience, and Female Support Groups: Mona Wilson at the Johns Hopkins Hospital School of Nursing, 1915–1918," *Bull. Hist. Med.*, 1995, 69: 599–619.

20.   Reverby, *Ordered to Care* (n. 9), pp. 77–90.

21.   For an analysis of the changes that led to working women's increasing economic and social dependence within patriarchal families, see Thomas Dublin, *Transforming Women's Work: New England Lives in the Industrial Revolution* (Ithaca: Cornell University Press, 1994).

22.   Thomas Olsen, Apprenticeship and Exploitation: An Analysis of the Work Patterns of Nurses in Training, 1897–1937," *Soc. Sci. Hist.*, 1993, 17: 559–76; Reverby, *Ordered to Care* (n. 9); Melosh, *Physician's Hand* (n. 9).

23.   May Ayres Burgess, ed., *Nurses, Patients, and Pocketbooks: Report of a Study of the Economics of Nursing Conducted by the Committee on the Grading of Nursing Schools* (New York: Committee on the Grading of Training Schools, 1928), pp. 48–53. For arguments about respectability and schooling as contributing to women's valuation of work options, see Ileen A. DeVault, "'Give the Boys a Trade': Gender and Job Choice in the 1890s," in Baron, *Work Engendered* (n. 15), pp. 191–215; Patricia Cooper, "The Faces of Gender: Sex Segregation and Work Relations at Philco, 1928–1938," in ibid., pp. 320–50.

24.   See, for example, the stories of Florence Blake, Jane Delano, Sara Parsons, Mary Roberts Rinehart, and Emma Edmonds Seelye in Bullough, Church, and Stein, *American Nursing* (n. 14).

25.   The issues of ambition, power, and status have been addressed more frankly in studies of religious nursing orders. See, for example, Mary Tarbox, "A Fierce Tenderness: Florence Nightingale Encounters the Sisters of Mercy," in *Florence Nightingale and Her Era: A Collection of New Scholarship,* ed. Vern L. Bullough, Bonnie Bullough, and Marietta P. Stanton (New York: Garland Publishing, 1990), pp. 274–87; Judith Moore, *A Zeal for Responsibility: The Struggle for Professional Nursing in Victorian England, 1868–1883* (Athens: University of Georgia Press, 1988).

26.   Charles E. Rosenberg, "From Almshouse to Hospital: The Shaping of Philadelphia General Hospital," *Milbank Quart.,* 1982, 60:108–54; quotation on p. 123.

27.   Patricia D'Antonio, "Staff Needs and Patient Care: Seclusion and Restraint in a Nineteenth-Century Insane Asylum," *Trans. Stud. Coll. Physicians Philadelphia,* 1991, 13: 411–23.

28.   Lois A. Monteiro, "Insights from the Past," *Nursing Outlook,* 1987, 35: 65–69.

29.   Martha Vicinus, *Independent Women: Work and Community for Single Women 1850–1920* (Chicago: University of Chicago Press, 1985), pp. 3–85.

30.   Judith Walzer Leavitt, "Strange Young Women on Errands," *Nursing Hist. Rev.,* 1998, 6: 3–24.

31.   Meryn Stuart, "'Half a Loaf Is Better Than No Bread': Public Health Nurses and Physicians in Ontario, 1920–1925," *Nursing Res.,* 1992, 41: 21–27, see especially p. 26.

32.   Barbara Melosh, "Doctors, Patients, and 'Big Nurse': Work and Gender in the Postwar Hospital," in Lagemann, *Nursing History* (n. 2), pp. 157–79. Claire Fagin and Donna Diers argue that social ambivalence about the work of nurses persists today: "Nursing as Metaphor," *N. Engl. J. Med.,* 1983, 309:116–17.

33.   Reverby, *Ordered to Care* (n. 9). See also her shorter synopsis: Susan Reverby, "A Caring Dilemma: Womanhood and Nursing in Historical Perspective," *Nursing Res.,* 1987, 36: 5–1 1.

34.   See Reverby, *Ordered to Care* (n. 9); Melosh, *Physician's Hand* (n. 9).

35.   Burgess, *Nurses, Patients* (n. 23), pp. 48–53.

36.   See Melosh, *Physician's Hand* (n. 9), p. 66; Everett C. Hughes, Helen MacGill Hughes, and Irwin Deutscher, *Twenty Thousand Nurses Tell Their Story: A Report on Studies of Nursing Functions, Sponsored by the American Nurses' Association* (Philadelphia: Lippincott, 1958), pp. 49–60. For a more current take, one might note that an analysis of the political style and policy positions of Sheila Burke, then-Senator Robert Dole's chief-of-staff, contextualized them in light of her history as a "former nurse" Jason DeParle, "Sheila Burke Is the Militant Feminist Commie Peacenik Who's Telling Bob Dole How to Think," *New York Times Magazine,* 12 November 1995, p. 32).

37.   See, for example, the oral histories in Sara Wuthnow, "Our Mothers' Stories," *Nursing Outlook,* 1990, 38: 218–22; quotation on p. 221. See also Vern Bullough, Bonnie Bullough, and Yow-Wu Wu's analysis of the biographies of American nursing leadership, "Achievement of Eminent American Nurses of the Past: A Prosopographical Study," *Nursing Res.,* 1992, 41: 120–24. A surprising

number of women had what, for lack of a better term, can be best described as working-class backgrounds, and yet had access to the more prestigious training schools.

38. Henriette Donner, "Under the Cross—Why V.A.D's Performed the Filthiest Task in the Dirtiest War: Red Cross Women Volunteers, 1914–1918," *J. Soc. Hist.*, 1997, 3: 667–704.

39. For descriptive studies of nursing and ethnicity, see Evelyn R. Benson, "Public Health Nursing and the Jewish Contribution," *Pub. Health Nursing*, 1993, 10: 55–57; Evelyn R. Benson and Janice Selekman, Jewish Women and Nursing: An Overview of Early History," *J. N. Y. State Nurses Assoc.*, 1992, 23: 16–19; Ina J. Bramadat and Marion I. Saydak, "Nursing on the Canadian Prairies, 1900–1930: Effects of Immigration," *Nursing Hist. Rev.*, 1993, 1: 105–17. See also Barbara Brush, "'Exchangees' or Employees? The Exchange Visitor Program and Foreign Nurse Immigration to the United States, 1945–1990," ibid., pp. 171–80.

40. This line of reasoning was first argued by Jo Ann Ashley in *Hospitals, Paternalism, and the Role of the Nurse* (New York: Teachers College Press, 1976), and it has been reworked in a more nuanced way by Stuart in "Half a Loaf" (n. 31).

41. For a general discussion of the fight for military rank, see Philip A. Kalish and Beatrice J. Kalish, *The Advance of American Nursing* (Boston: Little, Brown, 1978), pp. 452–55. See also Linda Beeber, "To Be One of the Boys: Aftershocks of the World War I Nursing Experience," *Adv. Nursing Sci.*, 1990, 12: 32–43; Mary Sarnecky, "Julia Catherine Stimson: Nurse and Feminist," *Image*, 1993, 25: 113–19.

42. This notion of conservatism, I must note, draws significantly from that constructed by Evelyn Brooks Higginbotham in *Righteous Discontent: The Women's Movement in the Black Baptist Church, 1880–1920* (Cambridge: Harvard University Press, 1993). See also Joan Lynaugh, "Nursing's History: Looking Backwards and Seeing Forward," in *Charting Nursing's Future: Agenda for the 1990s*, ed. Linda Aiken and Claire Fagin (Philadelphia: Lippincott, 1992), pp. 435–47.

43. Elizabeth D. Leonard, *Yankee Women: Gender Battles in the Civil War* (New York: W. W. Norton, 1994); Jane E. Schultz, "The Inhospitable Hospital: Gender and Professionalism in Civil War Medicine," *Signs*, 1992, 17: 363–92; idem, "Race, Gender, and Bureaucracy: Civil War Army Nurses and the Pension Bureau," *J. Women's Hist.*, 1994: 6: 45–69.

44. See Karen Buhler-Wilkerson, "Guarded by Standards and Directed by Strangers: Charleston, South Carolina's Response to a National Health Care Agenda, 1920–1930," *Nursing Hist. Rev.*, 1993, 1: 139–54; idem, "Caring in Its 'Proper Place': Race and Benevolence in Charleston, SC, 1813–1930," *Nursing Res.*, 1992, 41:14–20; idem, "Left Carrying the Bag: Experiments in Visiting Nursing, 1877–1909," *Nursing Res.*, 1987, 36: 42–47; idem, "False Dawn: The Rise and Decline of Public Health Nursing in America, 1900–1930," in Lagemann, *Nursing History* (n. 2), pp. 89–106. See also Diane Hamilton, "Research and Reform: Community Nursing and the Framingham Tuberculosis Project, 1914–1923," *Nursing Res.*, 1992, 41: 8–13; idem, 'The Cost of Caring: The Metropolitan Life Insurance Company's Visiting Nurse Service, 1909–1953," *Bull. Hist. Med.*, 1989, 63: 414–34; idem, "Faith and Finance," *Image*, 1988, 20: 124–27.

45. Frances Patai, "Heroines of the Good Fight: Testimonies of U.S. Volunteer

Nurses in the Spanish Civil War, 1936–1939," *Nursing Hist. Rev.*, 1995, 3: 79–104. Besides constructing social communities, Diane Hamilton argues, nursing constructed intellectual communities as well: see "Constructing the Mind of Nursing," ibid., 1994, 2: 3–28.

46. Carroll Smith-Rosenberg, "The New Woman as Androgyne: Social Disorder and Gender Crisis, 1870–1936," in idem, *Disorderly Conduct: Visions of Gender in Victorian America* (New York: Knopf, 1985), pp. 245–96. I am grateful to Karen Buhler-Wilkerson for calling my attention to this work.

47. A similar argument might be made for Lavinia Dock, Wald's friend and colleague, and another avowedly feminist early-twentieth-century nursing leader. Even then, Elizabeth Temkin suggests in an intriguing study that grounds Dock's feminism in the social mores of her time, there were limits that even the most radical of all nursing leaders accepted in the battle for gendered transformation: see Elizabeth Temkin, "Turn-of-the-Century Nursing Perspectives on Venereal Disease," *Image*, 1994, 26: 207–11. See also Carole A. Estabrooks, "Lavinia Dock: The Henry Street Years," *Nursing Hist. Rev.*, 1995, 3: 143–72.

48. Hine, *Black Women in White* (n. 9).

49. Vanessa Northington Gamble, *Making a Place for Ourselves: The Black Hospital Movement 1920–1945* (New York: Oxford University Press, 1995); Susan L. Smith, *Sick and Tired of Being Sick and Tired: Black Women's Health Activism in America, 1890–1950* (Philadelphia: University of Pennsylvania Press, 1995).

50. Susan Reverby, "Rethinking the Tuskegee Syphilis Study: Nurse Rivers, Silence, and the Meaning of Treatment," *Nursing Hist. Rev.*, 1999, 7: 3–28; Shula Marks, *Divided Sisterhood: Race, Class, and Gender in the South African Nursing Profession* (New York: St. Martin's Press, 1994).

51. On the conceptual importance of treating women's choices as meaningful despite their place within patriarchal structures, see Judith McGaw, "No Passive Victims, No Separate Spheres: A Feminist Perspective on Technology's History," in *In Context: History and the History of Technology: Essays in Honor of Melvin Kranzberg*, ed. Stephen H. Cutliffe and Robert C. Post (Bethlehem, Pa.: Lehigh University Press, 1989). I am grateful to Julie Fairman for sharing McGaw's work with me. For an empirical approach, see Ruth Schwartz Cowan, *More Work for Mother: The Ironies of Household Technology from the Open Hearth to the Microwave* (New York: Basic Books, 1983).

52. Linda V. Walsh, "Midwives as Wives and Mothers: Urban Midwives in the Early Twentieth Century," *Nursing Hist. Rev.*, 1994, 2: 51–66. Other descriptions of midwifery include Marie O. Pitts Mosley, "Satisfied to Carry the Bag: Three Black Community Health Nurses' Contributions to Health Care Reform," ibid., 1996, 4: 65–82; Susan L. Smith, "White Nurses, Black Midwives, and Public Health in Mississippi, 1920–1950," ibid., 1994, 2: 29–49; Pegge L. Bell, "'Making Do' with the Midwife: Arkansas's Mamie O. Hale in the 1940s," ibid., 1993, 1: 155–69; and Jane Pacht Brickman, "Public Health, Midwives, and Nurses, 1880–1930," in Lagemann, *Nursing History* (n. 2), pp. 65–88.

53. Borst, *Catching Babies* (n.16). See also Charlotte Borst, "The Training and Practice of Midwives: A Wisconsin Study," *Bull. Hist. Med.*, 1988, 62: 606–27.

54. Walsh, "Midwives as Wives and Mothers" (n. 52), p. 63.

55. In her later years, with too few expectant mothers to sustain her profes-

sionally and financially, Carastro turned her ambition toward their children and opened a day nursery.

56.   Christine Stansell, *City of Women: Sex and Class in New York, 1789–1860* (Urbana: University of Illinois Press, 1987); Emily Abel, "Family Caregiving in the Nineteenth Century: Emily Hawley Gillespie and Sarah Gillespie, 1858–1888," *Bull. Hist. Med.*, 1994, 68: 573–99.

57.   Abel, "Family Caregiving" (n. 56).

58.   Reverby, *Ordered to Care* (n. 9), pp. 177–79.

59.   Drew Gilpin Faust, *Mothers of Invention: Women of the Slaveholding South in the American Civil War* (Chapel Hill: University of North Carolina Press, 1996); John F. Marszalek, ed., *The Diary of Miss Emma Holmes, 1861–1866* (Baton Rouge: Louisiana State University Press, 1994).

60.   Linda Sabin, "Unheralded Nurses: Male Caregivers in the Nineteenth-Century South," *Nursing Hist. Rev.*, 1997, 5:131–48.

61.   Buhler-Wilkerson, "Guarded by Standards" (n. 44).

62.   Such touchstones have already, of course, been analyzed and dismissed as having been in no way instrumental in helping nursing women create paths, if not from "rags to riches," then from working-class to middle-class respectability. And, when we focus only on the health-care labor market's exploitation of nursing women's hopes and aspirations, we must admit their impotence.

63.   Ulrich, *Midwife's Tale* (n. 16), p. 62; Reverby, *Ordered to Care* (n. 9), chap. 1.

64.   Mary Neth, "Gender and the Family Labor System: Defining Work in the Rural Midwest," *J. Soc. Hist.*, 1994, 27: 563–78.

65.   Shirley Veith, "The Beginning of Baccalaureate Nursing Education at the University of Kansas: A Midwestern Experience," *Adv. Nursing Sci.*, 1990, 12: 63–73.

66.   Borst, *Catching Babies* (n. 16), pp. 68–89.

67.   Baron, "Gender and Labor History" (n. 15), pp. 27–32.

68.   See Susan Rimby Leighow, *Nurses' Questions/Women's Questions: The Impact of the Demographic Revolution and Feminism on United States Working Women, 1946–1986* (New York: Peter Lang, 1996).

69.   See Julie Fairman,, 'Watchful Vigilance: Nursing Care, Technology, and the Development of Intensive Care Units," *Nursing Res.*, 1992, 41: 56–60. See also Margarete Sandelowski, "'Making the Best of Things': Technology in American Nursing, 1870–1940," *Nursing Hist. Rev.*, 1997, 5: 3–22. It may also be argued of the 1950s that class became a less divisive issue: that nurses' skills were often more important than their backgrounds. This was not always the case. As Anne Summers suggests in another work on nursing in early-nineteenth-century British homes, the wish for a certain "refinement" among those nursing bourgeois families overrode any acknowledgment of their quite impressive skills: see "The Mysterious Demise of Sarah Gamp: The Domiciliary Nurse and Her Detractors, c. 1830–1860," *Victorian Studies*, 1989, 32: 365–86.

Appendix

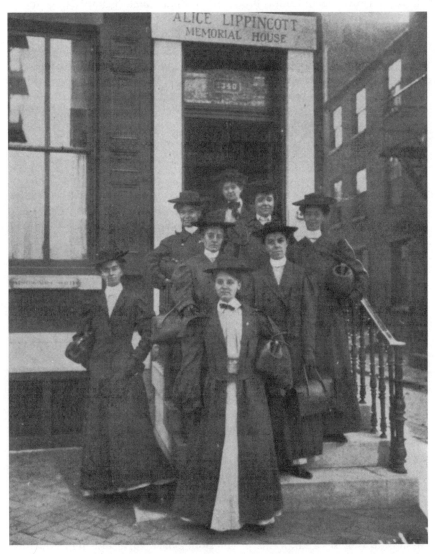

Visiting Nurses Leaving for Work, circa 1900. Courtesy of the Center for the Study of the History of Nursing, University of Pennsylvania.

Appendix: Suggestions for Further Reading

The following books and articles serve only to illustrate the depth and breath of recent scholarship on both the history of nursing and the history of health care. Those interested in exploring other themes and topics might turn to the *Nursing History Review*, the offical publication of the American Association of the History of Nursing, the *Bulletin of the History of Medicine*, the *Journal of the History of Medicine and Allied Sciences*, the *Journal of Social History*, and the *Journal of Women's History*.

The websites of both the American Association for the History of Nursing (http://www.aahn.org) and that of the History of Medicine division of the National Library of Medicine (http://www.nlm.nih.gov/hmd/ hmd.html) contain links to other relevant primary and secondary sources in the history of nursing and the history of health care.

Abel, Emily. "Family Caregiving in the Nineteenth Century: Emily Hawley Gillespie and Sarah Gillespie, 1858–1888." *Bulletin of the History of Medicine* 68 (1994): 573–599.

Aronowitz, Robert. *Making Sense of Illness: Science, Society and Disease.* Cambridge and New York: Cambridge University Press, 1998.

Baer, Ellen. "A Cooperative Venture" in Pursuit of Professional Status: A Research Journal for Nursing." *Nursing Research* 36, no. 1 (1987): 18–25.

Bates, Barbara. *Bargaining for Life: A Social History of Tuberculosis, 1876–1938.* Philadelphia: University of Pennsylvania, 1992.

Borst, Charlotte. *Catching Babies: The Professionalization of Childbirth, 1870–1920.* Cambridge: Harvard University Press, 1995.

Brown, Thomas. *Dorothea Dix: New England Reformer.* Cambridge: Harvard University Press, 1998.

Boschma, Geertje. "The Gender Specific Role of Male Nurses in Dutch Asylums, 1890–1910." *International Nursing History Journal* 4, no. 3 (1999): 13–19.

Brush, Barbara and Joan Lynaugh, eds, with Geertje Boschma, Anne Marie Rafferty, Meryn Stuart, and Nancy Tomes. *Nurses of All Nations: A History of the International Council of Nurses, 1899–1999.* Hagerstown, MD: Lippincott Williams & Wilkins, 1999.

Buhler-Wilkerson, Karen. "False Dawn: The Rise and Decline of Public Health Nursing in America, 1900–1930." In *Nursing History: New Perspectives, New*

Possibilities, ed. Ellen Condliffe Lageman, 89–106. New York: Teachers College Press, 1983.

Bullough, Vern, Bonnie Bullough, and Marietta Stanton, eds. *Florence Nightingale and Her Era: A Collection of New Scholarship.* New York: Garland Publishing, 1990.

Bullough, Vern, Olga Church, and Alice Stein, eds. *American Nursing: A Biographical Dictionary.* New York: Garland Publishing, 1988.

Bullough, Vern, Lilli Sentz, and Alice Stein, eds. *American Nursing: A Biographical Dictionary.* Vol. 2. New York: Garland Reference Library of the Social Sciences, 1992.

Bullough, Vern, and Lillian Sentz, eds. *American Nursing: A Biographical Dictionary.* Vol. 3. New York: Springer, 1999.

Carnegie, M. Elizabeth. *The Path We Tread: Blacks in Nursing, 1854–1984.* Philadelphia: Lippincott, 1986.

Chesler, Ellen. *Woman of Valor: Margaret Sanger and the Birth Control Movement in America.* New York: Doubleday, 1992.

Connolly, Cynthia. "Hampton, Nutting, and Rival Gospels at the Johns Hopkins Hospital and Training School for Nurses, 1889–1906." *Image* 30, no. 1 (1998): 23–30.

D'Antonio, Patricia. "The Legacy of Domesticity: Nursing in Early Nineteenth Century America." *Nursing History Review* 1 (1993): 229–246.

D'Antonio, Patricia. "Towards a History of Research in Nursing." *Nursing Research* 46 (1997): 105–110.

Dieckmann, Janna. "From Almshouse to City Nursing Home: Philadelphia's Riverview Home for the Aged, 1945–1965." *Nursing History Review* 1 (1993): 217–228.

Ettinger, Laura E. "Nurse-Midwives, the Mass Media, and the Politics of Maternal Health Care in the United States, 1925–1955." *Nursing History Review* 7 (1999): 47–66.

Fairman, Julie, and Joan Lynaugh. *Critical Care Nursing: A History.* Philadelphia: University of Pennsylvania, 1998.

Faust, Drew Gilpin. *Mothers of Invention: Women of the Slaveholding South in the Civil War.* Chapel Hill, NC: University of North Carolina Press, 1996.

Gamble, Vanessa Northington. *Making a Place for Ourselves: The Black Hospital Movement, 1920–1945.* New York: Oxford University Press, 1995.

Ginzberg, Lori. *Women and the Work of Benevolence: Morality, Politics and Class in Nineteenth Century America.* New Haven: Yale University Press, 1990.

Haase, Patricia. *The Origins and Rise of Associate Degree Nursing Education.* Durham, N.C.: Duke University Press in cooperation with the National League for Nursing, 1990.

Hamilton, Diane. "Faith and Finance." *Image* 20, no. 3 (1988): 124–127.

Hamilton, Diane. "The Idea of History and the History of Ideas." *Image* 25, no. 1 (1993): 45–48.

Hine, Darlene Clark. *Black Women in White: Racial Conflict and Cooperation in the Nursing Profession, 1890–1950.* Bloomington: University of Indiana Press, 1989.

Howell, Joel. *Technology in the Hospital: Transforming Patient Care in the Early Twentieth Century.* Baltimore: Johns Hopkins University Press, 1995.

Kramer, Susan. "The Nature of History: Meditations on Clio's Craft." *Nursing Research* 41, no. 1 (1992): 4–7.

Leavitt, Judith Walker. *Brought to Bed: A History of Childbearing in America, 1750–1950.* New York: Oxford Unviersity Press, 1986.

Ludmerer, Kenneth M. *Time to Heal: American Medical Education from the Turn of the Century to the Era of Managed Care.* New York: Oxford University Press, 1999.

Ludmerer, Kenneth M. *Learning to Heal: The Development of American Medical Education.* New York: Basic Books, 1985.

Lynaugh, Joan, and Barbara Brush. *American Nursing: From Hospitals to Health Systems.* Cambridge, MA: Blackwell Publishers and the Milbank Memorial Fund, 1996.

Marks, Shula. *Divided Sisterhood: Race, Class and Gender in the South African Nursing Profession.* New York: St. Martin's Press, 1994.

Mosley, Marie O. Pitts. "Satisfied to Carry the Bag: Three Black Community Health Nurses' Contributions to Health Care Reform, 1900–1937." *Nursing History Review* 4 (1996): 65–82.

Nelson, Sioban. "Entering the Professional Domain: The Making of the Modern Nurse in 17th Century France." *Nursing History Review* 7 (1999): 171–188.

Norman, Elizabeth. *Women at War: The Story of Fifty Military Nurses Who Served in Vietnam.* Philadelphia: University of Pennsylvania Press, 1990.

Norman, Elizabeth. *We Band of Angels: The Untold Story of American Nurses Trapped on Bataan by the Japanese.* New York: Random House, 1999.

Patai, Frances. "Heroines of the Good Fight: Testimonies of U.S. Volunteer Nurses in the Spanish American Civil War, 1936–1939." *Nursing History Review* 3 (1995): 79–104.

Pryor, Elizabeth Brown. *Clara Barton: Professional Angel.* Philadelphia: University of Pennsylvania Press, 1987.

Rafferty, Anne Marie. *The Politics of Nursing Knowledge.* London and New York: Routledge, 1996.

Reverby, Susan. *Ordered to Care: The Dilemma of American Nursing.* Cambridge and New York: Cambridge University Press, 1987.

Reverby, Susan. "A Legitimate Relationship: Nursing, Hospitals, and Science in the Twentieth Century." In *The American General Hospital: Communities and Social Contexts,* ed. Diana Elizabeth Long and Janet Golden, 135–156. Ithica: Cornell University Press, 1989.

Reverby, Susan. "Rethinking the Tuskegee Syphilis Study: Nurse Rivers, Silence and the Meaning of Treatment." *Nursing History Review* 7 (1999): 3–28.

Rosenberg, Charles. "Florence Nightingale on Contagion: The Hospital as Moral Universe." In *Healing and History: Essays for George Rosen,* ed. Charles Rosenberg, 116–136. New York: Science History Publications, 1979.

Rosenberg, Charles E. *The Care of Strangers: The Rise of America's Hospital System.* New York: Basic Books, 1987.

Sabin, Linda. "Unheralded Nurses: Male Caregivers in the Nineteenth Century South." *Nursing History Review* 5 (1997): 131–148.

Sandelowski, Margarete. "Exploring the Gender-Technology Relation in Nursing." *Nursing Inquiry* 4 (1997): 219–228.

Sarnecky, Mary. *A History of the U.S. Army Nurse Corps.* Philadelphia: University of Pennsylvania Press, 1999.

Smith, Susan L. *Sick and Tired of Being Sick and Tired: Black Women's Health Activism in America, 1890–1950.* Philadelphia: University of Pennsylvania Press, 1995.

Stevens, Rosemary. *In Sickness and in Wealth: American Hospitals in the Twentieth Century.* 2nd ed. New York: Basic Books, 1999.

Summers, Anne. *Angels and Citizens: British Women as Military Nurses, 1854–1914.* London: Routledge & Kegan Paul, 1988.

Tomes, Nancy. *The Gospel of Germs: Men, Women and the Microbe in American Life.* Cambridge: Harvard University Press, 1998.

Ulrich, Laurel Thatcher. *A Midwife's Tale: The Life of Martha Ballard, Based on Her Diary, 1785–1812.* New York: Knopf, 1990.

Walsh, Linda V. "Midwives as Wives and Mothers: Urban Midwives in the Early Twentieth Century." *Nursing History Review* 2 (1994).

Index

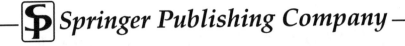
Springer Publishing Company

Nurses in the Political Arena
The Public Face of Nursing
Harriet R. Feldman, PhD, RN, FAAN and
Sandra B. Lewenson, EdD, RN

"The thrilling stories in the book tell of the way nurses work and the way they bring their experiences and knowledge to bear on political issues....The background presented in this book and the wonderful stories it tells will inform, stimulate and inspire current and future nurses. This book fills an important gap in the nursing literature."
— from the Foreword by **Claire Fagin**

This book was written to encourage nurses to become involved in the political process–by running for office, seeking appointments, or becoming active on some level in local government. The authors interviewed over 40 nurses who hold or have run for public office–from Members of Congress to local aldermen. These nurses share their experiences on everything from getting informed on the issues, to getting involved in a political party, to fundraising. A chapter on nurses who have made use of the public arena in the past includes figures such as Lillian Wald, Lavinia Dock, and Margaret Sanger. Nurses have inside knowledge of health issues and the trust of the public. Here is a handbook that can help them to realize their leadership potential.

Contents:
• Foreword by Claire Fagin• Nurses in the Political Process: The Face That No One Sees • Historical Perspective on Nurses Active in the Political Process • Nurses in the Political Arena: The Face the Public Sees • Nurses' Action on Social Issues • Negotiating the Political Process: Lessons Learned • Creating Political Opportunities • Appendix A: Individuals Interviewed for This Book • Appendix B: Political Action Databases and Audiovisuals on Nurses and Politics • Appendix C: Campaign Posters and Photographs • Index

2000   200pp.   0-8261-1331-1 hard

536 Broadway, New York, NY 10012 • (212)431-4370 • Fax: (212)941-7842
Order Toll-Free: 1-877-687-7476 • *www.springerpub.com*

Springer Publishing Company

American Nursing
A Biographical Dictionary, Volume 3

Vern L. Bullough, RN, PhD, and
Lilli Sentz, Editors

Sharon Richardson, Bonnie Bullough, Olga Church,
Contributing Editors

"For only a few of the nurses in this volume was achievement an easy process. Their lives emphasize what it was like to be a nurse, what kinds of difficulties they encountered, and how they overcame them. The reader will certainly find out a great deal about the nursing presence and about what individual nurses have done to make nursing what it is today."

—Vern L. Bullough, from the Introduction

This exciting collection traces the development of the nursing profession through the biographies of individual nurses since 1925. The list of several hundred names, compiled through the help of nurse historians and volunteers from the American Association for the History of Nursing, features notable nurses Faye Abdellah, Virginia Henderson, Margaret Kerr, and Thelma Schorr. It gives nurses a real sense of their history which is not available anywhere else. The contributors of the biographies, in an act of scholarly devotion, preserve a sense of the profession's past.

American Nursing: A Biographical Dictionary, Volume Three is an invaluable reference work for students and librarians. Fully illustrated with many one-of-a-kind photographs.

2000 328pp. 0-8261-1296-X hard

536 Broadway, New York, NY 10012-3955 • (212) 431-4370 • Fax (212) 941-7842
Order Toll-Free: 1-877-687-7476 • *www.springerpub.com*

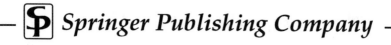
Springer Publishing Company

A Virginia Henderson Reader
Excellence in Nursing
Edward J. Halloran, RN, PhD, FAAN, Editor
Foreword by **Angela McBride,** PhD, RN, FAAN

"No nurse interested in our history, our theories, or our development as a scientific profession, will want to be without this book."
—Nurse Leadership Forum

This book provides a sampling of Virginia Henderson's classic writings in patient care, nursing education, nursing research, and nursing's role in the larger health care system. Ms. Henderson was an early advocate of autonomy for nurses and the importance of nursing scholarship. Her writings have much to say to today's nurses.

Partial Contents

I. Patient Care • Excellence in Nursing • The Essence of Nursing in High Technology • The Art and Science of Health Assessment • The Importance of Observation • Preserving the Essence of Nursing in a Technological Age

II. Nursing Education • Preparation for General Nursing • Suggestions for Basic Nursing Curricula • Preparation for Specialized Nursing Graduate Programs • The Nursing Process—Is the Title Right? • The Nature of Nursing

III. Nursing Research • Research in Nursing Practice—When? • An Overview of Nursing Research • We've "Come a Long Way," but What of the Direction? • Basis for the Selection of Method: Research as a Means of Improving Nursing Practice

IV. Nursing in Society • Nursing as an Aspect of Health Care • Nursing as a Constant Factor in Health Services • The Nurse's Role in Promoting Health Programs • Some Observations on the Health Care "Industry"

1995   416pp   0-8261-8830-3   hard

536 Broadway, New York, NY 10012-3955 • (212) 431-4370 • Fax (212) 941-7842
Order Toll-Free: 1-877-687-7476 • *www.springerpub.com*